RN Maternal Newborn Nursing Review Module Edition 9.0

CONTRIBUTORS

Sheryl Sommer, PhD, RN, CNE
VP Nursing Education & Strategy

Janean Johnson, MSN, RN
Nursing Education Strategist

Karin Roberts, PhD, MSN, RN, CNE
Nursing Education Coordinator

Sharon R. Redding, EdD, RN, CNE
Nursing Education Specialist and Content Project Coordinator

Lois Churchill, MN, RN
Nursing Education Specialist

EDITORIAL AND PUBLISHING

Derek Prater
Spring Lenox
Michelle Renner
Mandy Tallmadge
Kelly Von Lunen

CONSULTANTS

Christi Blair, MSN, RN
Mary Kay Smid, EdD, MSN, RN, CNE

Intellectual Property Notice

Important Notice to the Reader

User's Guide

Welcome to the Assessment Technologies Institute® RN Maternal Newborn Nursing Review Module Edition 9.0. The mission of ATI's Content Mastery Series® review modules is to provide user-friendly compendiums of nursing knowledge that will:

- Help you locate important information quickly.

- Assist in your learning efforts.

- Provide exercises for applying your nursing knowledge.

- Facilitate your entry into the nursing profession as a newly licensed RN.

Organization

This review module is organized into units covering antepartum, intrapartum, postpartum, and newborn nursing care. Chapters within these units conform to one of three organizing principles for presenting the content:

- Nursing concepts

- Procedures

- Complications of pregnancy

Nursing concepts chapters begin with an overview describing the central concept and its relevance to nursing. Subordinate themes are covered in outline form to demonstrate relationships and present the information in a clear, succinct manner.

Procedures chapters include an overview describing the procedure(s) covered in the chapter. These chapters will provide you with nursing knowledge relevant to each procedure, including indications, interpretations of findings, nursing actions, and complications.

Complications of pregnancy chapters include an overview describing the complication, followed by risk factors. These chapters will cover assessment, including subjective and objective data, and patient-centered care, including nursing care, medications, and health promotion.

Application Exercises

Questions are provided at the end of each chapter so you can practice applying your knowledge. The Application Exercises include NCLEX-style questions, such as multiple-choice and multiple-select items, and questions that ask you to apply your knowledge in other formats, such as by using an ATI Active Learning Template. After the Application Exercises, an answer key is provided, along with rationales for the answers.

NCLEX® Connections

To prepare for the NCLEX-RN, it is important for you to understand how the content in this review module is connected to the NCLEX-RN test plan. You can find information on the detailed test plan at the National Council of State Boards of Nursing's Web site: https://www.ncsbn.org/. When reviewing content in this review module, regularly ask yourself, "How does this content fit into the test plan, and what types of questions related to this content should I expect?"

To help you in this process, we've included NCLEX Connections at the beginning of each unit and with each question in the Application Exercises Answer Keys. The NCLEX Connections at the beginning of each unit will point out areas of the detailed test plan that relate to the content within that unit. The NCLEX Connections attached to the Application Exercises Answer Keys will demonstrate how each exercise fits within the detailed content outline.

These NCLEX Connections will help you understand how the detailed content outline is organized, starting with major client needs categories and subcategories and followed by related content areas and tasks. The major client needs categories are:

- Safe and Effective Care Environment
  - Management of Care
  - Safety and Infection Control
- Health Promotion and Maintenance
- Psychosocial Integrity
- Physiological Integrity
  - Basic Care and Comfort
  - Pharmacological and Parenteral Therapies
  - Reduction of Risk Potential
  - Physiological Adaptation

An NCLEX Connection might, for example, alert you that content within a unit is related to:

- Health Promotion and Maintenance
  - Ante/Intra/Postpartum and Newborn Care
    - Assess client psychosocial response to pregnancy.

QSEN Competencies

As you use the review modules, you will note the integration of the Quality and Safety Education for Nurses (QSEN) competencies throughout the chapters. These competencies are integral components of the curriculum of many nursing programs in the United States and prepare you to provide safe, high-quality care as a newly licensed RN. Icons appear to draw your attention to the six QSEN competencies:

- Safety: The minimization of risk factors that could cause injury or harm while promoting quality care and maintaining a secure environment for clients, self, and others.
- Patient-Centered Care: The provision of caring and compassionate, culturally sensitive care that addresses clients' physiological, psychological, sociological, spiritual, and cultural needs, preferences, and values.

- Evidence-Based Practice: The use of current knowledge from research and other credible sources, on which to base clinical judgment and client care.
- Informatics: The use of information technology as a communication and information-gathering tool that supports clinical decision-making and scientifically based nursing practice.
- Quality Improvement: Care related and organizational processes that involve the development and implementation of a plan to improve health care services and better meet clients' needs.
- Teamwork and Collaboration: The delivery of client care in partnership with multidisciplinary members of the health care team to achieve continuity of care and positive client outcomes.

Icons

Icons are used throughout the review module to draw your attention to particular areas. Keep an eye out for these icons:

 This icon is used for NCLEX connections.

 This icon is used for content related to safety. When you see this icon, take note of safety concerns or steps that nurses can take to ensure client safety and a safe environment.

 This icon is a QSEN competency that indicates the importance of a holistic approach to providing care.

 This icon, a QSEN competency, points out the integration of research into clinical practice.

 This icon is a QSEN competency and highlights the use of information technology to support nursing practice.

 This icon is used to focus on the QSEN competency of integrating planning processes to meet clients' needs.

 This icon highlights the QSEN competency of care delivery using an interprofessional approach.

 This icon indicates that a media supplement, such as a graphic, animation, or video, is available. If you have an electronic copy of the review module, this icon will appear alongside clickable links to media supplements. If you have a hardcopy version of the review module, visit www.atitesting.com for details on how to access these features.

Feedback

ATI welcomes feedback regarding this review module. Please provide comments to: comments@atitesting.com.

TABLE OF CONTENTS

UNIT 1   Antepartum Nursing Care

SECTIONS

› Human Reproduction
› Low-Risk, Uncomplicated Pregnancy: Changes During Pregnancy
› Complications of Pregnancy

NCLEX® CONNECTIONS

When reviewing the chapters in this unit, keep in mind the relevant sections of the NCLEX® outline, in particular:

Client Needs: Health Promotion and Maintenance

› Relevant topics/tasks include:
  » Ante/Intra/Postpartum and Newborn Care
    › Provide prenatal care and education.
  » Developmental Stages and Transitions
    › Identify expected body image changes associated with the client's developmental age.
  » Lifestyle Choices
    › Assess the client's need/desire for contraception.

Client Needs: Reduction of Risk Potential

› Relevant topics/tasks include:
  » Diagnostic Tests
    › Monitor the results of maternal and fetal diagnostic tests.
  » Potential for Complications of Diagnostic Tests/Treatments/Procedures
    › Monitor the client for signs of bleeding.
  » System Specific Assessment
    › Perform focused assessment.

Client Needs: Basic Care and Comfort

› Relevant topics/tasks include:
  » Nonpharmacological Comfort Interventions
    › Assess the client's need for alternative and/or complementary therapy.

Client Needs: Physiological Adaptation

› Relevant topics/tasks include:
  » Alterations in Body Systems
    › Identify signs of potential prenatal complications.

chapter 1

Overview

- Contraception refers to strategies or devices used to reduce the risk of fertilization or implantation in an attempt to prevent pregnancy.

- A nurse should assess clients' need/desire for contraception, as well as their preferences. A thorough discussion of benefits, risks, and alternatives of each method should be discussed.

- Sexual partners often make a joint decision regarding a desired preference (vasectomy or tubal ligation). Postpartum discharge instructions should include the discussion of future contraceptive plans.

- Expected outcomes for family planning methods consist of preventing pregnancy until a desired time.

- Nurses should support clients in making the decision that is best for their individual situations.

- Methods of contraception include natural family planning, barrier, hormonal, and intrauterine methods, as well as surgical procedures.

Natural Family Planning Methods

ABSTINENCE	
Definition	› Abstaining from having sexual intercourse eliminates the possibility of sperm entering a woman's vagina.
Client Instructions	› Refrain from sexual intercourse. This method can be associated with saying "no," but it also can incorporate saying "yes" to other gratifying sexual activities, such as affectionate touching, communication, holding hands, kissing, massage, and oral and manual stimulation.
Advantages	› Most effective method of birth control. › Abstinence during fertile periods (rhythm method) can be used, but it requires an understanding of the menstrual cycle and fertility awareness. › Can eliminate the risk of STIs if there is no genitalia contact.
Disadvantages	› Requires self-control
Risks/possible complications/ contraindications	› If complete abstinence is maintained, there are no risks.

COITUS INTERRUPTUS (WITHDRAWAL)

Definition	› Man withdraws penis from vagina prior to ejaculation.
Client Instructions	› Be aware of fluids leaking from the penis.
Advantages	› Possible choice for monogamous couples with no other option for birth control, such as those opposed to birth control due to religious conviction.
Disadvantages	› Most ineffective method of contraception. › No protection against STIs.
Risks/possible complications/ contraindications	› Male partner's control can make this an effective method. › Leakage of fluid that contains spermatozoa prior to ejaculation can be deposited in vagina. › Risk of pregnancy.

CALENDAR METHOD

Definition	› A woman records her menstrual cycle by calculating her fertile period based on the assumption that ovulation occurs about 14 days before the onset of her next menstrual cycle, and avoids intercourse during that period. Also taken into account is the timing of intercourse with this method because sperm are viable for 48-120 hr, and the ovum is viable for 24 hr.
Client Instructions	› Accurately record the number of days in each cycle counting from the first day of menses for a period of at least six cycles. › The start of the fertile period is figured by subtracting 18 days from the number of days in the woman's shortest cycle. › The end of the fertile period is established by subtracting 11 days from the number of days of the longest cycle. For example: » Shortest cycle, 26 – 18 = 8th day » Longest cycle, 30 – 11 = 19th day » Fertile period is days 8 through 19. › Refrain from intercourse during these days to avoid conception.
Advantages	› Most useful when combined with basal body temperature or cervical mucus method. › Inexpensive
Disadvantages	› Not a very reliable technique. › Requires accurate record keeping. › Requires compliance in regard to abstinence during fertile periods.
Risks/possible complications/ contraindications	› Various factors can affect and change the time of ovulation and cause unpredictable menstrual cycles. › Risk of pregnancy.

BASAL BODY TEMPERATURE (BBT)

Definition	› Temperature can drop slightly at the time of ovulation. This can be used to facilitate conception, or be used as a natural contraceptive.
Client Instructions	› A woman is instructed to measure oral temperature prior to getting out of bed each morning to monitor ovulation.
Advantages	› Inexpensive, convenient, and no side effects
Disadvantages	› BBT reliability can be influenced by many variables that can cause inaccurate interpretation of temperature changes, such as stress, fatigue, illness, alcohol, and warmth or coolness of sleeping environment.
Risks/possible complications/ contraindications	› Risk of pregnancy

SYMPTOM-BASED METHOD (CERVICAL MUCUS)

Definition	› Fertility awareness method based on ovulation. Ovulation occurs approximately 14 days prior to the next menstrual cycle, which is when a woman is fertile. Following ovulation, the cervical mucus becomes thin and flexible under the influence of estrogen and progesterone to allow for sperm viability and motility. The ability for the mucus to stretch between the fingers is greatest during ovulation. This is referred to as spinnbarkeit sign.
Client Instructions	› Engage in good hand hygiene prior to and following assessment. › Begin examining mucus from the last day of the menstrual cycle. › Mucus is obtained from the vaginal introitus. It is not necessary to reach into the vagina to the cervix. › Do not douche prior to assessment.
Advantages	› A woman can become knowledgeable in recognizing her own mucus characteristics at ovulation, and self-evaluation can be very accurate. › Self-evaluation of cervical mucus can also be diagnostically helpful in determining the start of ovulation while breastfeeding, in noting the commencement of menopause, and in planning a desired pregnancy.
Disadvantages	› Some women may be uncomfortable with touching their genitals and mucus and, therefore, will find this method objectionable.
Risks/possible complications/ contraindications	› Assessment of cervical mucus characteristics may be inaccurate if mucus is mixed with semen, blood, contraceptive foams, or discharge from infections. › Risk of pregnancy

Barrier Methods

CONDOMS	
Definition	› A thin flexible sheath worn on the penis during intercourse to prevent semen from entering the uterus.
Client Instructions	› A man places a condom on his erect penis, leaving an empty space at the tip for a sperm reservoir. › Following ejaculation, a man withdraws his penis from the woman's vagina while holding the rim of the condom to prevent any semen spillage to the woman's vulva or vaginal area. › May be used in conjunction with spermicidal gel or cream to increase effectiveness.
Advantages	› Protects against STIs and involves the male in the birth control method.
Disadvantages	› High rate of noncompliance. › May reduce spontaneity of intercourse. › The penis must be erect to apply a condom. › If the penis is withdrawn while still erect, this can interfere with sexual intercourse.
Risks/possible complications/ contraindications	› Condoms can rupture or leak, thus potentially resulting in an unwanted pregnancy. › Condoms have a one-time usage, which creates a replacement cost. › Condoms made of latex should not be worn by those who are sensitive or allergic to latex. › Only water-soluble lubricants should be used with latex condoms to avoid condom breakage.

DIAPHRAGM AND SPERMICIDE	
Definition	› A dome-shaped cup with a flexible rim made of latex or silicone that fits snugly over the cervix with spermicidal cream or gel placed into the dome and around the rim.
Client Instructions	› A female client should be fitted with a diaphragm properly by a provider. › A client must be refitted by the provider every 2 years, if there is a 7 kg (15 lb) weight change, full-term pregnancy, or second-term abortion. › Requires proper insertion and removal. Prior to coitus, the diaphragm is inserted vaginally over the cervix with spermicidal jelly or cream that is applied to the cervical side of the dome and around the rim. The diaphragm must remain in place for at least 6 hr after coitus. › Spermicide must be reapplied with each act of coitus. › A client should empty her bladder prior to insertion of the diaphragm.
Advantages	› This barrier method eliminates surgery and gives a woman more control over contraception.

DIAPHRAGM AND SPERMICIDE	
Disadvantages	› Diaphragms are inconvenient, interfere with spontaneity, and require reapplication with spermicidal gel, cream, or foam with each act of coitus to be effective.
	› Requires a prescription and a visit to a provider.
	› Must be inserted correctly to be effective.
Risks/possible complications/ contraindications	› A diaphragm is not recommended for clients who have a history of toxic shock syndrome (TSS), or frequent, recurrent urinary tract infections.
	› Increased risk of acquiring TSS.
	› TSS is caused by a bacterial infection. Signs and symptoms include high fever, a faint feeling and drop in blood pressure, watery diarrhea, headache, and muscle aches.
	› Proper hand hygiene aids in prevention of TSS, as well as removing diaphragm promptly at 6 hr following coitus.
	› Diaphragms made of latex should not be worn by those who are sensitive or allergic to latex.

Hormonal Methods

COMBINED ORAL CONTRACEPTIVES	
Definition	› Hormonal contraception containing estrogen and progestin, which acts by suppressing ovulation, thickening the cervical mucus to block semen, and altering the uterine decidua to prevent implantation.
Client Instructions	› Medication that requires a prescription and follow-up appointments with the provider.
	› Medication requires consistent and proper use to be effective.
	› A client is instructed in observing for side effects and danger signs of medication. Signs include chest pain, shortness of breath, leg pain from a possible clot, headache, or eye problems from a stroke, or hypertension.
	› In the event of a client missing a dose, the nurse should instruct the client that if one pill is missed, take one as soon as possible; if two or three pills are missed, instruct the client to follow the manufacturer's instructions. Instruct the client on the use of alternative forms of contraception or abstinence to prevent pregnancy until regular dosing is resumed.
Advantages	› Highly effective if taken correctly and consistently.
	› Medication can alleviate dysmenorrhea by decreasing menstrual flow and menstrual cramps.
	› Reduces acne.

COMBINED ORAL CONTRACEPTIVES

Disadvantages	› Oral contraceptives do not protect against STIs. › Birth control pills can increase the risk of thromboses, breast tenderness, scant or missed menstruation, stroke, nausea, headaches, and hormone-dependent cancers. › Exacerbates conditions affected by fluid retention such as migraine, epilepsy, asthma, kidney, or heart disease.
Risks/possible complications/ contraindications	› Women with a history of blood clots, stroke, cardiac problems, breast or estrogen-related cancers, pregnancy, or smoking (if over 35 years of age), are advised not to take oral contraceptive medications. › Oral contraceptive effectiveness decreases when taking medications that affect liver enzymes, such as anticonvulsants and some antibiotics.

MINIPILL

Definition	› Oral progestins that provide the same action as combined oral contraceptives.
Client Instructions	› A client should take the pill at the same time daily to ensure effectiveness secondary to a low dose of progestin. › A client cannot miss a pill. › A client may need another form of birth control during the first month of use to prevent pregnancy.
Advantages	› The minipill has fewer side effects when compared with a combined oral contraceptive. › Considered safe to take while breastfeeding.
Disadvantages	› Less effective in suppressing ovulation than combined oral contraceptives. › Pill increases occurrence of ovarian cysts. › Pill does not protect against STIs. › Users frequently report breakthrough, irregular, vaginal bleeding, and decreased libido. › Increases appetite
Risks/possible complications/ contraindications	› Oral contraceptive effectiveness decreases when taking medications that affect liver enzymes, such as anticonvulsants and some antibiotics.

EMERGENCY ORAL CONTRACEPTIVE

Definition	› Morning after pill that prevents fertilization from taking place.
Client Instructions	› Pill is taken within 72 hr after unprotected coitus. › A provider will recommend an over-the-counter antiemetic to be taken 1 hr prior to each dose to counteract the side effects of nausea that can occur with high doses of estrogen and progestin. › Advise a woman to be evaluated for pregnancy if menstruation does not begin within 21 days. › Provide client with counseling about contraception and modification of sexual behaviors that are risky. › Is considered a form of "emergency birth control."
Advantages	› Pill is not taken on a regular basis. › Can be obtained without a prescription by women 17 years and older.
Disadvantages	› Nausea, heavier than normal menstrual bleeding, lower abdominal pain, fatigue, and headache. › Does not provide long-term contraception. › Does not terminate an established pregnancy. › Does not protect against STIs.
Risks/possible complications/ contraindications	› Contraindicated if a client is pregnant or has undiagnosed abnormal vaginal bleeding. › If menstruation does not start within 1 week of expected date, a client may be pregnant.

TRANSDERMAL CONTRACEPTIVE PATCH

Definition	› Contains norelgestromin (progesterone) and ethinyl estradiol, which is delivered at continuous levels through the skin into subcutaneous tissue.
Client Instructions	› A client applies the patch to dry skin overlying subcutaneous tissue of the buttock, abdomen, upper arm, or torso, excluding breast area. › Requires patch replacement once a week. › Patch is applied the same day of the week for 3 weeks with no application of the patch on the fourth week.
Advantages	› Maintains consistent blood levels of hormone. › Avoids liver metabolism of medication because it is not absorbed in the gastrointestinal tract. › Decreases risk of forgetting daily pill.
Disadvantages	› Patch does not protect against STIs. › Poses same side effects as oral contraceptives. › Skin reaction may occur from patch application.
Risks/possible complications/ contraindications	› Same as those of oral contraceptives › Avoid applying of patch to skin rashes or lesions.

INJECTABLE PROGESTINS (DEPO-PROVERA)

Definition	› An intramuscular injection given to a female client every 11 to 13 weeks.
Client Instructions	› Start of injections should be during the first 5 days of a client's menstrual cycle and every 11 to 13 weeks thereafter. Injections in postpartum nonbreastfeeding women should begin within 5 days following delivery. For breastfeeding women, injections should start in the sixth week postpartum. › Advise clients to keep follow-up appointments. › A client should maintain an adequate intake of calcium and vitamin D.
Advantages	› Very effective and requires only four injections per year. › Does not impair lactation.
Disadvantages	› Can prolong amenorrhea. › Irregular or unpredictable bleeding or spotting. › Increases the risk of thromboembolism. › Decreases bone mineral density (loss of calcium). › Does not protect against STIs. › Should only be used as a long-term method of birth control (more than 2 years) if other birth control methods are inadequate.
Risks/possible complications/ contraindications	› Avoid massaging injection site following administration to avoid accelerating medication absorption, which will shorten the duration of its effectiveness.

CONTRACEPTIVE VAGINAL RING (NUVARING)

Definition	› Contains etonogestrel and ethinyl estradiol that is delivered at continuous levels vaginally.
Client Instructions	› A client inserts the ring vaginally. › Requires ring replacement after 3 weeks, and placement of new vaginal ring within 7 days. Insertion should occur on the same day of the week monthly.
Advantages	› Vaginal ring does not have to be fitted. › Decreases the risk of forgetting to take the pill.
Disadvantages	› Vaginal ring does not protect against STIs. › Poses the same side effects as oral contraceptives. › Some clients report discomfort during intercourse.
Risks/possible complications/ contraindications	› Blood clots, hypertension, stroke, heart attack. › Vaginal irritation, increased vaginal secretions, headache, weight gain, and nausea.

IMPLANTABLE PROGESTIN ETONOGESTREL (IMPLANON)

Definition	› Requires a minor surgical procedure to subdermally implant and remove a single rod containing etonogestrel on the inner side of the upper aspect of the arm.
Client Instructions	› Avoid trauma to the area of implantation.
Advantages	› Effective continuous contraception for 3 years. › Reversible. › Can be used by mothers who are breastfeeding after 4 weeks postpartum.
Disadvantages	› Etonogestrel can cause irregular menstrual bleeding. › Etonogestrel does not protect against STIs. › Most common side effect is irregular and unpredictable menstruation. › Headache.
Risks/possible complications/ contraindications	› Increased risk of ectopic pregnancy if pregnancy occurs.

INTRAUTERINE DEVICE (IUD)

Definition	› A chemically active T-shaped device that is inserted through a woman's cervix and placed in the uterus by the provider. Releases a chemical substance that damages sperm in transit to the uterine tubes and prevents fertilization.
Client Instructions	› The device must be monitored monthly by clients after menstruation to ensure the presence of the small string that hangs from the device into the upper part of the vagina to rule out migration or expulsion of the device.
Advantages	› An IUD can maintain effectiveness for 1 to 10 years. › Contraception can be reversed. › Does not interfere with spontaneity. › Safe for mothers who are breastfeeding. › It is 99% effective in preventing pregnancy.
Disadvantages	› An IUD can increase the risk of pelvic inflammatory disease, uterine perforation, or ectopic pregnancy. › A client should report to the provider late or abnormal spotting or bleeding, abdominal pain or pain with intercourse, abnormal or foul-smelling vaginal discharge, fever, chills, a change in string length, or if IUD cannot be located. › An IUD does not protect from STIs.
Risks/possible complications/ contraindications	› Best used by women in a monogamous relationship due to the risks of STIs. › May cause irregular menstrual bleeding. › A risk of bacterial vaginosis, uterine perforation, or uterine expulsion. › Must be removed in the event of pregnancy.

Transcervical Sterilization

ESSURE	
Definition	› Insertion of small flexible agents through the vagina and cervix into the fallopian tubes. This results in the development of scar tissue in the tubes preventing conception. › Examination must be done after 3 months to ensure fallopian tubes are blocked.
Client Instruction	› Normal activities may be resumed by most clients within 1 day of the procedure.
Advantages	› Quick procedure that requires no general anesthesia. › Nonhormonal means of birth control. › Essure is 99.8% effective in preventing pregnancy. › Rapid return to normal activities of daily living.
Disadvantages	› Not reversible. › Not intended for use in the client who is postpartum. › Delay in effectiveness for 3 months. Therefore, an alternative means of birth control should be used until confirmation of blocked fallopian tubes occurs. › Changes in menstrual patterns.
Risks/possible complications/ contraindications	› Perforation can occur › Unwanted pregnancy can occur if a client has unprotected sexual intercourse during the first 3 months following the procedure. › Increased risk of ectopic pregnancy if pregnancy occurs.

Surgical Methods

FEMALE STERILIZATION (BILATERAL TUBAL LIGATION SALPINGECTOMY)	
Definition	› A surgical procedure consisting of severance and/or burning or blocking the fallopian tubes to prevent fertilization.
Procedure	› The cutting, burning, or blocking of the fallopian tubes to prevent the ovum from being fertilized by the sperm.
Advantages	› Permanent contraception. › Sexual function is unaffected.
Disadvantages	› A surgical procedure carrying risks related to anesthesia, complications, infection, hemorrhage, or trauma. › Considered irreversible in the event that a client desires conception.
Risks/ possible complications/ contraindications	› Risk of ectopic pregnancy if pregnancy occurs.

MALE STERILIZATION (VASECTOMY)	
Definition	› A surgical procedure consisting of ligation and severance of the vas deferens.
Procedure	› The cutting of the vas deferens in the male as a form of permanent sterilization. Reinforce the need for alternate forms of birth control for approximately 20 ejaculations or 1 week to several months to allow all of the sperm to clear the vas deferens. This will ensure complete male infertility.
Client Instruction	› Following the procedure, scrotal support and moderate activity for a couple of days is recommended to reduce discomfort. › Sterility is delayed until the proximal portion of the vas deferens is cleared of all remaining sperm (approximately 20 ejaculations). › Alternate forms of birth control must be used until the vas deferens is cleared of sperm. › Follow up is important for sperm count.
Advantages	› A vasectomy is a permanent contraceptive method. › Procedure is short, safe, and simple. › Sexual function is not impaired.
Disadvantages	› Requires surgery. › Considered irreversible in the event that a client desires conception.
Risks/ possible complications/ contraindications	› Complications are rare, but may include bleeding, infection, and anesthesia reaction.

 View Images
> Bilateral Tubal Ligation > Vasectomy

PLICATION EXERCISES

A nurse in a health clinic is reviewing contraceptive use with a group of adolescent clients. Which of the llowing statements by an adolescent requires clarification?

   A. "A water-soluble lubricant should be used with condoms."

   B. "Spermicide is applied once when using a diaphragm."

   C. "Oral contraceptives can improve a case of acne."

   D. "A contraceptive patch is worn for a week."

2. A nurse is instructing a client who has been prescribed oral contraceptives about danger signs. The nurse evaluates that the client understands the teaching regarding side effects when she states the need to report

   A. reduced menstrual flow or amenorrhea.

   B. weight gain or breast tenderness.

   C. chest pain or shortness of breath.

   D. mild hypertension or headaches.

3. A nurse in an obstetrical clinic is providing education about contraception to a 21-year-old client. Which of the following statements by the client requesting information regarding an IUD indicates a need for additional teaching?

   A. "An IUD may increase my risk for an ectopic pregnancy."

   B. "I will wait until I have a child before I can have an IUD."

   C. "I might have irregular bleeding after I get an IUD."

   D. "A change in the string length of my IUD is expected."

4. A nurse in a clinic is teaching a client about her new prescription for medroxyprogesterone (Depo-Provera). Which of the following should be included in the teaching?

   A. "Weight loss can occur."

   B. "You are protected against STIs."

   C. "You should be taking calcium also."

   D. "You should avoid taking antibiotics when using this contraceptive."

5. Which of the following should the nurse include when teaching a client about the potential disadvantages of the minipill? (Select all that apply.)

_____ A. Amenorrhea

_____ B. Irregular vaginal bleeding

_____ C. Increased appetite

_____ D. Decreased libido

_____ E. Ovarian cysts

6. A nurse is reviewing teaching with a male client who is considering a vasectomy. Which of the following should be included in the teaching? Use the ATI Active Learning Template: Basic Concept to complete this item to include the following sections:

A. Topic Descriptor: Define the procedure.

B. Related Content: Describe one advantage and one disadvantage of this form of contraception.

C. Underlying Principles: Describe two teaching points for this client.

    D. INCORRECT: Contraceptive patches are replaced once a week.

     NCLEX® Connection: Health Promotion and Maintenance, Lifestyle Choices

2. A. INCORRECT: Reduced menstrual flow, or amenorrhea, is a common side effect of oral contraceptives and usually subsides after a few months of use.

    B. INCORRECT: Weight gain or breast tenderness is a common side effect of oral contraceptives and usually subsides after a few months of use.

    C. **CORRECT:** Chest pain or shortness of breath may indicate a pulmonary embolus or myocardial infarction.

    D. INCORRECT: Mild hypertension or headaches are a common side effect of oral contraceptives and usually subside after a few months of use.

     NCLEX® Connection: Health Promotion and Maintenance, Lifestyle Choices

3. A. INCORRECT: An IUD may increase the risk for an ectopic pregnancy.

    B. INCORRECT: Clients should have at least one child to be a candidate for an IUD.

    C. INCORRECT: An IUD may cause irregular vaginal bleeding.

    D. **CORRECT:** A change in the length of the string of an IUD may indicate expulsion and should be reported to the provider.

     NCLEX® Connection: Health Promotion and Maintenance, Lifestyle Choices

4. A. INCORRECT: Weight gain can occur.

    B. INCORRECT: Depo-Provera does not provide protection against STIs.

    C. **CORRECT:** Clients should take calcium and vitamin D to prevent loss of bone density, which can occur when taking Depo-Provera.

    D. INCORRECT: Antibiotics are not contraindicated when taking Depo-Provera.

     NCLEX® Connection: Pharmacological and Parenteral Therapies, Adverse Effects/Contraindications/ Side Effects/Interactions

B. **CORRECT:** Irregular vaginal bleeding is a disadvantage of the minipill.

C. **CORRECT:** Increased appetite is a disadvantage of the minipill.

D. **CORRECT:** Decreased libido is a disadvantage of the minipill.

E. **CORRECT:** The increased occurrence of ovarian cysts is a disadvantage of the minipill.

(N) NCLEX® Connection: Pharmacological and Parenteral Therapies, Adverse Effects/Contraindications/ Side Effects/Interactions

6. *Using the ATI Active Learning: Basic Concept*

A. Topic Descriptor
- Surgical procedure involving ligation and severance of the vas deferens.

B. Related Content
- Advantages
  - A permanent contraceptive method
  - Procedure is short, safe, and simple
  - Sexual function is not impaired
- Disadvantages
  - A surgical procedure; considered irreversible.

C. Underlying Principles
- Scrotal support and moderate activity are recommended for several days after the procedure to improve comfort.
- An alternate form of contraception should be used for approximately 20 ejaculations to ensure that the vas deferens is cleared of remaining sperm.
- A follow-up sperm count should be done.

(N) NCLEX® Connection: Reduction of Risk Potential, Therapeutic Procedures

chapter 2

Overview

- Infertility is defined as an inability to conceive despite engaging in unprotected sexual intercourse for a prolonged period of time or at least 12 months.
- Common factors associated with infertility may include decreased sperm production, endometriosis, ovulation disorders, and tubal occlusions.
- Partners who experience infertility may experience stress related to:
  - Physical inability to conceive
  - Expense
  - Effect on the couple's relationship
  - Lack of family support
- Infertility assessments, diagnostic procedures, and genetic counseling may be undertaken.

Infertility Assessments

- Female
  - Age – age greater than 35 years may affect fertility.
  - Duration of infertility – more than 1 year of coitus without contraceptives.
  - Medical history – atypical secondary sexual characteristic such as abnormal body fat distribution or hair growth, which is indicative of an endocrine disorder.
  - Surgical history – particularly, pelvic and abdominal procedures.
  - Obstetric history – past episodes of spontaneous abortions.
  - Gynecologic history – abnormal uterine contours or any history of disorders that may contribute to the formation of scar tissue that can cause blockage of ovum or sperm.
  - Sexual history – intercourse frequency, number of partners across the lifespan, and any history of STIs.
  - Occupational/environmental exposure risk assessment – exposure to hazardous teratogenic materials in the home or at a place of employment.
  - Weight – overweight or underweight.
- Male
  - Mumps during adolescence
  - Substance use (alcohol, cigarettes, heroin, marijuana [cannabis])
  - Exposure to hazardous teratogenic materials in home or work environment

Infertility Diagnostic Procedures

- Semen analysis – In 40% of couples who are infertile, inability to conceive is due to male infertility. This test is the first in an infertility workup because it is less expensive and less invasive compared with female infertility testing. It may need to be repeated.

- Pelvic examination – assesses for uterine or vaginal anomalies.

- Hormone analysis – evaluate hypothalamic-pituitary-ovarian axis to include serum prolactin, FSH, LH, estradiol, progesterone, and thyroid hormones.

- Endometrial biopsy – evaluates endometrial response, secretory, and luteal phase of menstrual cycle.

- Postcoital test – evaluates coital technique and mucus secretions.

- Ultrasonography – a transvaginal or abdominal ultrasound procedure performed to visualize female reproductive organs.

- Hysterosalpingography – outpatient radiological procedure in which dye is used to assess the patency of the fallopian tubes. Assess for history of allergies to iodine and seafood.

- Hysteroscopy – a radiographic procedure in which the uterus is examined for signs of defect, distortion, or scar tissue that may impair successful impregnation.

- Laparoscopy – a procedure where gas insufflation under general anesthesia is used to observe internal organs.

Complications

- Ectopic Pregnancy
  - Ovum may implant in the fallopian tubes or abdominal cavity due to the presence of endometrial tissue.
  - As ovum increases in size, fallopian tube may rupture, and extensive bleeding occurs, resulting in surgical removal of the damaged tube.
  - If ectopic pregnancy is identified prior to rupture of the tube, surgical removal of the products of conception may be performed, or methotrexate (Rheumatrex) is prescribed to dissolve the pregnancy.
  - Client faces increased risk of recurrence of an ectopic pregnancy and infertility.

Nursing Interventions for Infertility

- Encourage couples to express and discuss their feelings and recognize infertility as a major life stressor. Assist the couple to consider options, and provide education to assist in decision-making.

- Explain role of genetic counselor, reproductive specialist, geneticist, and pharmacist in providing psychosocial and medical care.

- Monitor for adverse effects associated with medications to treat female and male infertility.

- Advise that the use of medications to treat female infertility may increase the risk of multiple births by more than 25%.

- Provide information regarding assisted reproductive therapies (in vitro fertilization and embryo transfer, intrafallopian gamete transfer, surrogate parenting, and reproductive alternatives such as adoption).

- Make referrals to grief and infertility support groups.

Genetic Counseling

- Genetic counseling may be recommended by the provider if there is a family history of birth defects.

- Identify clients who are in need of genetic counseling, such as a client who has a sickle cell trait or sickle cell anemia, or a client older than 35. Make referrals to genetic specialists as necessary.

- Prenatal assessment of genetic disorders (amniocentesis) can pose potential risks to the fetus.

- Provide and clarify information pertaining to the risk of or the occurrence of genetic disorders within a family preceding, during, and following a genetic counseling session.

Nursing Interventions for Genetic Counseling

- Assist in the construction of family medical histories of several generations.

- Provide emotional support. Client responses vary and include denial, anger, grief, guilt, and self-blame.

- Make referrals to support groups and provide follow-up.

APPLICATION EXERCISES

1. A nurse in a clinic is caring for a group of female clients who are being evaluated for infertility. Which of the following clients should the nurse anticipate the provider will refer to a genetic counselor?

    A. A client whose sister has alopecia

    B. A client whose partner has von Willebrand disease

    C. A client who has an allergy to sulfa

    D. A client who had rubella 3 months ago

2. A nurse is caring for a couple who is being evaluated for infertility. Which of the following statements by the nurse indicates understanding of the infertility assessment process?

    A. "You will need to see a genetic counselor as part of the assessment."

    B. "It is usually the woman who is 'having trouble,' so the man doesn't have to be involved."

    C. "The man is the easiest to assess, and the provider will usually begin there."

    D. "Think about adopting first because there are many babies that need good homes."

3. A nurse in an infertility clinic is providing care to a couple who has been unable to conceive for 18 months. Which of the following data should be included in the assessment? (Select all that apply.)

    _____ A. Occupation

    _____ B. Menstrual history

    _____ C. Childhood infectious diseases

    _____ D. History of falls

    _____ E. Recent blood transfusions

4. A nurse in a clinic is caring for a client who is to be seen by the provider for a postoperative appointment following a salpingectomy due to an ectopic pregnancy. Which of the following statements by the client requires clarification?

    A. "It is good to know that I won't have a tubal pregnancy in the future."

    B. "The doctor said that this surgery can affect my ability to get pregnant again."

    C. "I understand that one of my fallopian tubes had to be removed."

    D. "Ovulation can still occur because my ovaries were not affected."

5. A nurse is reviewing the health record of a client who is to undergo hysterosalpingography. Which of the following data alert the nurse that the client is at risk for a complication related to this procedure? (Refer to the chart below.)

Vital Signs	History and Physical	Laboratory Findings	Medications
› Temperature 37.2° C (98.9° F) › BMI 40.3	› Employed as a radiology technician › Allergy to shrimp › Tonsillectomy at age 18	› Glucose 103 mg/dL › Hgb 13.1 g/dL › Total cholesterol 265 mg/dL	› Rosuvastatin (Crestor) › Magnesium oxide (Mag-Ox) › Mafenide acetate (Sulfamylon)

    A. Vital signs

    B. History and physical

    C. Laboratory findings

    D. Medications

6. A nurse in an infertility clinic is caring for a client and her partner. The client asks about the assessments and diagnostic procedures that are done to determine whether infertility can be identified. What is an appropriate response by the nurse? Use the ATI Active Learning Template: Systems Disorder to complete this item to include the following sections:

    A. Description of Disorder/Disease Process: Define infertility.

    B. Assessments: Describe at least three.

    C. Diagnostic Procedures: Describe at least three.

APPLICATION EXERCISES KEY

1. A. INCORRECT: Alopecia is a nonhereditary disorder and does not warrant referral to a genetic counselor.

    B. **CORRECT:** Von Willebrand disease is an genetic bleeding disorder and warrants a client being referred to a genetic counselor.

    C. INCORRECT: Allergy to sulfa is a nonhereditary condition and does not warrant referral to a genetic counselor.

    D. INCORRECT: A recent episode of rubella in a non-pregnant female does not warrant a referral to a genetic counselor.

     NCLEX® Connection: Health Promotion and Maintenance, Health Screening

2. A. INCORRECT: A referral to a genetic counselor occurs if there is a reason to suspect birth defects or other physiological concerns. It is not included in all infertility assessment processes.

    B. INCORRECT: The cause of infertility is almost evenly divided between men and women.

    C. **CORRECT:** A sperm analysis is one of the first steps in the infertility assessment process and can identify a cause of infertility in a less-invasive and less-costly manner.

    D. INCORRECT: Adoption is an option for the infertile couple after identifying a possible cause for the infertility.

     NCLEX® Connection: Health Promotion and Maintenance, Health Screening

3. A. **CORRECT:** Occupational hazards may include exposure to teratogenic substances in the workplace, such as radiation, chemicals, herbicides, and pesticides.

    B. **CORRECT:** Menstrual history can identify hormone-related patterns, such as anovulation, pituitary disorders, and endometriosis.

    C. **CORRECT:** Childhood infectious diseases may identify the male partner having had the mumps.

    D. INCORRECT: A history of falls is not a consideration in the assessment.

    E. INCORRECT: A recent blood transfusion is not a consideration in the assessment.

     NCLEX® Connection: Health Promotion and Maintenance, Health Screening

4. A. **CORRECT:** The risk of recurrence of an ectopic pregnancy is increased following an ectopic pregnancy.

    B. INCORRECT: Infertility can occur as a result of an ectopic pregnancy.

    C. INCORRECT: A salpingectomy involves the removal of a fallopian tube.

    D. INCORRECT: A salpingectomy does not involve the removal of the ovaries.

    (N) NCLEX® Connection: Reduction of Risk Potential, Therapeutic Procedures

5. A. INCORRECT: The client is obese, but this does not place the client at risk for a complication related to the procedure.

    B. **CORRECT:** An allergy to seafood is a contraindication to the dye used in hysterosalpingography.

    C. INCORRECT: The client's total cholesterol is elevated, but this does not place the client at risk for a complication related to the procedure.

    D. INCORRECT: There are no contraindications related to the medications the client is taking.

    (N) NCLEX® Connection: Reduction of Risk Potential, Potential for Complications from Surgical Procedures and Health Alterations

6. *Using the ATI Active Learning: Systems Disorder*

    A. Description of Disorder/Disease Process
       - Inability to conceive despite engaging in unprotected sexual intercourse for a prolonged period of time or at least 12 months

    B. Assessments
       - Age
       - Weight
       - Duration of infertility
       - Medical history
       - Surgical history
       - Obstetric history
       - Gynecologic history
       - Occupational/environmental exposure risk

    C. Diagnostic Procedures
       - Semen analysis
       - Pelvic examination
       - Hormone analysis
       - Endometrial biopsy
       - Postcoital test
       - Ultrasonography
       - Hysterosalpingography
       - Hysteroscopy
       - Laparoscopy

    (N) NCLEX® Connection: Health Promotion and Maintenance, Health Promotion/Disease Prevention

chapter 3

Overview

- Recognizing changes during pregnancy is helpful for both clients and nurses. The nurse and provider assess findings during the client's initial prenatal visit.
- Signs of pregnancy are classified into three groups.
  - Presumptive
  - Probable
  - Positive
- Calculating delivery date, number of pregnancies, and evaluating the physiological status of a client who is pregnant are performed.

Signs of Pregnancy

- Presumptive signs – changes that the woman experiences that make her think that she may be pregnant. These changes may be subjective symptoms or objective signs. Signs also may be a result of physiological factors other than pregnancy (peristalsis, infections, and stress).
  - Amenorrhea
  - Fatigue
  - Nausea and vomiting
  - Urinary frequency
  - Breast changes – darkened areolae, enlarged Montgomery's glands
  - Quickening – slight fluttering movements of the fetus felt by a woman, usually between 16 to 20 weeks of gestation
  - Uterine enlargement
- Probable signs – changes that make the examiner suspect a woman is pregnant (primarily related to physical changes of the uterus). Signs can be caused by physiological factors other than pregnancy (pelvic congestion, tumors).
  - Abdominal enlargement related to changes in uterine size, shape, and position
  - Hegar's sign – softening and compressibility of lower uterus
  - Chadwick's sign – deepened violet-bluish color of cervix and vaginal mucosa
  - Goodell's sign – softening of cervical tip
  - Ballottement – rebound of unengaged fetus
  - Braxton Hicks contractions – false contractions; painless, irregular, and usually relieved by walking
  - Positive pregnancy test
  - Fetal outline felt by examiner

- Positive signs – signs that can be explained only by pregnancy.
  - Fetal heart sounds
  - Visualization of fetus by ultrasound
  - Fetal movement palpated by an experienced examiner

Verifying Possible Pregnancy Using Serum and Urine Pregnancy Testing

- Serum and urine tests provide an accurate assessment for the presence of human chorionic gonadotropin (hCG). hCG production can start as early as the day of implantation and can be detected as early as 7 to 10 days after conception.
- Production of hCG begins with implantation, peaks at about 60 to 70 days of gestation, declines until around 80 days of pregnancy, and then gradually increases until term.
- Higher levels of hCG can indicate multifetal pregnancy, ectopic pregnancy, hydatidiform mole (gestational trophoblastic disease), or a genetic abnormality such as Down syndrome. Lower blood levels of hCG may suggest a miscarriage.
- Some medications (anticonvulsants, diuretics, tranquilizers) can cause false-positive or false-negative pregnancy results.
- Urine samples should be first-voided morning specimens.

Calculating Delivery Date and Determining Number of Pregnancies for Pregnant Client

- Nägele's rule – Take the first day of the woman's last menstrual cycle, subtract 3 months, and then add 7 days and 1 year, adjusting for the year as necessary.
- Measurement of fundal height in centimeters from the symphysis pubis to the top of the uterine fundus (between 18 and 32 weeks of gestation).
  - Approximates the gestational age
- Gravidity – number of pregnancies.
  - Nulligravida – a woman who has never been pregnant
  - Primigravida – a woman in her first pregnancy
  - Multigravida – a woman who has had two or more pregnancies
  - Parity – number of pregnancies in which the fetus or fetuses reach viability (approximately 20 weeks) regardless of whether the fetus is born alive
    - Nullipara – no pregnancy beyond the stage of viability
    - Primipara – has completed one pregnancy to stage of viability
    - Multipara – has completed two or more pregnancies to stage of viability
- GTPAL acronym
  - Gravidity
  - Term births (38 weeks or more)
  - Preterm births (from viability up to 37 weeks)
  - Abortions/miscarriages (prior to viability)
  - Living children

Physiological Status of Pregnant Client

- Reproductive – Uterus increases in size and changes shape and position. Ovulation and menses cease during pregnancy.

- Cardiovascular – Cardiac output and blood volume increase (45 to 50% at term) to meet the greater metabolic needs. Heart rate increases during pregnancy.

- Respiratory – Maternal oxygen needs increase. During the last trimester, the size of the chest may enlarge, allowing for lung expansion, as the uterus pushes upward. Respiratory rate increases and total lung capacity decreases.

- Musculoskeletal – Body alterations and weight increase necessitate an adjustment in posture. Pelvic joints relax.

- Gastrointestinal – Nausea and vomiting may occur due to hormonal changes and/or an increase of pressure within the abdominal cavity as the pregnant client's stomach and intestines are displaced within the abdomen. Constipation may occur due to increased transit time of food through the gastrointestinal tract and, thus, increased water absorption.

- Renal – Filtration rate increases secondary to the influence of pregnancy hormones and an increase in blood volume and metabolic demands. The amount of urine produced remains the same. Urinary frequency is common during pregnancy.

- Endocrine – The placenta becomes an endocrine organ that produces large amounts of hCG, progesterone, estrogen, human placental lactogen, and prostaglandins. Hormones are very active during pregnancy and function to maintain pregnancy and prepare the body for delivery.

- Body Image Changes
  - Due to physical and psychological changes that occur, the pregnant woman requires support from her provider and family members.
  - In the first trimester of pregnancy, physiological changes are not obvious. Many women look forward to the changes so that pregnancy will be more noticeable.
  - During the second trimester, there are rapid physical changes due to the enlargement of the abdomen and breasts. Skin changes also occur, such as stretch marks and hyperpigmentation. These changes can affect a woman's mobility. She may find herself losing her balance and feeling back or leg discomfort and fatigue. These factors may lead to a negative body image. The client may make statements of resentment toward the pregnancy and express anxiousness for the pregnancy to be over soon.

- Expected Vital Signs
  - Blood pressure measurements are within the prepregnancy range during the first trimester.
  - Blood pressure decreases 5 to 10 mm Hg for both the diastolic and the systolic during the second trimester.
  - Blood pressure should return to the prepregnancy baseline range after approximately 20 weeks of gestation.
  - Position of the pregnant woman also may affect blood pressure. In the supine position, blood pressure may appear to be lower due to the weight and pressure of the gravid uterus on the vena cava, which decreases venous blood flow to the heart. Maternal hypotension and fetal hypoxia may occur, which is referred to as supine hypotensive syndrome or supine vena cava syndrome. Signs and symptoms include dizziness, lightheadedness, and pale, clammy skin. Encourage the client to engage in maternal positioning on the left-lateral side, semi-Fowler's position, or, if supine, with a wedge placed under one hip to alleviate pressure to the vena cava.

- Pulse increases 10 to 15/min around 20 weeks of gestation and remains elevated throughout the remainder of the pregnancy.
- Respirations increase by 1 to 2/min. Respiratory changes in pregnancy are attributed to the elevation of the diaphragm by as much as 4 cm, as well as changes to the chest wall to facilitate increased maternal oxygen demands. Some shortness of breath may be noted.
- Expected Physical Assessment Findings
  - Fetal heart tones are heard at a normal baseline rate of 110 to 160/min with reassuring FHR accelerations noted, which indicates an intact fetal CNS.
  - The client's heart changes in size and shape with resulting cardiac hypertrophy to accommodate increased blood volume and increased cardiac output. Heart sounds also change to accommodate the increase in blood volume with a more distinguishable splitting of S_1 and S_2, with S_3 more easily heard following 20 weeks of gestation. Murmurs also may be auscultated. Heart size and shape should return to normal shortly after delivery.
  - Uterine size changes from a uterine weight of 50 to 1,000 g (0.1 to 2.2 lb). By 36 weeks of gestation, the top of the uterus and the fundus will reach the xiphoid process. This may cause the pregnant woman to experience shortness of breath as the uterus pushes against the diaphragm.
  - Cervical changes are obvious as a purplish-blue color extends into the vagina and labia, and the cervix becomes markedly soft.
  - Breast changes occur due to hormones of pregnancy, with the breasts increasing in size and the areolas darkening.
  - Skin changes
    - Chloasma – Pigmentation increases on the face.
    - Linea nigra – Dark line of pigmentation from the umbilicus extending to the pubic area.
    - Striae gravidarum – Stretch marks most notably found on the abdomen and thighs.

Nursing Interventions for the Pregnant Client

- Acknowledge the client's concerns about pregnancy, and encourage sharing of these feelings while providing an atmosphere free of judgment.
- Discuss with the client the expected physiological changes and a possible timeline for a return to the prepregnant state.
- Assist the client in setting goals for the postpartum period in regard to self-care and newborn care.
- Refer the client to counseling if body image concerns appear to have a negative impact on the pregnancy.
- Provide education about the expected physiological and psychosocial changes. Common discomforts of pregnancy and ways to resolve those discomforts are reviewed during prenatal visits.
- The client is encouraged to keep all follow-up appointments and to contact the provider immediately if there is any bleeding, leakage of fluid, or contractions at any time during the pregnancy.

APPLICATION EXERCISES

1. A nurse is caring for a client who is pregnant and states that her last menstrual period was April 1, 2013. Which of the following is the client's estimated date of delivery?

    A. Jan. 8, 2014

    B. Jan. 15, 2014

    C. Feb. 8, 2014

    D. Feb. 15, 2014

2. A nurse in a prenatal clinic is caring for a client who is in the first trimester of pregnancy. The client's health record includes this data: G3 T1 P0 A1 L1. How should the nurse interpret this information? (Select all that apply.)

_____ A. Client has delivered one newborn at term.

_____ B. Client has experienced no preterm labor.

_____ C. Client has been through active labor.

_____ D. Client has had two prior pregnancies.

_____ E. Client has one living child.

3. A nurse is reviewing the health record of a client who is pregnant. The provider indicated the client exhibits probable signs of pregnancy. Which of the following would be included? (Select all that apply.)

_____ A. Montgomery's glands

_____ B. Goodell's sign

_____ C. Ballottement

_____ D. Chadwick's sign

_____ E. Quickening

4. A nurse in a prenatal clinic is caring for a client who is pregnant and experiencing episodes of maternal hypotension. The client asks the nurse what causes these episodes. Which of the following is an appropriate response by the nurse?

    A. "This is due to an increase in blood volume."

    B. "This is due to pressure from the uterus on the diaphragm."

    C. "This is due to the weight of the uterus on the vena cava."

    D. "This is due to increased cardiac output."

5. A nurse in a clinic receives a phone call from a client who believes she is pregnant and would like to be tested in the clinic to confirm her pregnancy. Which of the following information should the nurse provide to the client?

    A. "You should wait until 4 weeks after conception to be tested."

    B. "You should be off any medications for 24 hours prior to the test."

    C. "You should be NPO for at least 8 hours prior to the test."

    D. "You should collect urine from the first morning void."

6. A nurse is caring for a client who is in the fourth week of gestation. The client asks about skin and breast changes that can occur during pregnancy. What is an appropriate response by the nurse? Use the ATI Active Learning Template: Basic Concept to complete this item to include the following:

    A. Related Content: Describe at least three changes that occur to skin and breasts during pregnancy.

    B. Underlying principles: Describe the basis for these changes.

APPLICATION EXERCISES KEY

1. A. **CORRECT:** April 1, 2013, minus 3 months plus 7 days and 1 year equals an estimated date of delivery of Jan. 8, 2014.

   B. INCORRECT: This is incorrect using Nägele's rule.

   C. INCORRECT: This is incorrect using Nägele's rule.

   D. INCORRECT: This is incorrect using Nägele's rule.

   N NCLEX® Connection: Health Promotion and Maintenance, Ante/Intra/Postpartum and Newborn Care

2. A. **CORRECT:** T1 indicates the client has delivered one newborn at term.

   B. INCORRECT: P0 indicates the client has had no preterm deliveries.

   C. INCORRECT: A1 indicates the client has had one miscarriage.

   D. **CORRECT:** G3 indicates the children has had two prior pregnancies and the client is currently pregnant

   E. **CORRECT:** L1 indicates the client has one living child.

   N NCLEX® Connection: Health Promotion and Maintenance, Ante/Intra/Postpartum and Newborn Care

3. A. INCORRECT: Montgomery's glands are a presumptive sign of pregnancy.

   B. **CORRECT:** Goodell's sign is a probable sign of pregnancy.

   C. **CORRECT:** Ballottement is a probable sign of pregnancy.

   D. **CORRECT:** Chadwick's sign is a probable sign of pregnancy.

   E. INCORRECT: Quickening is a presumptive sign of pregnancy.

   N NCLEX® Connection: Health Promotion and Maintenance, Developmental Stages and Transitions

4.   A. INCORRECT: An increase in blood volume during pregnancy results in cardiac hypertrophy.

     B. INCORRECT: Pressure from the gravid uterus on the diaphragm may cause the client to experience shortness of breath.

     C. **CORRECT:** Maternal hypotension occurs when the client is lying in the supine position, and the weight of the gravid uterus places pressure on the vena cava, decreasing venous blood flow to the heart.

     D. INCORRECT: An increase in cardiac output during pregnancy results in cardiac hypertrophy.

     (N) NCLEX® Connection: Reduction of Risk Potential, Changes/Abnormalities in Vital Signs

5.   A. INCORRECT: The production of hCG can be detected as early as 7 to 10 days after conception.

     B. INCORRECT: Clients are not advised to stop taking medications in preparation for pregnancy tests. Medications should be reviewed to determine whether they can affect the results.

     C. INCORRECT: Clients are not advised to remain NPO prior to pregnancy testing. Serum or blood tests are not affected by food or fluid intake.

     D. **CORRECT:** Urine pregnancy tests should be done on a first-voided morning specimen to provide the most accurate results.

     (N) NCLEX® Connection: Reduction of Risk Potential, Laboratory Values

6.   *Using the ATI Active Learning Template: Basic Concept*

     A. Related Content
         - Skin changes: hyperpigmentation; linea nigra; chloasma (mask of pregnancy) on the face; striae gravidarum (stretch marks), most pronounced on abdomen and thighs
         - Breast changes: darkening of the areola, enlarged Montgomery's glands, increase in size and heaviness, increased sensitivity

     B. Underlying principles
         - Increase in estrogen and progesterone occurring during pregnancy

     (N) NCLEX® Connection: Health Promotion and Maintenance, Developmental Stages and Transitions

chapter 4

Overview

- Prenatal care involves nursing assessments and client education for expectant mothers. When providing prenatal care, nurses must take into account cultural considerations.

- Prenatal education encompasses information provided to a client who is pregnant. Major areas of focus include assisting the client in self-care of the discomforts of pregnancy, promoting a safe outcome to pregnancy, and fostering positive feelings by the pregnant woman and her family regarding the childbearing experience.

- Prenatal care dramatically reduces infant and maternal morbidity and mortality rates by early detection and treatment of potential problems. A majority of birth defects occur between 2 and 8 weeks of gestation.

Nursing Assessments

- Nurses play an integral role in assessing a client's current knowledge, previous pregnancies, and birthing experiences.

- Nursing assessment in prenatal care includes obtaining information regarding:

  ○ Reproductive and obstetrical history (contraception use, gynecological diagnoses, and obstetrical difficulties).

  ○ Medical history, including the woman's immune status (rubella and hepatitis B).

  ○ Family history, such as genetic disorders.

  ○ Any recent or current illnesses or infections.

  ○ Current medications, including substance use and alcohol consumption. The nurse should display a nonjudgmental, matter-of-fact demeanor when interviewing a client regarding substance abuse and observe for signs and symptoms such as lack of grooming.

  ○ Psychosocial history (a client's emotional response to pregnancy, adolescent pregnancy, spouse, support system, history of depression, domestic violence issues).

  ○ Any hazardous environmental exposures; current work conditions.

  ○ Current exercise and diet habits as well as lifestyle.

- A nurse ascertains what a client's goals are for the birthing process. The nurse should discusses birthing methods, such as Lamaze, and pain control options (epidural, natural childbirth).

- Prenatal care begins with an initial assessment and continues throughout pregnancy. In an uneventful pregnancy, prenatal visits are scheduled monthly for 7 months, every 2 weeks during the eighth month, and every week during the last month.
  - At the initial prenatal visit:
    - Determine estimated date of birth based on the last menstrual period.
    - Obtain medical and nursing history to include social supports, and review of systems (to determine risk factors).
    - Perform a physical assessment to include a client's baseline weight, vital signs, and pelvic examination. Assess for costovertebral angle tenderness to identify kidney infection.
    - Obtain initial laboratory tests.
  - Ongoing prenatal visits include the following:
    - Monitoring weight, blood pressure, and urine for glucose, protein, and leukocytes.
    - Monitoring for the presence of edema.
    - Monitoring fetal development.
      - FHR can be heard by Doppler at 10 to 12 weeks of gestation or heard with an ultrasound stethoscope at 16 to 20 weeks of gestation. Listen at the midline, right above the symphysis pubis, by holding the stethoscope firmly on the abdomen.
      - Measure fundal height after 12 weeks of gestation.

 View Video: Measuring Fundal Height

      - Begin assessing for fetal movement between 16 and 20 weeks of gestation.
    - Providing education for self-care to include management of common discomforts and concerns of pregnancy (nausea and vomiting, fatigue, backache, varicosities, heartburn, activity, sexuality).

PRENATAL CARE: ROUTINE LABORATORY TESTS
Blood type, Rh factor, and presence of irregular antibodies
› Determines the risk for maternal-fetal blood incompatibility (erythroblastosis fetalis) or neonatal hyperbilirubinemia. Indirect Coombs' test identifies clients sensitized to Rh-positive blood. For clients who are Rh-negative and not sensitized, the indirect Coombs' test is repeated between 24 to 28 weeks of gestation.
CBC with differential, Hgb, and Hct
› Detects infection and anemia.
Hgb electrophoresis
› Identifies hemoglobinopathies (sickle cell anemia and thalassemia).
Rubella titer
› Determines immunity to rubella.
Hepatitis B screen
› Identifies carriers of hepatitis B.
Group B Streptococcus (GBS)
› Obtained at 35 to 37 weeks of gestation.

PRENATAL CARE: ROUTINE LABORATORY TESTS

Urinalysis with microscopic examination of pH, specific gravity, color, sediment, protein, glucose, albumin, RBCs, WBCs, casts, acetone, and human chorionic gonadotropin

› Identifies pregnancy, diabetes mellitus, gestational hypertension, renal disease, and infection.

One-hour glucose tolerance (Oral ingestion or IV administration of concentrated glucose with venous sample taken 1 hr later [fasting not necessary])

› Identifies hyperglycemia; done at initial visit for at-risk clients, and at 24 to 28 weeks of gestation for all pregnant women (> 140 mg/dL requires follow up).

Three-hour glucose tolerance (Fasting overnight prior to oral ingestion or IV administration of concentrated glucose with a venous sample taken 1, 2, and 3 hr later)

› Used in clients with elevated 1-hr glucose test as a screening tool for diabetes mellitus. A diagnosis of gestational diabetes requires two elevated blood-glucose readings.

Papanicolaou (PAP) test

› Screening tool for cervical cancer, herpes simplex type 2, and/or human papillomavirus.

Vaginal/cervical culture

› Detects streptococcus ß-hemolytic, bacterial vaginosis, or sexually transmitted infections (gonorrhea and chlamydia).

PPD (tuberculosis screening), chest x-ray after 20 weeks of gestation with PPD test

› Identifies exposure to tuberculosis.

Venereal disease research laboratory (VDRL)

› Syphilis screening mandated by law.

HIV

› Detects HIV infection (the Centers for Disease Control and Prevention and the American Congress of Obstetricians and Gynecologists recommend testing all clients who are pregnant unless the client refuses testing).

Toxoplasmosis, other infections, rubella, cytomegalovirus, and herpes virus (TORCH) screening when indicated

› Screening for a group of infections capable of crossing the placenta and adversely affecting fetal development.

Maternal serum alpha-fetoprotein (MSAFP)

› Screening occurs between 15 to 22 weeks of gestation. Used to rule out Down syndrome (low level) and neural tube defects (high level). The provider may decide to use a more reliable indicator and opt for the Quad screen instead of the MSAFP at 16 to 18 weeks of gestation. This includes AFP, inhibin-A, a combination analysis of human chorionic gonadotropin, and estriol.

- ○ Perform or assist with Leopold maneuvers to palpate presentation and position of the fetus.
- ○ Assist the provider with the gynecological examination. This examination is performed to determine the status of a client's reproductive organs and birth canal. Pelvic measurements determine whether the pelvis will allow for the passage of the fetus at delivery.
  - ▪ The nurse has the client empty her bladder and take deep breaths during the examination to decrease discomfort.
- ○ Administer RhO(D) immune globulin (RhoGAM) IM around 28 weeks of gestation for clients who are Rh-negative.

Client Education

- Prenatal education includes health promotion, preparation for pregnancy and birth, common discomforts of pregnancy, and warning/danger signs to report.

- Health Promotion

  - Preconception and prenatal education emphasizes healthy behaviors that promote the health of the pregnant woman and her fetus.

    - A client is instructed to avoid all over-the-counter medications, supplements, and prescription medications unless the provider who is supervising her care has knowledge of this practice.

    - Alcohol (birth defects) and tobacco (low birth weight) are contraindicated during pregnancy.

    - Substance use of any kind is to be avoided during pregnancy and lactation. Strategies to reduce or eliminate substance use are reviewed.

  - The nurse educates a client about the following:

    - Need for flu immunization

    - Smoking cessation

    - Treatment of current infections

    - Genetic testing and counseling

    - Exposure to hazardous materials

  - Exercise during pregnancy yields positive benefits and should consist of 30 min of moderate exercise (walking or swimming) daily if not medically or obstetrically contraindicated.

    - Avoid the use of hot tubs or saunas.

    - Consume at least 2 to 3 L of water each day from food and beverage sources.

- Preparation for Pregnancy and Birth

  - Nurses provide anticipatory teaching to the pregnant client and her family about the following:

    - Physical and emotional changes during pregnancy and interventions that can be implemented to provide relief.

    - Signs and symptoms of complications to report to the provider.

    - Birthing options available to enhance the birthing process.

  - Maternal adaptation to pregnancy and the attainment of the maternal role – whereby the idea of pregnancy is accepted and assimilated into the client's way of life – includes hormonal and psychological aspects.

    - Emotional lability is experienced by many women with unpredictable mood changes and increased irritability, tearfulness, and anger alternating with feelings of joy and cheerfulness. This may result from hormonal changes.

    - A feeling of ambivalence about the pregnancy, which is a normal response, may occur early in the pregnancy and resolve before the third trimester. It consists of conflicting feelings (joy, pleasure, sorrow, hostility) about the pregnancy. These feelings can occur simultaneously, whether the pregnancy was planned or not.

Q
PCC

- The nurse anticipates reviewing prenatal education topics with a client based on her current knowledge and previous pregnancy and birth experiences. The client's readiness to learn is enhanced when the nurse provides teaching during the appropriate trimester based on learning needs. Using a variety of educational methods, such as pamphlets and videos, and having the client verbalize and demonstrate learned topics will ensure that learning has taken place.

  - First Trimester
    - Physical and psychosocial changes
    - Common discomforts of pregnancy and measures to provide relief
    - Lifestyle: exercise, stress, nutrition, sexual health, dental care, over-the-counter and prescription medications, tobacco, alcohol, substance use, and STIs (encourage safe sexual practices)
    - Possible complications and signs to report (preterm labor)
    - Fetal growth and development
    - Prenatal exercise
    - Expected laboratory testing

  - Second Trimester
    - Benefits of breastfeeding
    - Common discomforts and relief measures

Q
S

    - Lifestyle: sex and pregnancy, rest and relaxation, posture, body mechanics, clothing, and seat belt safety and travel
    - Fetal movement
    - Complications (preterm labor, gestational hypertension, gestational diabetes mellitus, premature rupture of membranes)
    - Preparation for childbirth and childbirth education classes
    - Review of birthing methods
    - Development of a birth plan (verbal or written agreement about what client wishes during labor and delivery)

Q
EBP

  - Third Trimester
    - Childbirth preparation
      - Childbirth classes or birth plan.
      - Breathing and relaxation techniques
      - Use of effleurage and counterpressure
      - Application of heat/cold, touch and massage, and water therapy
      - Use of transcutaneous electrical nerve stimulation (TENS)
      - Acupressure and acupuncture
      - Music and aromatherapy
      - Discussion regarding pain management during labor and birth (natural childbirth, epidural)
      - Signs and symptoms of preterm labor and labor
      - Labor process
      - Infant care
      - Postpartum care

- Fetal movement/kick counts to ascertain fetal well-being. A client should be instructed to count and record fetal movements or kicks daily.
  - ▸ Mothers should count fetal activity two or three times a day for 60 min each time. Fetal movements of less than 3 per hr or movements that cease entirely for 12 hr indicate a need for further evaluation.
  - Diagnostic testing for fetal well-being (nonstress test, biophysical profile, ultrasound, and contraction stress test).
- Common Discomforts of Pregnancy
  - Nausea and vomiting may occur during the first trimester. The client should eat crackers or dry toast 30 min to 1 hr before rising in the morning to relieve discomfort. Instruct the client to avoid having an empty stomach and ingesting spicy, greasy, or gas-forming foods. Encourage the client to drink fluids between meals.
  - Breast tenderness may occur during the first trimester. The client should wear a bra that provides adequate support.
  - Urinary frequency may occur during the first and third trimesters. The client should empty her bladder frequently, decrease fluid intake before bedtime, and use perineal pads. The client is taught how to perform Kegel exercises (alternate tightening and relaxation of pubococcygeal muscles) to reduce stress incontinence (leakage of urine with coughing and sneezing).
  - Urinary tract infections (UTIs) are common during pregnancy because of renal changes and the vaginal flora becoming more alkaline.

    - UTI risks can be decreased by encouraging the client to wipe the perineal area from front to back after voiding; avoiding bubble baths; wearing cotton underpants; avoiding tight-fitting pants; and consuming plenty of water (8 glasses per day).
    - The client should urinate before and after intercourse to flush bacteria from the urethra that are present or introduced during intercourse.
    - Advise the client to urinate as soon as the urge occurs because retaining urine provides an environment for bacterial growth.
    - Advise the client to notify her provider if her urine is foul-smelling, contains blood, or appears cloudy.
  - Fatigue may occur during the first and third trimesters. The client is encouraged to engage in frequent rest periods.
  - Heartburn may occur during the second and third trimesters due to the stomach being displaced by the enlarging uterus and a slowing of gastrointestinal tract motility and digestion brought about by increased progesterone levels. The client should eat small frequent meals, not allow the stomach to get too empty or too full, sit up for 30 min after meals, and check with her provider prior to using any over-the-counter antacids.
  - Constipation may occur during the second and third trimesters. The client is encouraged to drink plenty of fluids, eat a diet high in fiber, and exercise regularly.
  - Hemorrhoids may occur during the second and third trimesters. A warm sitz bath, witch hazel pads, and application of topical ointments will help relieve discomfort.
  - Backaches are common during the second and third trimesters. The client is encouraged to exercise regularly, perform pelvic tilt exercises (alternately arching and straightening the back), use proper body mechanics by using the legs to lift rather than the back, and use the side-lying position.
  - Shortness of breath and dyspnea may occur because of the enlarged uterus, which limits inspiration. The client should maintain good posture, sleep with extra pillows, and contact her provider if symptoms worsen.

○ Leg cramps during the third trimester may occur due to the compression of lower-extremity nerves and blood vessels by the enlarging uterus. This can result in poor peripheral circulation as well as an imbalance in the calcium/phosphorus ratio. The client should extend the affected leg, keeping the knee straight, and dorsiflex the foot (toes toward head). Application of heat over the affected muscle or a foot massage while the leg is extended can help relieve cramping. The client should notify her provider if frequent cramping occurs.

○ Varicose veins and lower-extremity edema can occur during the second and third trimesters. The client should rest with her legs elevated, avoid constricting clothing, wear support hose, avoid sitting or standing in one position for extended periods of time, and not sit with her legs crossed at the knees. She should sleep in the left-lateral position and exercise moderately with frequent walking to stimulate venous return.

○ Gingivitis, nasal stuffiness, and epistaxis (nosebleed) can occur as a result of elevated estrogen levels causing increased vascularity and proliferation of connective tissue. The client should gently brush her teeth, observe good dental hygiene, use a humidifier, and use normal saline nose drops or spray.

○ Braxton Hicks contractions, which occur from the first trimester onward, may increase in intensity and frequency during the third trimester. Inform the client that a change of position and walking should cause contractions to subside. If contractions increase in intensity and frequency (true contractions) with regularity, the client should notify her provider.

○ Supine hypotension occurs when a woman lies on her back and the weight of the gravid uterus compresses her vena cava. This reduces blood supply to the fetus. The client may experience feelings of lightheadedness and faintness. Teach the client to lie in a side-lying or semi-sitting position with her knees slightly flexed.

• Danger Signs During Pregnancy

○ The following indicate potential dangerous situations that should be reported to the provider immediately.

 View Video: Danger Signs of Pregnancy

- Gush of fluid from the vagina (rupture of amniotic fluid) prior to 37 weeks of gestation
- Vaginal bleeding (placental problems such as abruption or previa)
- Abdominal pain (premature labor, abruptio placentae, or ectopic pregnancy)
- Changes in fetal activity (decreased fetal movement may indicate fetal distress)
- Persistent vomiting (hyperemesis gravidarum)
- Severe headaches (gestational hypertension)
- Elevated temperature (infection)
- Dysuria (urinary tract infection)
- Blurred vision (gestational hypertension)
- Edema of face and hands (gestational hypertension)
- Epigastric pain (gestational hypertension)
- Concurrent occurrence of flushed dry skin, fruity breath, rapid breathing, increased thirst and urination, and headache (hyperglycemia)
- Concurrent occurrence of clammy pale skin, weakness, tremors, irritability, and lightheadedness (hypoglycemia)

APPLICATION EXERCISES

1. A nurse is teaching a group of women who are pregnant about measures to relieve backache during pregnancy. The nurse should teach the women which of the following? (Select all that apply.)

_____ A. Avoid any lifting.

_____ B. Perform Kegel exercises twice a day.

_____ C. Perform the pelvic rock exercise every day.

_____ D. Use proper body mechanics.

_____ E. Avoid constrictive clothing.

2. A client who is at 8 weeks of gestation tells the nurse that she isn't sure she is happy about being pregnant. Which of the following is an appropriate response by the nurse to the client's statement?

A. "I will inform the provider that you are having these feelings."

B. "It is normal to have these feelings during the first few months of pregnancy."

C. "You should be happy that you are going to bring new life into the world."

D. "I am going to make an appointment with the counselor for you to discuss these thoughts."

3. A nurse is caring for a client who is pregnant and reviewing signs of complications that should be promptly reported to the provider. Which of the following should be included?

A. Vaginal bleeding

B. Swelling of the ankles

C. Heartburn after eating

D. Lightheadedness when lying on back

4. A client who is at 7 weeks of gestation is experiencing nausea and vomiting in the morning. The nurse in the prenatal clinic provides teaching that should include which of the following?

A. Eat crackers or plain toast before getting out of bed.

B. Awaken during the night to eat a snack.

C. Skip breakfast, and eat lunch after nausea has subsided.

D. Eat a large evening meal.

5. A nurse is teaching a group of clients who are pregnant about behaviors to avoid during pregnancy. Which of the following statements by a client indicates a need for further instruction?

    A. "I can have a glass of wine with dinner."

    B. "Smoking is a cause of low birth weight in babies."

    C. "Signs of infection should be reported to my doctor."

    D. "I should not take over-the-counter medications without checking with my obstetrician."

6. A nurse is caring for a client at 14 weeks of gestation and is reviewing self-care concepts regarding the prevention of urinary tract infections (UTIs). Which of the following should be included in the teaching? Use the ATI Active Learning Template: Basic Concept to complete this item to include the following sections:

    A. Underlying Principles: Describe two.

    B. Nursing Interventions: Describe two actions that decrease the risk of UTIs as they relate to each of the following types of interventions – When? Why? and How?

APPLICATION EXERCISES KEY

1. A. INCORRECT: Lifting may be done by using the legs, rather than the back.

    B. INCORRECT: Kegel exercises are done to strengthen the perineal muscles and do not relieve backache.

    C. **CORRECT:** The pelvic rock or tilt exercise stretches the muscles of the lower back and helps relieve lower-back pain.

    D. **CORRECT:** The use of proper body mechanics prevents back injury due to the incorrect use of muscles when lifting.

    E. INCORRECT: Avoiding constrictive clothing helps prevent urinary tract infections, vaginal infections, varicosities, and edema of the lower extremities.

    (N) NCLEX® Connection: Health Promotion and Maintenance, Ante/Intra/Postpartum and Newborn Care

2. A. INCORRECT: This is a nontherapeutic response by the nurse and does not acknowledge the client's concerns.

    B. **CORRECT:** Feelings of ambivalence about pregnancy are normal during the first trimester.

    C. INCORRECT: This is a nontherapeutic response by the nurse and indicates disapproval.

    D. INCORRECT: This is a nontherapeutic response by the nurse and does not acknowledge the client's feelings.

    (N) NCLEX® Connection: Health Promotion and Maintenance, Health Promotion/Disease Prevention

3. A. **CORRECT:** Vaginal bleeding indicates a potential complication of the placenta such as placenta previa and should be reported to the provider immediately.

    B. INCORRECT: Swelling of the ankles is a common occurrence during pregnancy and can be relieved by sitting with the legs elevated.

    C. INCORRECT: Heartburn occurs during pregnancy due to pressure on the stomach by the enlarging uterus. It can be relieved by eating small meals.

    D. INCORRECT: Supine hypotension can be experienced by the client who feels lightheaded or faint when lying on her back. The client should be instructed about the side-lying position to remove pressure of the uterus on the vena cava.

    (N) NCLEX® Connection: Health Promotion and Maintenance, Ante/Intra/Postpartum and Newborn Care

4. A. **CORRECT:** Nausea and vomiting during the first trimester may be relieved by eating crackers or plain toast 30 to 60 min prior to rising in the morning.

    B. INCORRECT: Eating during the night can cause heartburn and does not relieve nausea and vomiting during the first trimester.

    C. INCORRECT: Instruct the client to avoid an empty stomach for prolonged periods to reduce nausea and vomiting.

    D. INCORRECT: Eating a large meal in the evening can cause heartburn and does not relieve morning nausea and vomiting.

     NCLEX® Connection: Physiological Adaptations, Alterations in Body Systems

5. A. **CORRECT:** Alcohol should not be consumed during pregnancy due to the risk of birth defects.

    B. INCORRECT: Smoking during pregnancy results in low birth weight infants.

    C. INCORRECT: Signs of complications, such as infection, should be reported to the provider.

    D. INCORRECT: All medications should be reviewed with and approved by the provider.

     NCLEX® Connection: Health Promotion and Maintenance, Ante/Intra/Postpartum and Newborn Care

6. *Using ATI Active Learning Template: Basic Concept*

    A. Underlying Principles
    - UTIs are common because of renal changes during pregnancy and the vaginal flora becoming more alkaline.

    B. Nursing Interventions
    - Decrease risk of UTIs by:
      - How, When: Encouraging client to wipe the perineal area from front to back after voiding.
      - How: Avoiding bubble baths.
      - How: Wearing cotton underpants, avoiding tight-fitting pants.
      - How: Consuming at least 8 glasses of water per day.
      - How, Why: Instructing client to urinate before and after intercourse to flush bacteria from the urethra that are present or introduced during intercourse.
      - How, Why: Advising client to urinate as soon as the urge occurs because retaining urine provides an environment for bacterial growth.
      - When, Why: Advising client to notify her provider if her urine is foul-smelling, contains blood, or is cloudy so evaluation and early treatment can be initiated.

     NCLEX® Connection: Health Promotion and Maintenance, Ante/Intra/Postpartum and Newborn Care

chapter 5

Overview

- Adequate nutritional intake during pregnancy is essential to promoting fetal and maternal health.

- Recommended weight gain during pregnancy is usually 11.2 to 15.9 kg (25 to 35 lb). The general rule is that clients should gain 1 to 2 kg (2.2 to 4.4 lb) during the first trimester and after that, a weight gain of approximately 0.4 kg (1 lb) per week for the last two trimesters. Underweight woman are advised to gain 28 to 40 lb; overweight women, 15 to 25 lb.

- It is important for the nurse to evaluate the pregnant client's nutritional choices, possible risk factors, and diet history. The nurse also should review specific nutritional guidelines for at-risk clients. Assistance is given to clients to develop a postpartum nutritional plan.

Nursing Assessment and Interventions

- Obtain subjective and objective dietary information.
  - Journal of client's food habits, eating pattern, and cravings
  - Nutrition-related questionnaires
  - Client's weight on first prenatal visit and follow-up visits
  - Laboratory findings, such as Hgb and iron levels

- Determine client's caloric intake.
  - Have client record everything eaten. The nurse, dietician, or client can identify the caloric value of each item. This record can provide better objective data about the client's nutrition status.

PLAN OF CARE FOR A PREGNANT CLIENT	
Expected Outcomes	› The client will consume the recommended dietary allowances/nutrients during her pregnancy.
Interventions	› The nurse assesses the client's dietary journal on the next prenatal visit.
	› The nurse provides educational materials regarding nutritional benefits to the mother and her newborn.
	› The nurse provides encouragement and answers questions that the client has regarding her dietary plans.
	› The nurse weighs the client and monitors for signs of inadequate weight gain.
	› The nurse makes a referral if needed.
Evaluation of the Plan	› Is there adequate weight gain?
	› Is the client compliant with the nursing plan of care?

- Instruct the client to adhere to and maintain the following during pregnancy.

  ○ An increase of 340 calories/day is recommended during the second trimester. An increase of 452 calories/day is recommended during the third trimester.

  ○ If the client is breastfeeding during the postpartum period, an additional intake of 330 calories/day is recommended during the first 6 months, and an additional intake of 400 calories/day is recommended during the second 6 months.

  ○ Increasing protein intake is essential to basic growth. Also, the intake of foods high in folic acid is crucial for neurological development and the prevention of fetal neural tube defects. Foods high in folic acid include leafy vegetables, dried peas and beans, seeds, and orange juice. Breads, cereals, and other grains are fortified with folic acid. Increased intake of folic acid is encouraged for clients who wish to become pregnant and clients of childbearing age. It is recommended that 600 mcg of folic acid should be taken during pregnancy. Current recommendations for clients who are lactating include consuming 500 mcg of folic acid.

  ○ Iron supplements are often added to the prenatal plan to facilitate an increase of the maternal RBC mass. Iron is best absorbed between meals and when given with a source of vitamin C. Milk and caffeine interfere with the absorption of iron supplements. Food sources of iron include beef liver, red meats, fish, poultry, dried peas and beans, and fortified cereals and breads. A stool softener may need to be added to decrease constipation experienced with iron supplements.

  ○ Calcium, which is important to a developing fetus, is involved in bone and teeth formation.

    ▪ Sources of calcium include milk, calcium-fortified soy milk, fortified orange juice, nuts, legumes, and dark green leafy vegetables. Daily recommendation is 1,000 mg/day for pregnant and nonpregnant women over the age of 19, and 1,300 mg/day for those under 19 years of age.

  ○ 2 to 3 L of fluids is recommended daily. Preferred fluids are water, fruit juice, and milk.

  ○ Caffeine intake should be limited to 300 mg/day. The equivalent of 500 to 750 mL/day of coffee may increase the risk of a spontaneous abortion or fetal intrauterine growth restriction.

  ○ It is recommended that women abstain from alcohol consumption during pregnancy.

Risk Factors to Ensuring Adequate Nutrition During Pregnancy

- Age, culture, education, and socioeconomic issues may affect adequate nutrition during pregnancy. Also, certain conditions specific to each client may inhibit adequate caloric intake.

  ○ Adolescents may have poor nutritional habits (a diet low in vitamins and protein, not taking prescribed iron supplements).

  ○ Vegetarians may have low protein, calcium, iron, zinc, and vitamin B_{12}.

  ○ Nausea and vomiting during pregnancy.

  ○ Anemia.

  ○ Eating disorders such as anorexia nervosa or bulimia nervosa.

  ○ Pregnant clients diagnosed with the appetite disorder pica (craving to eat nonfood substances such as dirt or red clay). This disorder may diminish the amount of nutritional foods ingested.

  ○ Excessive weight gain can lead to macrosomia and labor complications.

  ○ Inability to gain weight may result in low birth weight of the newborn.

  ○ Financially unable to purchase/access food. Therefore, the nurse should advise the client about the Women, Infants and Children (WIC) programs, which are federally funded state programs for pregnant women and their children (up to 5 years old).

Dietary Complications During Pregnancy

- Nausea and constipation are common during pregnancy.
    - For nausea, tell the client to eat dry crackers or toast, and avoid alcohol, caffeine, fats, and spices. Also avoid drinking fluids with meals, and DO NOT take a medication to control nausea without first checking with her provider.
    - For constipation, increase fluid consumption, and include extra fiber in the diet. Fruits, vegetables, and whole grains all contain fiber.
- Maternal phenylketonuria (PKU) is a maternal genetic disease in which high levels of phenylalanine pose a danger to the fetus.
    - It is important for the client to resume the PKU diet for at least 3 months prior to pregnancy and continue the diet throughout pregnancy.
    - The diet includes foods that are low in phenylalanine. Foods high in protein, such as fish, poultry, meat, eggs, nuts, and dairy products, must be avoided due to high phenylalanine levels.
    - The client's blood phenylalanine levels are monitored during pregnancy.
    - These interventions can prevent fetal complications such as mental retardation and behavioral problems.

Creating a Postpartum Nutritional Plan

- A lactating woman's nutritional plan includes the following instructions:
    - Increase protein and calorie intake while adhering to a recommended, well-balanced diet.
    - Increase oral fluids, but avoid alcohol and caffeine.
    - Avoid food substances that do not agree with the newborn (foods that may cause altered bowel function).
    - The client should take calcium supplements if she consumes an inadequate amount of dietary calcium.
- A nutritional plan for a woman who is not breastfeeding should include resumption of a previously recommended well-balanced diet.

APPLICATION EXERCISES

1. A nurse in a prenatal clinic is providing education to a client who is in the 8th week of gestation. The client states that she does not like milk. What is a good source of calcium that the nurse can recommend to the client?

    A. Dark green, leafy vegetables

    B. Deep red or orange vegetables

    C. White breads and rice

    D. Meat, poultry, and fish

2. A nurse in a prenatal clinic is caring for a group of clients. Which of the following clients should the nurse be concerned about regarding weight gain?

    A. 1.8 kg (4 lb) weight gain and is in her first trimester

    B. 3.6 kg (8 lb) weight gain and is in her first trimester

    C. 6.8 kg (15 lb) weight gain and is in her second trimester

    D. 11.3 kg (25 lb) weight gain and is in her third trimester

3. A nurse in a clinic is teaching a client of childbearing age about recommended folic acid supplements. Which of the following defects can occur in the fetus or neonate as a result of folic acid deficiency?

    A. Iron deficiency anemia

    B. Poor bone formation

    C. Macrosomic fetus

    D. Neural tube defects

4. A nurse is reviewing a new prescription for iron supplements with a client who is in the 8th week of gestation and has iron deficiency anemia. The nurse should advise the client to take the iron supplements with which of the following?

    A. Ice water

    B. Low-fat or whole milk

    C. Tea or coffee

    D. Orange juice

5. A nurse is reviewing postpartum nutrition needs with a group of new mothers who are breastfeeding their newborns. Which of the following statements by a member of the group requires clarification?

    A. "I am glad I can have my morning coffee."

    B. "I know that certain foods that I eat will affect my baby."

    C. "I will continue adding 330 calories per day to my diet."

    D. "I will continue my calcium supplements because I don't like milk."

6. A nurse manager in a prenatal clinic is preparing an in-service education program for a group of newly licensed nurses about risk factors to ensuring adequate nutrition during pregnancy. Which of the following should be included in this presentation? Use the ATI Active Learning Template: Basic Concept to answer this item and include the following:

    A. Underlying principles:

        • Identify one that is age-related.

        • Identify two that are related to culture/lifestyle.

        • Identify one that is related to a socioeconomic factor.

        • Identify two that are related to dietary complications during pregnancy.

    B. Nursing Intervention: Describe a federal program that is available to woman and children to provide nutrition support.

APPLICATION EXERCISES KEY

1. A. **CORRECT:** Good sources of calcium for bone and teeth formation include low-oxalate, dark green, leafy vegetables, such as kale, artichokes, and turnip greens.

    B. INCORRECT: Deep red or orange vegetables are good sources of vitamins C and A.

    C. INCORRECT: White breads and rice do not contain high levels of calcium.

    D. INCORRECT: Meat, poultry, and fish are sources of protein but do not contain high levels of calcium.

     NCLEX® Connection: Basic Care and Comfort, Nutrition and Oral Hydration

2. A. INCORRECT: This client has gained the appropriate weight of 3 to 4 lb for a client in the first trimester.

    B. **CORRECT:** The nurse should be concerned about this client because she has exceeded the expected 3- to 4-lb weight gain of a client in the first trimester.

    C. INCORRECT: This client has gained the appropriate weight of 3 to 4 lb in the first trimester and approximately 1 pound per week in the second trimester.

    D. INCORRECT: This client is within the recommended weight gain of 25 to 35 lb during the third trimester.

     NCLEX® Connection: Health Promotion and Maintenance, Health Promotion/Disease Prevention

3. A. INCORRECT: Iron deficiency anemia is the result of a lack of iron-rich dietary sources, such as meat, chicken, and fish.

    B. INCORRECT: Calcium deficiency can result in poor bone and teeth formation.

    C. INCORRECT: Maternal obesity can lead to a macrosomic fetus.

    D. **CORRECT:** Neural tube defects are caused by folic acid deficiency. Food sources of folic acid include fresh green, leafy vegetables, liver, peanuts, cereals, and whole-grain breads.

     NCLEX® Connection: Health Promotion and Maintenance, Health Promotion/Disease Prevention

4. A. INCORRECT: Water does not promote absorption of iron, but drinking plenty of water can prevent constipation, which is an adverse effect of iron supplements.

    B. INCORRECT: Milk interferes with iron absorption.

    C. INCORRECT: Caffeine, found in tea and coffee, can interfere with iron absorption. It should also be limited to 300 mg/day because it increases the risk of spontaneous abortion or fetal intrauterine growth restriction.

    D. **CORRECT:** Orange juice contains vitamin C, which aids in the absorption of iron.

     NCLEX® Connection: Pharmacological and Parenteral Therapies, Medication Administration

5. A. **CORRECT:** Women who are breastfeeding should avoid caffeine intake because it affects iron absorption and infant weight gain.

    B. INCORRECT: Foods ingested by the mother, especially gas-producing foods, can affect breast milk and the breastfeeding infant.

    C. INCORRECT: Women who are breastfeeding require an additional 330 calories per day to support adequate nutrition during the first 6 months of lactation.

    D. INCORRECT: Postpartum women who are at risk for inadequate dietary calcium should continue taking calcium supplements during lactation.

    NCLEX® Connection: Health Promotion and Maintenance, Ante/Intra/Postpartum and Newborn Care

6. *Using the ATI Active Learning Template: Basic Concept*

    A. Underlying Principles
    - Age-related: Adolescents may have poor nutritional habits during pregnancy.
    - Culture/lifestyle: Vegetarians may have diets low in protein, calcium, zinc, and vitamin B_{12}. Excessive weight gain can lead to macrosomia and labor complications.
    - Socioeconomic factor: Inability to purchase or access foods can limit nutrition during pregnancy.
    - Dietary complications: Nausea and vomiting during pregnancy, anemia, eating disorders (anorexia nervosa or bulimia nervosa), inability to gain weight, presence of the appetite disorder pica.

    B. Nursing Interventions
    - Women, Infants and Children (WIC) is a federally funded state program that provides nutritional support to pregnant women and their children (up to 5 years old).

    NCLEX® Connection: Health Promotion and Maintenance, Ante/Intra/Postpartum and Newborn Care

chapter 6

Overview

- This chapter includes the assessments that determine the well-being of a fetus during pregnancy.
- The diagnostic procedures to be reviewed include ultrasound (abdominal, transvaginal, Doppler), biophysical profile, nonstress test, contraction stress test (nipple, oxytocin [Pitocin])and amniocentesis. Additional diagnostic procedures for high-risk pregnancy include percutaneous umbilical cord blood sampling, chorionic villus sampling, quad marker screening, and maternal serum alpha-fetoprotein.

DIAGNOSTIC PROCEDURE AND NURSING MANAGEMENT: ULTRASOUND (ABDOMINAL, TRANSVAGINAL, DOPPLER)

Overview

- Ultrasound – a procedure lasting approximately 20 min that consists of high-frequency sound waves used to visualize internal organs and tissues by producing a real-time, three-dimensional image of the developing fetus and maternal structures (FHR, pelvic anatomy). An ultrasound allows for early diagnosis of complications, permits earlier interventions, and thereby decreases neonatal and maternal morbidity and mortality. There are three types of ultrasound: external abdominal, transvaginal, and Doppler.
    - External abdominal ultrasound – a safe, noninvasive, painless procedure whereby an ultrasound transducer is moved over a client's abdomen to obtain an image. An abdominal ultrasound is more useful after the first trimester when the gravid uterus is larger.
    - Internal transvaginal ultrasound – an invasive procedure in which a probe is inserted vaginally to allow for a more accurate evaluation. An advantage of this procedure is that it does not require a full bladder.
        - It is especially useful in clients who are obese and those in the first trimester to detect an ectopic pregnancy, identify abnormalities, and to establish gestational age.
        - A transvaginal ultrasound also may be used in the third trimester in conjunction with abdominal scanning to evaluate for preterm labor.
    - Doppler ultrasound blood flow analysis – a noninvasive external ultrasound method to study the maternal-fetal blood flow by measuring the velocity at which RBCs travel in the uterine and fetal vessels using a handheld ultrasound device that reflects sound waves from a moving target. It is especially useful in fetal intrauterine growth restriction (IUGR) and poor placental perfusion, and as an adjunct in pregnancies at risk because of hypertension, diabetes mellitus, multiple fetuses, or preterm labor.
- Indications for the use of an ultrasound during pregnancy
    - Potential diagnoses for:
        - Confirming pregnancy
        - Confirming gestational age by biparietal diameter (side-to-side) measurement
        - Identifying multifetal pregnancy

- Site of fetal implantation (uterine or ectopic)
- Assessing fetal growth and development
- Assessing maternal structures
- Confirming fetal viability or death
- Ruling out or verifying fetal abnormalities
- Locating the site of placental attachment
- Determining amniotic fluid volume
- Fetal movement observation (fetal heartbeat, breathing, and activity)
- Placental grading (evaluating placental maturation)
- Adjunct for other procedures (e.g., amniocentesis, biophysical profile)

○ Client presentation

- Vaginal bleeding evaluation
- Questionable fundal height measurement in relationship to gestational weeks
- Reports of decreased fetal movements
- Preterm labor
- Questionable rupture of membranes

• Nursing actions for an ultrasound

○ Preparation of client

- Explain the procedure to the client and that it presents no known risk to her or her fetus.
- Advise the client to drink 1 to 2 quarts of fluid prior to the ultrasound to fill the bladder, lift and stabilize the uterus, displace the bowel, and act as an echolucent to better reflect sound waves to obtain a better image of the fetus.
- Assist the client into a supine position with a wedge placed under her right hip to displace the uterus (prevents supine hypotension).

○ Ongoing care

- Apply an ultrasonic/transducer gel to the client's abdomen before the transducer is moved over the skin to obtain a better fetal image, ensuring that the gel is at room temperature or warmer.
- Allow the client to empty her bladder at the termination of the procedure.

• Nursing actions for a transvaginal ultrasound

○ Preparation of client

- Assist the client into a lithotomy position. The vaginal probe is covered with a protective device, lubricated with a water-soluble gel, and the client or examiner inserts the probe.

○ Ongoing care

- During the procedure, the position of the probe or tilt of the table may be changed to facilitate the complete view of the pelvis.
- Inform the client that pressure may be felt as the probe is moved.

• Client education

○ Fetal and maternal structures may be pointed out to the client as the ultrasound procedure is performed.

DIAGNOSTIC PROCEDURE AND NURSING MANAGEMENT: BIOPHYSICAL PROFILE

Overview

- Biophysical profile (BPP) – uses a real-time ultrasound to visualize physical and physiological characteristics of the fetus and observe for fetal biophysical responses to stimuli.

- BPP assesses fetal well-being by measuring the following five variables with a score of 2 for each normal finding, and 0 for each abnormal finding for each variable.

  ○ Reactive FHR (reactive nonstress test) = 2; nonreactive = 0.

  ○ Fetal breathing movements (at least 1 episode of greater than 30 seconds duration in 30 min) = 2; absent or less than 30 seconds duration = 0.

  ○ Gross body movements (at least 3 body or limb extensions with return to flexion in 30 min) = 2; less than 3 episodes = 0.

  ○ Fetal tone (at least 1 episode of extension with return to flexion) = 2; slow extension and flexion, lack of flexion, or absent movement = 0.

  ○ Qualitative amniotic fluid volume (at least 1 pocket of fluid that measures at least 2 cm in 2 perpendicular planes) = 2; pockets absent or less than 2 cm = 0.

- Interpretation of findings

  ○ Total score of 8 to 10 is normal; low risk of chronic fetal asphyxia

  ○ 4 to 6 is abnormal; suspect chronic fetal asphyxia

  ○ < 4 is abnormal; strongly suspect chronic fetal asphyxia

- Potential diagnoses

  ○ Nonreactive stress test

  ○ Suspected oligohydramnios or polyhydramnios

  ○ Suspected fetal hypoxemia and/or hypoxia

- Client presentation

  ○ Premature rupture of membranes

  ○ Maternal infection

  ○ Decreased fetal movement

  ○ Intrauterine growth restriction

- Nursing Actions

  ○ Prepare the client following the same nursing management principles as those used for an ultrasound.

DIAGNOSTIC PROCEDURE AND NURSING MANAGEMENT:
NONSTRESS TEST (NST)

Overview

- Nonstress test (NST) – most widely used technique for antepartum evaluation of fetal well-being performed during the third trimester. It is a noninvasive procedure that monitors response of the FHR to fetal movement. A Doppler transducer, used to monitor the FHR, and a tocotransducer, used to monitor uterine contractions, are attached externally to a client's abdomen to obtain tracing strips. The client pushes a button attached to the monitor whenever she feels a fetal movement, which is then noted on the tracing. This allows a nurse to assess the FHR in relationship to the fetal movement.

- Indications for the use of an NST during pregnancy
  - Potential diagnoses for:
    - Assessing for an intact fetal CNS during the third trimester.
    - Ruling out the risk for fetal death in clients who have diabetes mellitus. Used twice a week or until after 28 weeks of gestation.
  - Client presentation
    - Decreased fetal movement
    - Intrauterine growth restriction
    - Postmaturity
    - Gestational diabetes mellitus
    - Gestational hypertension
    - Maternal chronic hypertension
    - History of previous fetal demise
    - Advanced maternal age
    - Sickle cell disease
    - Isoimmunization

- Interpretation of findings
  - The NST is interpreted as reactive if the FHR is a normal baseline rate with moderate variability, accelerates to 15 beats/min for at least 15 seconds and occurs two or more times during a 20-min period.

 View Image: Reactive NST

  - Nonreactive NST indicates that the fetal heart rate does not accelerate adequately with fetal movement. It does not meet the above criteria after 40 min. If this is so, a further assessment, such as a contraction stress test (CST) or biophysical profile (BPP), is indicated.

- Nursing actions
  - Preparation of client
    - Seat the client in a reclining chair, or place in a semi-Fowler's or left-lateral position.
    - Apply conduction gel to the client's abdomen.
    - Apply two belts to the client's abdomen, and attach the FHR and uterine contraction monitors.

- ○ Ongoing care
  - ▪ Instruct the client to press the button on the handheld event marker each time she feels the fetus move.
  - ▪ If there are no fetal movements (fetus sleeping), vibroacoustic stimulation (sound source, usually laryngeal stimulator) may be activated for 3 seconds on the maternal abdomen over the fetal head to awaken a sleeping fetus.
- Miscellaneous
  - ○ Disadvantages of a NST include a high rate of false nonreactive results with the fetal movement response blunted by sleep cycles of the fetus, fetal immaturity, maternal medications, and chronic smoking.

DIAGNOSTIC PROCEDURE AND NURSING MANAGEMENT: CONTRACTION STRESS TEST (CST)

Overview

- Nipple stimulated CST consists of a woman lightly brushing her palm across her nipple for 2 min, which causes the pituitary gland to release endogenous oxytocin, and then stopping the nipple stimulation when a contraction begins. The same process is repeated after a 5-min rest period.
  - ○ Analysis of the FHR response to contractions (which decrease placental blood flow) determines how the fetus will tolerate the stress of labor. A pattern of at least three contractions within a 10-min time period with duration of 40 to 60 seconds each must be obtained to use for assessment data.
  - ○ Hyperstimulation of the uterus (uterine contraction longer than 90 seconds or more frequent than every 2 min) should be avoided by stimulating the nipple intermittently with rest periods in between and avoiding bimanual stimulation of both nipples unless stimulation of one nipple is unsuccessful.
- Oxytocin (Pitocin) administration CST is used if nipple stimulation fails and consists of the IV administration of oxytocin to induce uterine contractions.
  - ○ Contractions started with oxytocin may be difficult to stop and can lead to preterm labor.
- Indications for the use of a contraction stress test during pregnancy
  - ○ Potential diagnoses
    - ▪ High-risk pregnancies (gestational diabetes mellitus, postterm pregnancy)
    - ▪ Nonreactive stress test
  - ○ Client presentation
    - ▪ Decreased fetal movement
    - ▪ Intrauterine growth restriction
    - ▪ Postmaturity
    - ▪ Gestational diabetes mellitus
    - ▪ Gestational hypertension

- Maternal chronic hypertension
- History of previous fetal demise
- Advanced maternal age
- Sickle-cell disease

- Interpretation of findings
  - A negative CST (normal finding) is indicated if within a 10-min period, with three uterine contractions, there are no late decelerations of the FHR.
  - A positive CST (abnormal finding) is indicated with persistent and consistent late decelerations on more than half of the contractions. This is suggestive of uteroplacental insufficiency. Variable deceleration may indicate cord compression, and early decelerations may indicate fetal head compression. Based on these findings, the provider may determine to induce labor or perform a cesarean birth.

 View Image: Positive CST

- Nursing Actions
  - Preparation of client
    - Obtain a baseline of the FHR, fetal movement, and contractions for 10 to 20 min, and document.
    - Explain the procedure to the client, and obtain informed consent.
    - Complete an assessment without artificial stimulation if contractions are occurring spontaneously.
  - Ongoing care
    - Initiate nipple stimulation if there are no contractions. Instruct the client to roll a nipple between her thumb and fingers or brush her palm across her nipple. The client should stop when a uterine contraction begins.
    - Monitor and provide adequate rest periods for the client to avoid hyperstimulation of the uterus.
  - Interventions
    - Initiate IV oxytocin administration if nipple stimulation fails to elicit a sufficient uterine contraction pattern. If hyperstimulation of the uterus and/or preterm labor occurs, do the following:
      - Monitor for contractions lasting longer than 90 seconds and/or occurring more frequently than every 2 min.
      - Provide administration of tocolytics as prescribed.
      - Maintain bed rest during the procedure.
      - Observe the client for 30 min afterward to see that contractions have ceased and preterm labor does not begin.

- Complications
  - Potential for preterm labor

DIAGNOSTIC PROCEDURE AND NURSING MANAGEMENT: AMNIOCENTESIS

Overview

- Amniocentesis – the aspiration of amniotic fluid for analysis by insertion of a needle transabdominally into a client's uterus and amniotic sac under direct ultrasound guidance locating the placenta and determining the position of the fetus. It may be performed after 14 weeks of gestation.

- Indications for the use of an amniocentesis during pregnancy

  - Potential diagnoses

    - Previous birth with a chromosomal anomaly

    - A parent who is a carrier of a chromosomal anomaly

    - A family history of neural tube defects

    - Prenatal diagnosis of a genetic disorder or congenital anomaly of the fetus

    - Alpha fetoprotein level for fetal abnormalities

    - Lung maturity assessment

    - Fetal hemolytic disease

    - Meconium in the amniotic fluid

- Interpretation of findings

  - Alpha-fetoprotein (AFP) can be measured from the amniotic fluid between 16 and 18 weeks of gestation and may be used to assess for neural tube defects in the fetus or chromosomal disorders. May be evaluated to follow up a high level of AFP in maternal serum.

    - High levels of AFP are associated with neural tube defects, such as anencephaly (incomplete development of fetal skull and brain), spina bifida (open spine), or omphalocele (abdominal wall defect). High AFP levels also may be present with normal multifetal pregnancies.

    - Low levels of AFP are associated with chromosomal disorders (Down syndrome) or gestational trophoblastic disease (hydatidiform mole).

  - Tests for fetal lung maturity may be performed if gestation is less than 37 weeks, in the event of a rupture of membranes, for preterm labor, or for a complication indicating a cesarean birth. Amniotic fluid is tested to determine whether the fetal lungs are mature enough to adapt to extrauterine life, or if the fetus will likely have respiratory distress. Determination is made whether the fetus should be removed immediately or if the fetus requires more time in utero with the administration of glucocorticoids to promote fetal lung maturity.

    - Fetal lung tests

      - Lecithin/sphingomyelin (L/S) ratio – a 2:1 ratio indicating fetal lung maturity (2.5:1 or 3:1 for a client who has diabetes mellitus).

      - Presence of phosphatidylglycerol (PG) – absence of PG is associated with respiratory distress

- Preprocedure for an amniocentesis

  - Nursing actions

    - Explain the procedure to the client, and obtain informed consent.

  - Client education

    - Instruct the client to empty her bladder prior to the procedure to reduce its size and reduce the risk of inadvertent puncture.

- Intraprocedure
  - Nursing actions
    - Obtain client's baseline vital signs and FHR, and document prior to the procedure.
    - Assist client into a supine position, and place a wedge under her right hip to displace the uterus off the vena cava, and place a drape over the client exposing only her abdomen.
    - Prepare client for an ultrasound to locate the placenta.
    - Cleanse client's abdomen with an antiseptic solution prior to the administration of a local anesthetic by the provider.
  - Client education
    - Advise the client that she will feel slight pressure as the needle is inserted. She should continue breathing because holding her breath will lower the diaphragm against the uterus and shift the intrauterine contents.
- Postprocedure
  - Nursing actions
    - Monitor the client's vital signs, FHR, and uterine contractions throughout and 30 min following the procedure.
    - Have the client rest for 30 min.
    - Administer $Rh_o(D)$ immune globulin (Rh_oGAM) to the client if she is Rh-negative (standard practice after an amniocentesis for all women who are Rh-negative to protect against Rh isoimmunization).
  - Client education
    - Advise the client to report to her provider if she experiences fever, chills, leakage of fluid, or bleeding from the insertion site, decreased fetal movement, vaginal bleeding, or uterine contractions after the procedure.
    - Encourage the client to drink plenty of liquids and rest for the 24 hr postprocedure.
  - Complications
    - Amniotic fluid emboli
    - Maternal or fetal hemorrhage
    - Fetomaternal hemorrhage with Rh isoimmunization
    - Maternal or fetal infection
    - Inadvertent fetal damage or anomalies involving limbs
    - Fetal death
    - Inadvertent maternal intestinal or bladder damage
    - Miscarriage or preterm labor
    - Premature rupture of membranes
    - Leakage of amniotic fluid
  - Nursing actions
    - Monitor the client's vital signs, temperature, respiratory status, FHR, uterine contractions, and vaginal discharge for amniotic fluid or bleeding.
    - Administer medication as prescribed.
    - Offer support and reassurance.

DIAGNOSTIC PROCEDURE AND NURSING MANAGEMENT (HIGH-RISK PREGNANCY): PERCUTANEOUS UMBILICAL BLOOD SAMPLING

Overview

- Percutaneous umbilical blood sampling (PUBS) – the most common method used for fetal blood sampling and transfusion. This procedure obtains fetal blood from the umbilical cord by passing a fine-gauge, fiber-optic scope (fetoscope) into the amniotic sac using the amniocentesis technique. The needle is advanced into the umbilical cord under ultrasound guidance, and blood is aspirated from the umbilical vein. Blood studies from the cordocentesis may consist of:
  - Kleihauer-Betke test that ensures that fetal blood was obtained.
  - CBC count with differential.
  - Indirect Coombs' test for Rh antibodies.
  - Karyotyping (visualization of chromosomes).
  - Blood gases.
- Indications for the use of PUBS
  - Potential diagnoses
    - Fetal blood type, RBC, and chromosomal disorders
    - Karyotyping of malformed fetuses
    - Fetal infection
    - Altered acid-base balance of fetuses with IUGR
- Interpretation of findings
  - Evaluates for isoimmune fetal hemolytic anemia and assesses the need for a fetal blood transfusion.
- Nursing actions
  - Administer medication as prescribed.
  - Offer support.
- Complications
  - Cord laceration
  - Preterm labor
  - Amnionitis
  - Hematoma
  - Fetomaternal hemorrhage

DIAGNOSTIC PROCEDURE AND NURSING MANAGEMENT (HIGH-RISK PREGNANCY): CHORIONIC VILLUS SAMPLING

Overview

- Chorionic villus sampling (CVS) – assessment of a portion of the developing placenta (chorionic villi), which is aspirated through a thin sterile catheter or syringe inserted through the abdominal wall or intravaginally through the cervix under ultrasound guidance and analyzed.
    - CVS is a first-trimester alternative to amniocentesis with one of its advantages being an earlier diagnosis of any abnormalities. CVS can be performed at 10 to 12 weeks of gestation.
- Indications for the use of CVS during pregnancy
    - Potential diagnoses
        - Women at risk for giving birth to a neonate who has a genetic chromosomal abnormality (cannot determine spina bifida or anencephaly)
    - Client education
        - Instruct the client to drink plenty of fluid to fill the bladder prior to the procedure to assist in positioning the uterus for catheter insertion.
        - Provide ongoing education and support.
- Complications
    - Spontaneous abortion (higher risk with CVS than with amniocentesis)
    - Risk for fetal limb loss
    - Miscarriage
    - Chorioamnionitis and rupture of membranes
- Miscellaneous
    - The advantage of an earlier diagnosis should be weighed against the increased risk of fetal anomalies and death.

DIAGNOSTIC PROCEDURE AND NURSING MANAGEMENT (HIGH-RISK PREGNANCY): QUAD MARKER AND ALPHA-FETOPROTEIN (AFP) SCREENING

Overview

- Description of procedure
  - Quad marker screening – a blood test that ascertains information about the likelihood of fetal birth defects. It does not diagnose the actual defect. It may be performed instead of the maternal serum alpha-fetoprotein yielding more reliable findings. Includes testing for:
    - Human chorionic gonadotropin (hCG) – a hormone produced by the placenta
    - Alpha-fetoprotein (AFP) – a protein produced by the fetus
    - Estriol – a protein produced by the fetus and placenta
    - Inhibin-A – a protein produced by the ovaries and placenta
- Indications
  - Client presentation
    - Preferred at 16-18 weeks gestation
    - Women at risk for giving birth to a neonate who has a genetic chromosomal abnormality
- Interpretation of findings
  - Low levels of AFP may indicate a risk for Down syndrome.
  - High levels of AFP may indicate a risk for neural tube defects.
  - Higher levels than the expected reference range of hCG and Inhibin-A indicates a risk for Down syndrome.
  - Lower levels than the expected reference range of estriol may indicate a risk for Down syndrome.
- Description of procedure
  - Maternal serum alpha-fetoprotein (MSAFP) is a screening tool used to detect neural tube defects. Clients who have abnormal findings should be referred for a quad marker screening, genetic counseling, ultrasound, and an amniocentesis.
- Indications
  - Potential diagnoses
    - All pregnant clients, preferably between 16-18 weeks of gestation
- Interpretation of findings
  - High levels may indicate a neural tube defect or open abdominal defect.
  - Lower levels may indicate Down syndrome.
- Nursing Actions
  - Preparation of a client
    - Discuss testing with the client.
    - Draw blood sample.
    - Offer support and education as needed.

APPLICATION EXERCISES

1. A nurse is caring for a client and reviewing the findings of the client's biophysical profile (BPP). Which of the following variables are included in this test? (Select all that apply.)

_____ A. Fetal weight

___X___ B. Fetal breathing movement

___X___ C. Fetal tone

___X___ D. Reactive FHR

___X___ E. Amniotic fluid volume

2. A nurse is caring for a client who is in preterm labor and is scheduled to undergo an amniocentesis to assess fetal lung maturity. Which of the following is a test for fetal lung maturity?

    A. Alpha-fetoprotein (AFP)

    B. Lecithin/sphingomyelin (L/S) ratio

    C. Kleihauer-Betke test

    D. Indirect Coombs' test

3. A nurse is caring for a client who is pregnant and undergoing a nonstress test. The client asks why the nurse is using an acoustic vibration device. Which of the following is an appropriate response by the nurse?

    A. "It is used to stimulate uterine contractions."

    B. "It will decrease the incidence of uterine contractions."

    C. "It lulls the fetus to sleep."

    D. "It awakens a sleeping fetus."

4. A nurse is teaching a client who is pregnant about the amniocentesis procedure. Which of the following statements by the client requires clarification?

    A. "I will report cramping or signs of infection to the physician."

    B. "I should drink lots of fluids during the 24 hours following the procedure."

    C. "I need to have a full bladder at the time of the procedure."

    D. "The test is done to detect genetic abnormalities."

5. A nurse is caring for a client who is pregnant and is to undergo a contraction stress test (CST). Which of the following findings are indications for this procedure? (Select all that apply.)

_____X_____ A. Decreased fetal movement

_____X_____ B. Intrauterine growth restriction (IUGR)

_____X_____ C. Postmaturity

_____X_____ D. Advanced maternal age

_____ E. Amniotic fluid emboli

6 A nurse in a prenatal clinic is orienting a recently hired nurse about how to perform a nonstress test (NST). What should be included in the orientation? Use the ATI Active Learning Template: Diagnostic Procedure to complete this item to include the following:

A. Indications: Identify three that relate to the status of the fetus.

B. Interpretation of findings: Describe a nonreactive NST.

C. Nursing Actions: Two preprocedure, one intraprocedure.

APPLICATION EXERCISES KEY

1. A. INCORRECT: Fetal weight is not one of the variables included in the BPP.

    B. **CORRECT:** Fetal breathing movements are a variable included in the BPP.

    C. **CORRECT:** Fetal tone is a variable included in the BPP.

    D. **CORRECT:** Reactive FHR is a variable included in the BPP.

    E. **CORRECT:** Amniotic fluid volume is a variable included in the BPP.

    Ⓝ NCLEX® Connection: Reduction of Risk Potential, Diagnostic Tests

2. A. INCORRECT: AFP is a test to assess for fetal neural tube defects or chromosome disorders.

    B. **CORRECT:** A test of the L/S ratio is done as a part of an amniocentesis to determine fetal lung maturity.

    C. INCORRECT: A Kleihauer-Betke test is used to verify that fetal blood is present during a percutaneous umbilical blood sampling procedure.

    D. INCORRECT: An indirect Coombs' test detects Rh antibodies in the mother's blood.

    Ⓝ NCLEX® Connection: Reduction of Risk Potential, Diagnostic Tests

3. A. INCORRECT: The acoustic vibration device does not stimulate the uterus.

    B. INCORRECT: The acoustic vibration device has no effect on the uterine muscles.

    C. INCORRECT: The acoustic vibration device stimulates a sleeping fetus.

    D. **CORRECT:** The acoustic vibration device is activated for 3 seconds on the maternal abdomen over the fetal head to awaken a sleeping fetus.

    Ⓝ NCLEX® Connection: Reduction of Risk Potential, Therapeutic Procedures

4. A. INCORRECT: Cramping and signs of infection following the procedure should be reported to the provider.

    B. INCORRECT: The client is encouraged to drink extra fluids and rest during the 24 hr following an amniocentesis.

    C. **CORRECT:** The client's bladder should be empty to avoid an inadvertent puncture during the procedure.

    D. INCORRECT: Amniotic fluid is tested to identify fetal genetic defects.

    (N) NCLEX® Connection: Reduction of Risk Potential, Therapeutic Procedures

5. A. **CORRECT:** Decreased fetal movement is an indication for a CST.

    B. **CORRECT:** IUGR is an indication for a CST.

    C. **CORRECT:** Postmaturity is an indication for a CST.

    D. **CORRECT:** Advanced maternal age is an indication for a CST.

    E. INCORRECT: Amniotic fluid emboli are a complication of an amniocentesis.

    (N) NCLEX® Connection: Reduction of Risk Potential, Diagnostic Tests

6. *Using the ATI Active Learning Template: Diagnostic Procedure*

    A. Indications

    - Assessment for intact fetal CNS during the third trimester
    - Rule out fetal death in a client who has diabetes mellitus

    - Decreased fetal movement
    - Intrauterine growth restriction
    - Postmaturity

    B. Interpretation of findings

    - Nonreactive NST: Fetal heart rate does not accelerate by 15 beats/min above the baseline FHR for at least 15 seconds at least two or more times during a period of 20 min.

    C. Nursing Actions

    - Preprocedure

      ○ Seat the client in a reclining chair in a semi-Fowler's or left-lateral position.

      ○ Apply conduction gel to the client's abdomen.

      ○ Apply the Doppler transducer and the tocotransducer.

    - Intraprocedure

      ○ Instruct the client to depress the event marker button each time she feels fetal movement.

    (N) NCLEX® Connection: Health Promotion and Maintenance, Ante/Intra/Postpartum and Newborn Care

UNIT 1   ANTEPARTUM NURSING CARE
SECTION: COMPLICATIONS OF PREGNANCY

CHAPTER 7   Bleeding During Pregnancy

Overview

- Vaginal bleeding during pregnancy is always abnormal and must be investigated to determine the cause. It can impair both the outcome of the pregnancy and the mother's life.

- The primary causes of bleeding are summarized in the following table according to common causes during each trimester of pregnancy.

SUMMARY OF CAUSES OF BLEEDING DURING PREGNANCY		
Time	Complication	Signs and symptoms
› First trimester	› Spontaneous abortion	› Vaginal bleeding, uterine cramping, and partial or complete expulsion of products of conception
	› Ectopic pregnancy	› Abrupt unilateral lower-quadrant abdominal pain with or without vaginal bleeding
› Second trimester	› Gestational trophoblastic disease	› Uterine size increasing abnormally fast, abnormally high levels of hCG, nausea and increased emesis, no fetus present on ultrasound, and scant or profuse dark brown or red vaginal bleeding
› Third trimester	› Placenta previa	› Painless vaginal bleeding
	› Abruptio placenta	› Vaginal bleeding, sharp abdominal pain, and tender rigid uterus

- Other Causes of Bleeding
  - Precurrent premature dilation of the cervix
    - Painless bleeding with cervical dilation leading to fetal expulsion
  - Preterm labor
    - Pink-stained vaginal discharge, uterine contractions becoming regular, cervical dilation and effacement

---

SPONTANEOUS ABORTION

Overview

- Spontaneous abortion is when a pregnancy is terminated before 20 weeks of gestation (the point of fetal viability) or a fetal weight less than 500 g.

- Types of abortion are clinically classified according to clinical manifestations and whether the products of conception are partially or completely retained or expelled. Types of abortions include threatened, inevitable, incomplete, complete, and missed.

Risk Factors

- Chromosomal abnormalities (account for 50%)
- Maternal illness, such as type 1 diabetes mellitus
- Advancing maternal age
- Premature cervical dilation
- Chronic maternal infections
- Maternal malnutrition
- Trauma or injury
- Anomalies in the fetus or placenta
- Substance use
- Antiphospholipid syndrome

Assessment

- Subjective and Objective Data
  - Backache and abdominal tenderness
  - Rupture of membranes, dilation of the cervix
  - Fever
  - Signs and symptoms of hemorrhage such as hypotension and tachycardia

SPONTANEOUS ABORTION (MISCARRIAGE) ASSESSMENT				
Type	Cramps	Bleeding	Tissue Passed	Cervical Opening
› Threatened	› With or without slight cramps	› Spotting to moderate	› None	› Closed
› Inevitable	› Moderate	› Mild to severe	› None	› Dilated with membranes or tissue bulging at cervix
› Incomplete	› Severe	› Continuous and severe	› Partial fetal tissue or placenta	› Dilated with tissue in cervical canal or passage of tissue
› Complete	› Mild	› Minimal	› Complete expulsion of uterine contents	› Closed with no tissue in cervical canal
› Missed	› None	› Brownish discharge	› None, prolonged retention of tissue	› Closed
› Septic	› Varies	› Malodorous discharge	› Varies	› Usually dilated
› Recurrent	› Varies	› Varies	› Yes	› Usually dilated

- ○ Laboratory Tests
  - ▪ Hgb and Hct, if considerable blood loss
  - ▪ Clotting factors monitored for disseminated intravascular coagulopathy (DIC) – a complication with retained products of conception
  - ▪ WBC for suspected infection
  - ▪ Serum human chorionic gonadotropin (hCG) levels to confirm pregnancy
- ○ Diagnostic and Therapeutic Procedures
  - ▪ Ultrasound – to determine the presence of a viable or dead fetus, or partial or complete products of conception within the uterine cavity.
  - ▪ Examination of the cervix – to observe whether it is opened or closed.
  - ▪ Dilation and curettage (D&C) – to dilate and scrape the uterine walls to remove uterine contents for inevitable and incomplete abortions.
  - ▪ Dilation and evacuation (D&E) – to dilate and evacuate uterine contents after 16 weeks of gestation.
  - ▪ Prostaglandins and oxytocin (Pitocin) – to augment or induce uterine contractions and expulse the products of conception.

Patient-Centered Care

- • Nursing Actions
  - ○ Observe color and amount of bleeding (counting pads).
  - ○ Perform a pregnancy test.
  - ○ Maintain client on bed rest; inform client of risk for falls due to sedative medications if prescribed.
  - ○ Avoid vaginal exams.
  - ○ Assist with an ultrasound.
  - ○ Administer medications and blood products as prescribed.
  - ○ Determine how much tissue has passed and save passed tissue for examination.
  - ○ Assist with termination of pregnancy (D&C, D&E, prostaglandin administration) as indicated.
- • Medications
  - ○ Analgesics and sedatives
  - ○ Prostaglandin – administered into the amniotic sac or as a vaginal suppository
  - ○ Oxytocin (Pitocin)
  - ○ Broad-spectrum antibiotics – in septic abortion
  - ○ $Rh_o(D)$ immune globulin (RhoGAM) – suppresses immune response of clients who are Rh-negative
- • Nursing Considerations
  - ○ Use the lay term "miscarriage" with clients because the medical term "abortion" can be misunderstood.
  - ○ Provide client education and emotional support.
  - ○ Provide referral for client and partner to pregnancy loss support groups.

- Health Promotion and Disease Prevention
  - Discharge instructions
    - Notify the provider of heavy, bright red vaginal bleeding; elevated temperature; or foul-smelling vaginal discharge.
    - A small amount of discharge is normal for 1 to 2 weeks.
    - Take prescribed antibiotics.
    - Refrain from tub baths, sexual intercourse, or placing anything into the vagina for 2 weeks.
    - Avoid becoming pregnant for 2 months.

ECTOPIC PREGNANCY

Overview

- Ectopic pregnancy is the abnormal implantation of a fertilized ovum outside of the uterine cavity usually in the fallopian tube, which can result in a tubal rupture causing a fatal hemorrhage.
- Ectopic pregnancy is the second most frequent cause of bleeding in early pregnancy and a leading cause of infertility.

Risk Factors

- Risk factors for an ectopic pregnancy include any factor that compromises tubal patency (STIs, assisted reproductive technologies, tubal surgery, and contraceptive intrauterine device [IUD]).

Assessment

- Subjective Data
  - Unilateral stabbing pain and tenderness in the lower-abdominal quadrant.
  - Delayed (1 to 2 weeks), lighter than usual, or irregular menses.
  - Scant, dark red, or brown vaginal spotting occurs 6 to 8 weeks after last normal menses; red, vaginal bleeding if rupture has occurred.
  - Referred shoulder pain due to blood in the peritoneal cavity irritating the diaphragm or phrenic nerve after tubal rupture.
  - Report of faintness and dizziness related to amount of bleeding in abdominal cavity.
- Objective Data
  - Signs of hemorrhage and shock (hypotension, tachycardia, pallor)
- Laboratory Tests
  - Serum levels of progesterone and hCG elevated rules out ectopic pregnancy.

- Diagnostic and Therapeutic Procedures
  - Transvaginal ultrasound showing an empty uterus
  - Caution used if vaginal and bimanual examination undertaken
  - Rapid surgical treatment
    - Salpingostomy is done to salvage the fallopian tube if not ruptured.
    - Laparoscopic salpingectomy (removal of the tube) is performed when the tube has ruptured.
    - Medical management if rupture has not occurred and tube preservation desired.
      - Methotrexate (MTX) – inhibits cell division and embryo enlargement, dissolving the pregnancy

Patient-Centered Care

- Nursing Actions
  - Replace fluids, and maintain electrolyte balance.
  - Provide client education and psychological support.
  - Administer medications as prescribed.
  - Prepare the client for surgery and postoperative nursing care.
  - Provide referral for client and partner to pregnancy loss support group.
- Nursing Considerations
  - Obtain serum hCG and progesterone levels, liver and renal function studies, CBC, and type and Rh.
- Health Promotion and Disease Prevention
  - Client education
    - Instruct the client who is prescribed methotrexate to avoid alcohol consumption and vitamins containing folic acid to prevent a toxic response to the medication.
    - Advise the client to protect herself from sun exposure (photosensitivity).

GESTATIONAL TROPHOBLASTIC DISEASE (HYDATIDIFORM MOLE, CHORIOCARCINOMA, AND MOLAR PREGNANCY)

Overview

- Gestational trophoblastic disease (GTD) is the proliferation and degeneration of trophoblastic villi in the placenta that becomes swollen, fluid-filled, and takes on the appearance of grape-like clusters. The embryo fails to develop beyond a primitive state and these structures are associated with choriocarcinoma, which is a rapidly metastasizing malignancy. Two types of molar growths are identified by chromosomal analysis.
- In the complete mole, all genetic material is paternally derived.
  - The ovum has no genetic material or the material is inactive.
  - The complete mole contains no fetus, placenta, amniotic membranes, or fluid.
  - There is no placenta to receive maternal blood; therefore, hemorrhage into the uterine cavity occurs and vaginal bleeding results.
  - Approximately 20% of complete moles progress toward a choriocarcinoma.

- In the partial mole, genetic material is derived both maternally and paternally.

  - A normal ovum is fertilized by two sperm or one sperm in which meiosis or chromosome reduction and division did not occur.

  - A partial mole often contains abnormal embryonic or fetal parts, an amniotic sac, and fetal blood, but congenital anomalies are present.

  - Approximately 6% of partial moles progress toward a choriocarcinoma.

Risk Factors

- Low carotene or animal fat intake

- Age – early teens or over age 40

- Ovulation stimulation with clomiphene (Clomid)

Assessment

- Subjective Data

  - Excessive vomiting (hyperemesis gravidarum) due to elevated hCG levels

- Objective Data

  - Physical assessment findings

    - Rapid uterine growth more than expected for the duration of the pregnancy due to the overproliferation of trophoblastic cells.

    - Bleeding is often dark brown resembling prune juice, or bright red that is either scant or profuse and continues for a few days or intermittently for a few weeks and may be accompanied by passage of vesicles.

    - Symptoms of preeclampsia that occur prior to 24 weeks of gestation.

  - Laboratory Tests

    - Serum level of hCG persistently high compared with expected decline after weeks 10 to 12 of pregnancy.

  - Diagnostic and Therapeutic Procedures

    - An ultrasound reveals a dense growth with characteristic vesicles, but no fetus in utero.

    - Suction curettage is done to aspirate and evacuate the mole.

    - Following mole evacuation, the client should undergo a baseline pelvic exam and ultrasound scan of the abdomen.

    - Serum hCG analysis following molar pregnancy to be done weekly for 3 weeks, then monthly for 6 months up to a year to detect GTD.

Patient-Centered Care

- Nursing Actions
  - Measure fundal height.
  - Assess vaginal bleeding and discharge.
  - Assess gastrointestinal status and appetite.
  - Monitor for signs and symptoms of preeclampsia.
  - Administer medications as prescribed.
    - $Rh_o(D)$ immune globulin (RhoGAM) to the client who is Rh-negative
    - Chemotherapeutic medications for findings of malignant cells indicating choriocarcinoma
  - Advise client to save clots or tissue for evaluation.
- Health Promotion and Disease Prevention
  - Client education
    - Provide client education and emotional support.
    - Offer referral for client and partner to pregnancy loss support group.
    - Instruct the client to use reliable contraception as a component of follow-up care.
    - Reinforce the importance of follow-up because of the increased risk of choriocarcinoma.

PLACENTA PREVIA

Overview

- Placenta previa occurs when the placenta abnormally implants in the lower segment of the uterus near or over the cervical os instead of attaching to the fundus. The abnormal implantation results in bleeding during the third trimester of pregnancy as the cervix begins to dilate and efface.

 View Image: Placenta Previa

- Placenta previa is classified into three types dependent on the degree to which the cervical os is covered by the placenta.
  - Complete or total – when the cervical os is completely covered by the placental attachment
  - Incomplete or partial – when the cervical os is only partially covered by the placental attachment
  - Marginal or low-lying – when the placenta is attached in the lower uterine segment but does not reach the cervical os

Risk Factors

- Previous placenta previa
- Uterine scarring (previous cesarean birth, curettage, endometritis)
- Maternal age greater than 35 to 40 years
- Multifetal gestation
- Multiple gestations or closely spaced pregnancies
- Smoking

Assessment

- Subjective Data
  - Painless, bright red vaginal bleeding during the second or third trimester
- Objective Data
  - Uterus soft, relaxed and nontender with normal tone
  - Fundal height greater than usually expected for gestational age
  - Fetus in a breech, oblique, or transverse position
  - Reassuring FHR
  - Vital signs within normal limits
  - Decreasing urinary output may be a better indicator of blood loss
- Laboratory Tests
  - Hgb and Hct for blood loss assessment
  - CBC
  - Blood type and Rh
  - Coagulation profile
  - Kleihauer-Betke test (used to detect fetal blood in maternal circulation)
- Diagnostic Procedures
  - Transabdominal or transvaginal ultrasound for placement of the placenta
  - Fetal monitoring for fetal well-being assessment

Patient-Centered Care

- Nursing Actions
  - Assess for bleeding, leakage, or contractions.
  - Assess fundal height.
  - Perform Leopold maneuvers (fetal position and presentation).

  - Refrain from performing vaginal exams (may exacerbate bleeding).
  - Administer IV fluids, blood products, and medications as prescribed.
    - Corticosteroids, such as betamethasone (Celestone), promote fetal lung maturation if delivery is anticipated (cesarean birth).
  - Have oxygen equipment available in case of fetal distress.
- Health Promotion and Disease Prevention
  - Discharge instructions
    - Bed rest
    - Nothing inserted vaginally

ABRUPTIO PLACENTA

Overview

- Abruptio placenta is the premature separation of the placenta from the uterus, which can be a partial or complete detachment. This separation occurs after 20 weeks of gestation, which is usually in the third trimester. It has significant maternal and fetal morbidity and mortality and is a leading cause of maternal death.

 View Image: Abruptio Placenta

- Coagulation defect, such as disseminated intravascular coagulopathy (DIC), is often associated with moderate to severe abruption.

Risk Factors

- Maternal hypertension (chronic or gestational)
- Blunt external abdominal trauma (motor-vehicle crash, maternal battering)
- Cocaine use resulting in vasoconstriction
- Previous incidents of abruptio placenta
- Cigarette smoking
- Premature rupture of membranes
- Multifetal pregnancy

Assessment

- Subjective Data
  - Sudden onset of intense localized uterine pain with dark red vaginal bleeding
- Objective Data
  - Area of uterine tenderness may be localized or diffuse over uterus and boardlike
  - Contractions with hypertonicity
  - Fetal distress
  - Signs of hypovolemic shock
- Laboratory Tests
  - Hgb and Hct decreased
  - Coagulation factors decreased
  - Clotting defects (disseminated intravascular coagulation)
  - Cross and type match for possible blood transfusions
  - Kleihauer-Betke test (used to detect fetal blood in maternal circulation)
- Diagnostic Procedures
  - Ultrasound for fetal well-being and placental assessment
  - Biophysical profile to ascertain fetal well-being

Patient-Centered Care

- Nursing Actions
  - Palpate the uterus for tenderness and tone.
  - Assess FHR pattern.
  - Administer IV fluids, blood products, and medications as prescribed.
    - Corticosteroids to promote fetal lung maturity
  - Administer oxygen 8 to 10 L/min via face mask.
  - Assess urinary output and monitor fluid balance.
- Client Education
  - Provide emotional support for the client and family.

APPLICATION EXERCISES

1. A nurse in the emergency department is caring for a client who reports abrupt, sharp, right-sided lower quadrant abdominal pain and bright red vaginal bleeding. The client states she missed one menstrual cycle and cannot be pregnant because she has an intrauterine device. The nurse should suspect which of the following?

    A. Missed abortion

    B. Ectopic pregnancy

    C. Severe preeclampsia

    D. Hydatidiform mole

2. A nurse at an antepartum clinic is caring for a client who is at 4 months of gestation. The client reports continued nausea and vomiting and scant, prune-colored discharge. She has experienced no weight loss and has a fundal height larger than expected. Which of the following complications should the nurse suspect?

    A. Hyperemesis gravidarum

    B. Threatened abortion

    C. Hydatidiform mole

    D. Preterm labor

3. A nurse is providing care for a client who is diagnosed with a marginal abruptio placenta. The nurse is aware that which of the following findings are risk factors for developing the condition? (Select all that apply.)

    _____ A. Maternal hypertension

    _____ B. Blunt abdominal trauma

    _____ C. Cocaine use

    _____ D. Maternal age

    _____ E. Cigarette smoking

4. A nurse is providing care for a client who is at 32 weeks of gestation and who has a placenta previa. The nurse notes that the client is actively bleeding. Which of the following types of medications should the nurse anticipate the provider will prescribe?

    A. Betamethasone (Celestone)

    B. Indomethacin (Indocin)

    C. Nifedipine (Adalat)

    D. Methylergonovine (Methergine)

5. A nurse is caring for a client who has a diagnosis of ruptured ectopic pregnancy. Which of the following is an expected finding?

    A. No alteration in menses

    B. Transvaginal ultrasound indicating a fetus in the uterus

    C. Serum progesterone greater than the expected reference range

    D. Report of severe shoulder pain

6. A nurse manager is presenting an educational program on placenta previa for a group of nurses. What should be included in this presentation? Use the ATI Active Learning Template: Systems Disorder to complete this item to include the following sections:

    A. Description of the disorder: Describe the three types.

    B. Risk Factors: Identify three.

    C. Diagnostic Procedures: Describe two.

    D. Nursing Actions: Describe one that is contraindicated.

APPLICATION EXERCISES KEY

1. A. INCORRECT: A client who experienced a missed abortion would report brownish discharge and no pain.

    B. **CORRECT:** Manifestations of an ectopic pregnancy include unilateral lower quadrant pain with or without bleeding. Use of an IUD is a risk factor associated with this condition.

    C. INCORRECT: A client who has severe preeclampsia does not have vaginal bleeding and presents with right upper quadrant epigastric pain.

    D. INCORRECT: A client who has a hydatidiform mole usually has dark brown vaginal bleeding in the second trimester that is not accompanied by abdominal pain.

    (N) NCLEX® Connection: Physiological Adaptations, Hemodynamics

2. A. INCORRECT: A client who has hyperemesis gravidarum will have weight loss and signs of dehydration.

    B. INCORRECT: A client who has a threatened abortion would be in the first trimester and report spotting to moderate bleeding with no enlarged uterus.

    C. **CORRECT:** A client who has a hydatidiform mole exhibits increased fundal height that is inconsistent with the week of gestation, and excessive nausea and vomiting due to elevated hCG levels. Scant, dark discharge occurs in the second trimester.

    D. INCORRECT: Preterm labor presents prior to 37 weeks of gestation and is accompanied by pink-stained vaginal discharge and uterine contractions that become more regular.

    (N) NCLEX® Connection: Physiological Adaptations, Illness Management

3. A. **CORRECT:** Maternal hypertension is a risk factor associated with abruptio placenta.

    B. **CORRECT:** Blunt abdominal trauma is a risk factor associated with abruptio placenta.

    C. **CORRECT:** Cocaine use is a risk factor associated with abruptio placenta.

    D. INCORRECT: Maternal age is not a risk factor associated with abruptio placenta.

    E. **CORRECT:** Cigarette smoking is a risk factor associated with abruptio placenta.

    (N) NCLEX® Connection: Physiological Adaptations, Illness Management

4. A. **CORRECT:** Betamethasone (Celestone) is given to promote lung maturity if delivery is anticipated.

    B. INCORRECT: Indomethacin (Indocin) is prescribed for the client in preterm labor.

    C. INCORRECT: Nifedicine (Adalat) is prescribed for the client in preterm labor.

    D. INCORRECT: Methylergonovine (Methergine) is prescribed for the client experiencing postpartum hemorrhage.

    Ⓝ NCLEX® Connection: Physiological Adaptations, Alterations in Body Systems

5. A. INCORRECT: A client experiencing a ruptured ectopic pregnancy has delayed, scant, or irregular menses.

    B. INCORRECT: A transvaginal ultrasound would indicate an empty uterus in a client who has a ruptured ectopic pregnancy.

    C. INCORRECT: A serum progesterone level lower than the expected reference range is an indication of ectopic pregnancy.

    D. **CORRECT:** A client's report of severe shoulder pain is a finding associated with a ruptured ectopic pregnancy due to the presence of blood in the abdominal cavity, which irritates the diaphragm and phrenic nerve.

    Ⓝ NCLEX® Connection: Physiological Adaptations, Alterations in Body Systems

6. *Using the ATI Active Learning Template: Systems Disorder*

    A. Description of the Disorder: Types of placenta previa
       ○ Complete or total – cervical os is covered by the placenta
       ○ Incomplete or partial – cervical os is only partially covered by the placenta
       ○ Marginal or low-lying – placenta is attached in the lower uterine segment but does not reach the cervical os

    B. Risk Factors
       • Previous placenta previa
       • Uterine scarring due to previous cesarean birth, curettage, or endometritis
       • Maternal age 35 to 40 years
       • Multifetal gestation
       • Multiple gestations or closely spaced pregnancies
       • Smoking

    C. Diagnostic procedures
       • Transabdominal or transvaginal ultrasound
       • Fetal monitoring

    D. Contraindicated Nursing Actions: Performing a vaginal exam

    Ⓝ NCLEX® Connection: Physiological Adaptations, Hemodynamics

chapter 8

Overview

- Maternal infections during pregnancy require prompt identification and treatment by a provider. This section will explore HIV, TORCH infections, Group B streptococcus ß-hemolytic, chlamydia, gonorrhea, and *Candida albicans*. Risk factors, assessment findings, and teamwork and collaboration will be discussed.

HIV/AIDS

Overview

- HIV is a retrovirus that attacks and causes destruction of T lymphocytes. It causes immunosuppression in a client. HIV is transmitted from the mother to a neonate perinatally through the placenta and postnatally through the breast milk.

- Routine laboratory testing in the early prenatal period includes testing for HIV. Early identification and treatment significantly decreases the incidence of perinatal transmission.

- Testing is recommended in the third trimester for clients who are at an increased risk, and rapid HIV testing should be done if a client is in labor and her HIV status is unknown.

- Procedures, such as amniocentesis and an episiotomy, should be avoided due to the risk of maternal blood exposure.

- Use of internal fetal monitors, vacuum extraction, and forceps during labor should be avoided because of the risk of fetal bleeding.

- Administration of injections and blood testing should not take place until the first bath is given to the newborn.

Risk Factors

- IV drug use
- Multiple sexual partners
- Bisexuality
- Maternal history of multiple STIs
- Blood transfusion (rare occurrence)

Assessment

- Subjective Data
  - Fatigue and influenzalike symptoms
- Objective Data
  - Physical assessment findings
    - Diarrhea and weight loss
    - Lymphadenopathy and rash
    - Anemia
  - Laboratory Tests
    - Obtain informed maternal consent prior to testing. Testing begins with an antibody screening test, such as enzyme immunoassay. Confirmation of positive results is confirmed by Western blot test or immunofluorescence assay.
    - Use rapid HIV antibody test (blood or urine sample) for a client in labor.
    - Screen the client for STIs such as gonorrhea, chlamydia, syphilis, and hepatitis B.
    - Obtain frequent viral load levels and CD4 cell counts throughout the pregnancy.

Teamwork and Collaboration

- Nursing Care
  - Provide counseling prior to and after testing.
  - Refer the client for a mental health consultation, legal assistance, and financial resources.
  - Use standard precautions.
  - Administer antiviral prophylaxis, triple-drug antiviral, or highly active antiretroviral therapy (HAART) as prescribed.
  - Obtain prescribed laboratory testing.
  - Encourage vaccination against hepatitis B, pneumococcal infection, *Haemophilus influenzae* type B and viral influenza.
  - Encourage use of condoms to minimize exposure if partner is the source of infection.
  - Review plan for scheduled cesarean birth at 38 weeks for maternal viral load of more than 1,000 copies/mL.
  - Infant should be bathed after birth before remaining with the mother.
- Medications
  - Retrovir (Zidovudine)
    - Antiretroviral agent
    - Nucleoside reverse transcriptase inhibitor
  - Nursing considerations
    - Administer retrovir at 14 weeks of gestation, throughout the pregnancy, and before the onset of labor or cesarean birth.
    - Administer retrovir to the infant at delivery and for 6 weeks following birth.

- Health Promotion and Disease Prevention
  - Discharge instructions
    - Instruct the client not to breastfeed.
    - Discuss HIV and safe sexual relations with the client.
    - Refer client and infant to providers specializing in the care of clients who have HIV.

TORCH INFECTIONS

Overview

- TORCH is an acronym for a group of infections that can negatively affect a woman who is pregnant. These infections can cross the placenta and have teratogenic affects on the fetus. TORCH does not include all the major infections that present risks to the mother and fetus.

Risk Factors

- Toxoplasmosis is caused by consumption of raw or undercooked meat or handling cat feces. The symptoms are similar to influenza or lymphadenopathy. Other infections can include hepatitis A and B, syphilis, mumps, parvovirus B19, and varicella-zoster. These are some of the most common and can be associated with congenital anomalies.

- Rubella (German measles) is contracted through children who have rashes or neonates who are born to mothers who had rubella during pregnancy.

- Cytomegalovirus (member of herpes virus family) is transmitted by droplet infection from person to person, a virus found in semen, cervical and vaginal secretions, breast milk, placental tissue, urine, feces, and blood. Latent virus may be reactivated and cause disease to the fetus in utero or during passage through the birth canal.

- The herpes simplex virus (HSV) is spread by direct contact with oral or genital lesions. Transmission to the fetus is greatest during vaginal birth if the woman has active lesions.

Assessment

- Subjective Data
  - Toxoplasmosis findings similar to influenza or lymphadenopathy
  - Malaise, muscle aches, (flulike symptoms)
  - Rubella joint and muscle pain
  - Cytomegalovirus has asymptomatic or mononucleosis-like manifestations

- Objective Data
  - Physical assessment findings
    - Manifestations of toxoplasmosis include fever and tender lymph nodes.
    - Manifestations of rubella include rash, mild lymphedema, fever, and fetal consequences, which include miscarriage, congenital anomalies, and death.
    - Herpes simplex virus initially presents with lesions and tender lymph nodes. Fetal consequences include miscarriage, preterm labor, and intrauterine growth restriction.
  - Laboratory Tests
    - For herpes simplex, obtain cultures from women who have HSV or are at or near term.
  - Diagnostic Procedures
    - A TORCH screen is an immunologic survey that is used to identify the existence of these infections in the mother (to identify fetal risks) or in her newborn (detection of antibodies against infections).
    - Prenatal screenings

Teamwork and Collaboration

- Nursing Care
  - Monitor fetal well-being.
  - Educate the client on prevention practices, including correct hand hygiene and cooking meat properly. Clients should be instructed to avoid contact with contaminated cat litter.
- Medications
  - Administer antibiotics as prescribed.
  - Treatment of toxoplasmosis includes sulfonamides or a combination of pyrimethamine and sulfadiazine (potentially harmful to the fetus, but parasitic treatment is essential).
- Health Promotion and Disease Prevention
  - Client Education
    - For rubella, vaccination of women who are pregnant is contraindicated because rubella infection may develop. These women should avoid crowds of young children. Women with low titers prior to pregnancy should receive immunizations.
    - Because no treatment for cytomegalovirus exists, tell the client to prevent exposure by frequent hand hygiene before eating, and avoiding crowds of young children.
    - Emphasize to the client the importance of compliance with prescribed treatment.
    - Provide client with emotional support.

GROUP B, STREPTOCOCCUS ß-HEMOLYTIC

Overview

- Group B streptococcus ß-hemolytic (GBS) is a bacterial infection that can be passed to a fetus during labor and delivery.

Risk Factors

- History of positive culture with previous pregnancy
- Risk factors for early-onset neonatal GBS
  - Maternal age less than 20 years
  - African American or Hispanic ethnicity
  - Positive culture with pregnancy
  - Prolonged rupture of membranes
  - Preterm delivery
  - Low birth weight
  - Use of intrauterine fetal monitoring
  - Intrapartum maternal fever (38° C [100.4° F])

Assessment

- Objective Data
  - Physical Assessment Findings
    - Positive GBS may have maternal and fetal effects, including premature rupture of membranes, preterm labor and delivery, chorioamnionitis, infections of the urinary tract, and maternal sepsis.
  - Laboratory Tests
    - Vaginal and rectal cultures are performed at 36 to 37 weeks of gestation.

Teamwork and Collaboration

- Nursing Care
  - Administer intrapartum antibiotic prophylaxis (IAP).
    - Client who delivered previous infant with GBS infection
    - Client who has GBS bacteriuria during current pregnancy
    - Client who has a GBS-positive screening during current pregnancy
    - Client who has unknown GBS status who is delivering at less than 37 weeks of gestation
    - Client who has maternal fever of 38° C (100.4° F)
    - Client who has rupture of membranes for 18 hr or longer

- Medications
  - Penicillin G or ampicillin (Principen) is most commonly prescribed for GBS.
    - Administer penicillin 5 million units initially IV bolus, followed by 2.5 million units intermittent IV bolus every 4 hr. The client may be prescribed ampicillin 2 grams IV initially, followed by 1 g every 4 hr.
    - Bactericidal antibiotic is used to destroy the GBS.
- Health Promotion and Disease Prevention
  - Client Education
    - Instruct the client to notify the labor and delivery nurse of GBS status.

CHLAMYDIA

Overview

- Chlamydia is a bacterial infection caused by *Chlamydia trachomatis*. It is the most common STI. The infection is often difficult to diagnose because it is typically asymptomatic. According to current guidelines from the Centers for Disease Control and Prevention, all women and adolescents ages 20 to 25 who are sexually active should be screened for STIs.

Risk Factors

- Multiple sexual partners
- Unprotected sexual practices

Assessment

- Subjective Data
  - Vaginal spotting
  - Vulvar itching
  - Postcoital bleeding and dysuria
- Objective Data
  - Physical Assessment Findings
    - White, watery vaginal discharge
  - Laboratory Tests
    - Endocervical culture

Teamwork and Collaboration

- Nursing Care
  - ○ Instruct the client to take the entire prescription as prescribed.
  - ○ Identify and treat all sexual partners.
  - ○ Clients who are pregnant should be retested 3 weeks after completing the prescribed regimen.
- Medications
  - ○ Azithromycin (Zithromax) and amoxicillin (Amoxil) are prescribed during pregnancy.
    - ■ Broad-spectrum antibiotic
    - ■ Bactericidal action
    - ■ Nursing Care
      - □ Administer erythromycin (Romycin) to all infants following delivery. This is the medication of choice for ophthalmia neonatorum. This antibiotic is both bacteriostatic and bactericidal, thus it provides prophylaxis against *Neisseria gonorrhoeae* and *Chlamydia trachomatis*.
    - ■ Client Education
      - □ Instruct the client to take all prescriptions as prescribed.
      - □ Educate the client about the possibility of decreasing effectiveness of oral contraceptives.

GONORRHEA

Overview

- *Neisseria gonorrhoeae* is the causative agent of gonorrhea. Gonorrhea is a bacterial infection that is primarily spread by genital-to-genital contact. However, it also can be spread by anal-to-genital contact or oral-to-genital contact. It can also be transmitted to a newborn during delivery. Women are frequently asymptomatic.

Risk Factors

- Multiple sexual partners
- Unprotected sexual practices

Assessment

- Subjective Data (Male)
  - ○ Urethral discharge
  - ○ Painful urination
  - ○ Frequency
- Subjective Data (Female)
  - ○ Lower abdominal pain
  - ○ Dysmenorrhea

- Objective Data – Male/Female
  - Physical Assessment Findings
    - Urethral discharge
    - Yellowish-green vaginal discharge
    - Reddened vulva and vaginal walls
    - If gonorrhea is left untreated, it can cause pelvic inflammatory disease, heart disease, and arthritis.
  - Laboratory Tests
    - Urethral and vaginal cultures
    - Urine culture

Teamwork and Collaboration

- Nursing Care
  - Provide client education regarding disease transmission.
  - Identify and treat all sexual partners.
- Medications
  - Ceftriaxone (Rocephin) IM and azithromycin (Zithromax) PO for gonorrhea
    - One dose prescription
    - Broad-spectrum antibiotic
    - Bactericidal action
  - Client Education
    - Instruct the client to take entire prescription as prescribed.
    - Instruct the client to repeat the culture to assess for medication effectiveness.
    - Educate the client regarding safe sex practices.

CANDIDA ALBICANS

Overview

- A fungal infection caused by *Candida albicans*.

Risk Factors

- Diabetes mellitus
- Oral contraceptives
- Recent antibiotic treatment

Assessment

- Subjective Data
  - Vulvar itching
- Objective Data
  - Physical Assessment Findings
    - Thick, creamy, white vaginal discharge
    - Vulvar redness
    - White patches on vaginal walls
    - Gray-white patches on the tongue and gums (neonate)
  - Laboratory Tests
    - Wet prep
  - Diagnostic Procedures
    - Potassium hydroxide (KOH) prep
    - Presence of hyphae and pseudohyphae indicates positive findings.

Teamwork and Collaboration

- Nursing Care
  - Medications
    - Fluconazole (Diflucan)
      - Antifungal agent
      - Fungicidal action
      - Over-the-counter treatments, such as clotrimazole (Monistat), are available to treat candidiasis. However, it is important for the provider to diagnosis candidiasis initially.
- Health Promotion and Disease Prevention
  - Client Education
    - Instruct the client to avoid tight-fitting clothing.
    - Instruct the client to wear cotton-lined underpants.
    - Instruct the client to limit wearing damp clothing.
    - Instruct the client to void before and after intercourse and avoid douching.
    - Instruct the client to increase dietary intake of yogurt with active cultures.

APPLICATION EXERCISES

1. A nurse on the obstetrical unit is admitting a client who is in labor. The client has a positive HIV status. The nurse is aware that which of the following is contraindicated for this client? (Select all that apply.)

_____X_____ A. Episiotomy

_____X_____ B. Vacuum extraction

_____X_____ C. Forceps

_____ D. Cesarean birth

_____X_____ E. Internal fetal monitoring

2. A nurse in an antepartum clinic is providing care for a client. Which of the following clinical findings are suggestive of a TORCH infection? (Select all that apply.)

_____X_____ A. Joint pain

_____X_____ B. Malaise

_____X_____ C. Rash

_____ D. Urinary frequency

_____X_____ E. Tender lymph nodes

3. A nurse is caring for a client who has a diagnosis of gonorrhea. Which of the following medications should the nurse anticipate the provider will prescribe?

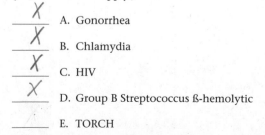

A. Ceftriaxone (Rocephin)

B. Fluconazole (Diflucan)

C. Metronidazole (Flagyl)

D. Zidovudine (Retrovir)

4. A nurse is caring for a client who is in labor. The nurse is aware that which of the following conditions have medications that can be prescribed as prophylactic treatment during labor or immediately following delivery? (Select all that apply.)

_____X_____ A. Gonorrhea

_____X_____ B. Chlamydia

_____X_____ C. HIV

_____X_____ D. Group B Streptococcus ß-hemolytic

_____ E. TORCH

5. A nurse manager in a prenatal clinic is reviewing ways to prevent a TORCH infection during pregnancy with a group of newly licensed nurses during an education program. Which of the following statements by a nurse indicates understanding of the teaching?

    A. "Obtain a vaccination against rubella early in pregnancy."

    B. "Seek prophylactic treatment if cytomegalovirus is detected."

    C. "A woman should avoid handling dog feces."

    D. "A woman should avoid consuming undercooked meat."

6. A nurse is planning care for a client who is pregnant and positive for group B streptococcus ß-hemolytic. Use the ATI Active Learning Template: Systems Disorder to complete this item to include:

    A. Laboratory Test: Describe the test and when it is performed.

    B. Risk Factors: Describe two maternal risk factors and three fetal risk factors.

    C. Medications: Describe three clients who should receive intrapartum antibiotic prophylaxis.

APPLICATION EXERCISES KEY

1.   A. **CORRECT:** An episiotomy should be avoided for a client who is HIV positive due to the risk of maternal blood exposure.

   B. **CORRECT:** Vacuum extraction during delivery should be avoided because of the risk of fetal bleeding.

   C. **CORRECT:** The use of forceps during delivery should be avoided because of the risk of fetal bleeding.

   D. INCORRECT: A cesarean birth is not contraindicated for this client.

   E. **CORRECT:** Internal fetal monitoring should be avoided because of the risk of fetal bleeding.

   Ⓝ NCLEX® Connection: Physiological Adaptations, Illness Management

2.   A. **CORRECT:** TORCH infections are flulike in presentation, such as joint pain.

   B. **CORRECT:** TORCH infections are flulike in presentation, such as malaise.

   C. **CORRECT:** TORCH infections may include findings such as a rash.

   D. INCORRECT: Urinary frequency is not a symptom associated with a TORCH infection.

   E. **CORRECT:** TORCH infections are flulike in presentation, such as tender lymph nodes.

   Ⓝ NCLEX® Connection: Physiological Adaptations, Alterations in Body Systems

3.   A. **CORRECT:** Ceftriaxone IM or doxycycline (Vibramycin) orally for 7 days is prescribed for the treatment of gonorrhea.

   B. INCORRECT: Fluconazole is used to treat candidiasis.

   C. INCORRECT: Metronidazole is used in the treatment of bacterial vaginosis and trichomoniasis.

   D. INCORRECT: Zidovudine is used to treat HIV/AIDS.

   Ⓝ NCLEX® Connection: Physiological Adaptations, Illness Management

4.   A. **CORRECT:** Erythromycin (Romycin) is administered to the infant immediately following delivery to prevent *Neisseria gonorrhoeae*.

   B. **CORRECT:** Erythromycin (Romycin) is administered to the infant immediately following delivery to prevent *Chlymydia trachomatis*.

   C. **CORRECT:** Retrovir (Zidovudine) is prescribed to the client in labor who is HIV positive.

   D. **CORRECT:** Penicillin G or ampicillin (Principen) may be prescribed to treat positive GBS.

   E. INCORRECT: A TORCH infection may be treated during pregnancy depending upon the infection.

   Ⓝ NCLEX® Connection: Health Promotion and Maintenance, Ante/Intra/Postpartum and Newborn Care

5. A. INCORRECT: Vaccination against rubella is contraindicated during pregnancy due to the risk of fetal congenital anomalies.

    B. INCORRECT: There is no treatment for cytomegalovirus.

    C. INCORRECT: Toxoplasmosis, a TORCH infection, is contracted by handling cat feces.

    D. **CORRECT:** Toxoplasmosis, a TORCH infection, is contracted by consuming undercooked meat.

    (N) NCLEX® Connection: Health Promotion and Maintenance, Ante/Intra/Postpartum and Newborn Care

6. *Using the ATI Active Learning Template: Systems Disorder*

    A. Laboratory Test
      - Vaginal and rectal cultures performed at 36 to 37 weeks of gestation

    B. Risk Factors
      - Maternal
        ○ History of positive culture with previous pregnancy
        ○ Maternal age less than 20 years
        ○ African American or Hispanic ethnicity
      - Fetal
        ○ Positive during with pregnancy
        ○ Prolonged rupture of membranes
        ○ Preterm delivery
        ○ Low birth weight
        ○ Use of intrauterine fetal monitoring
        ○ Intrapartum maternal fever (38° C [100.4° F])

    C. Medications
      - Client who delivered previous infant with GBS infection
      - Client who has GBS bacteriuria during current pregnancy
      - Client who has a GBS-positive screening during current pregnancy
      - Client who has unknown GBS status who is delivering at less than 37 weeks of gestation
      - Client who has maternal fever of 38° C (100.4° F)
      - Client who has rupture of membranes for 18 hr or longer

    (N) NCLEX® Connection: Physiological Adaptations, Alterations in Body Systems

chapter 9

Overview

- Unexpected medical conditions may occur during pregnancy. Awareness, early detection, and interventions are crucial components to ensure fetal well-being and maternal health.

- Unexpected medical conditions include recurrent premature dilation of the cervix, hyperemesis gravidarum, anemia, gestational diabetes mellitus, and gestational hypertension.

RECURRENT PREMATURE DILATION OF THE CERVIX (INCOMPETENT CERVIX)

Overview

- Recurrent premature dilation of the cervix or cervical insufficiency is a variable condition whereby expulsion of the products of conception occurs. It is thought to be related to tissue changes and alterations in the length of the cervix.

Risk Factors

- History of cervical trauma (previous lacerations, excessive dilations, and curettage for biopsy), short labors, pregnancy loss in early gestation, or advanced cervical dilation at earlier weeks of gestation

- In utero, exposure to diethylstilbestrol (ingested by the client's mother during pregnancy)

- Congenital structural defects of the uterus or cervix

Assessment

- Subjective Data
  - Increase in pelvic pressure or urge to push
- Objective Data
  - Physical assessment findings
    - Pink-stained vaginal discharge or bleeding
    - Possible gush of fluid (rupture of membranes)
    - Uterine contractions with the expulsion of the fetus
    - Postoperative (cerclage) monitoring for uterine contractions, rupture of membranes, and signs of infection

○ Diagnostic and therapeutic procedures

- An ultrasound showing a short cervix (less than 25 mm in length), the presence of cervical funneling (beaking), or effacement of the cervical os indicates reduced cervical competence.

- Prophylactic cervical cerclage is the surgical reinforcement of the cervix with a heavy ligature that is placed submucosally around the cervix to strengthen it and prevent premature cervical dilation. Best results occur if this is done before 23 to 24 weeks of gestation. The cerclage is removed at 37 weeks of gestation or when spontaneous labor occurs.

Patient-Centered Care

- Nursing Care

  ○ Evaluate the client's support systems and availability of assistance if activity restrictions and/or bed rest are prescribed.

  ○ Assess vaginal discharge.

  ○ Monitor client reports of pressure and contractions.

  ○ Check vital signs.

- Medications

  ○ Administer tocolytics prophylactically to inhibit uterine contractions.

- Health Promotion and Disease Prevention

  ○ Discharge instructions

    - Place the client on activity restriction/bed rest.

    - Encourage hydration to promote a relaxed uterus. (Dehydration stimulates uterine contractions.)

    - Advise the client to refrain from intercourse and to monitor for cervical/uterine changes.

  ○ Client education

    - Provide client education about signs and symptoms to report to the provider for preterm labor, rupture of membranes, infection, strong contractions less than 5 min apart, severe perineal pressure, and an urge to push.

    - Instruct the client about using the home uterine activity monitor to evaluate uterine contractions.

    - Arrange for the client to follow up with a home health agency for close observation and supervision.

    - Plan for removal of the cerclage around 37 weeks of gestation.

HYPEREMESIS GRAVIDARUM

Overview

- Hyperemesis gravidarum is excessive nausea and vomiting (possibly related to elevated hCG levels) that is prolonged past 12 weeks of gestation and results in a 5% weight loss from prepregnancy weight, electrolyte imbalance, acetonuria, and ketosis.
- Hyperemesis gravidarum may be associated with altered thyroid function.
- There is a risk to the fetus for intrauterine growth restriction (IUGR) or preterm birth if the condition persists.

Risk Factors

- Maternal age younger than 20 years
- History of migraines
- Obesity
- First pregnancy
- Multifetal gestation
- Gestational trophoblastic disease or fetus with chromosomal anomaly
- Psychosocial issues and high levels of emotional stress
- Transient hyperthyroidism

Assessment

- Objective Data
  - Physical Assessment Findings
    - Excessive vomiting for prolonged periods and diarrhea
    - Dehydration with possible electrolyte imbalance
    - Weight loss
    - Increased pulse rate
    - Decreased blood pressure
    - Poor skin turgor and dry mucous membranes
  - Laboratory Tests
    - Urinalysis for ketones and acetones (breakdown of protein and fat) is the most important initial laboratory test.
    - Elevated urine specific gravity.
    - Chemistry profile revealing electrolyte imbalances, such as:
      - Sodium, potassium, and chloride reduced from low intake
      - Acidosis resulting from excessive vomiting
      - Elevated liver enzymes
    - Thyroid test indicating hyperthyroidism.
    - Hct concentration is elevated because inability to retain fluid results in hemoconcentration.

Patient-Centered Care

- Nursing Care
  - Monitor the client's I&O.
  - Assess the client's skin turgor and mucous membranes.
  - Monitor the client's vital signs.
  - Monitor the client's weight.
  - Have the client remain NPO for 24 to 48 hr.
- Medications
  - Give the client IV fluids of lactated Ringer's for hydration.
  - Give pyridoxine (Vitamin B_6) and other vitamin supplements as tolerated.
  - Use antiemetic medications cautiously for uncontrollable nausea and vomiting (ondansetron [Zofran], metoclopramide [Reglan]).
  - Use corticosteroids to treat refractory hyperemesis gravidarum.
- Health Promotion and Disease Prevention
  - Discharge instructions
    - Advance the client to clear liquids after 24 hr if no vomiting.
    - Advance the client's diet, as tolerated, with frequent, small meals. Start with dry toast, crackers, or cereal; then move to a soft diet; and finally to a normal diet as tolerated.
    - In severe cases, or if vomiting returns, enteral nutrition per feeding tube or total parental nutrition (TPN) may be considered.

ANEMIA

Overview

- Iron-deficiency anemia occurs during pregnancy due to inadequacy in maternal iron stores and consuming insufficient amounts of dietary iron.

Risk Factors

- Risk Factors
  - Less than 2 years between pregnancies
  - Heavy menses
  - Diet low in iron

Assessment

- Subjective Data
  - Fatigue
  - Irritability
  - Headache
  - Shortness of breath with exertion
  - Palpitations
  - Craving unusual food (pica)
- Objective Data
  - Physical Assessment Findings
    - Pallor
    - Brittle nails
    - Shortness of breath
  - Laboratory Tests
    - Hgb less than 11 mg/dL in the first and third trimesters and less than 10.5 mg/dL in the second trimester
    - Hct less than 33%

Patient-Centered Care

- Nursing Care
  - Prophylactic treatment using prenatal supplements with 60 mg of iron is suggested.
  - Increase dietary intake of foods rich in iron (legumes, fruit, green, leafy vegetables, and meat).
  - Educate the client about ways to minimize gastrointestinal adverse effects.
- Medications
  - Ferrous sulfate (325 mg) iron supplements twice daily
    - Nursing Considerations and Client Education
      - Instruct the client to take the supplement on an empty stomach.
      - Encourage a diet rich in vitamin C-containing foods to increase absorption.
      - Suggest that the client increase roughage and fluid intake in diet to assist with discomforts of constipation.
  - Iron dextran (Imferon)
    - Used in the treatment of iron-deficiency anemia when oral iron supplements cannot be tolerated by the client who is pregnant.

GESTATIONAL DIABETES MELLITUS

Overview

- Gestational diabetes mellitus is an impaired tolerance to glucose with the first onset or recognition during pregnancy. The ideal blood glucose level during pregnancy should fall between 70 and 110 mg/dL.

- Symptoms of diabetes mellitus may disappear a few weeks following delivery. However, approximately 50% of women will develop diabetes mellitus within 5 years.

- Gestational diabetes mellitus causes increased risks to the fetus including the following:

  - Spontaneous abortion, which is related to poor glycemic control.

  - Infections (urinary and vaginal), which are related to increased glucose in the urine and decreased resistance because of altered carbohydrate metabolism.

  - Hydramnios, which can cause overdistention of the uterus, premature rupture of membranes, preterm labor, and hemorrhage.

  - Ketoacidosis from diabetogenic effect of pregnancy (increased insulin resistance), untreated hyperglycemia, or inappropriate insulin dosing.

  - Hypoglycemia, which is caused by overdosing in insulin, skipped or late meals, or increased exercise.

  - Hyperglycemia, which can cause excessive fetal growth (macrosomia).

Risk Factors

- Obesity
- Maternal age older than 25 years
- Family history of diabetes mellitus
- Previous delivery of an infant that was large or stillborn

Assessment

- Subjective Data

  - Hypoglycemia (nervousness, headache, weakness, irritability, hunger, blurred vision, tingling of mouth or extremities)

  - Hyperglycemia (thirst, nausea, abdominal pain, frequent urination, flushed dry skin, fruity breath)

- Objective Data

  - Physical Assessment Findings

    - Hypoglycemia

    - Shaking

    - Clammy pale skin

    - Shallow respirations

CHAPTER 9 MEDICAL CONDITIONS

- Rapid pulse
- Hyperglycemia
- Vomiting
- Excess weight gain during pregnancy
- ○ Laboratory Tests
  - Routine urinalysis with glycosuria

  - A glucola screening test/1-hr glucose tolerance test (50 g oral glucose load, followed by plasma glucose analysis 1 hr later performed at 24 to 28 weeks of gestation – fasting not necessary; a positive blood glucose screening is 130 to 140 mg/dL or greater; additional testing with a 3-hr oral glucose tolerance test [OGTT] is indicated)
  - An OGTT (following overnight fasting, avoidance of caffeine, and abstinence from smoking for 12 hr prior to testing; a fasting glucose is obtained, a 100 g glucose load is given, and serum glucose levels are determined at 1, 2, and 3 hr following glucose ingestion)
  - Presence of ketones in urine is tested to assess the severity of ketoacidosis
- ○ Diagnostic Procedures
  - Biophysical profile to ascertain fetal well-being
  - Amniocentesis with alpha-fetoprotein
  - Nonstress test to assess fetal well-being

Patient-Centered Care

- Nursing Care
  - ○ Monitor the client's blood glucose.
  - ○ Monitor the fetus.
- Medications
  - ○ Administer insulin as prescribed.
    - Most oral hypoglycemic agents are contraindicated for gestational diabetes mellitus, but there is limited use of glyburide (DiaBeta) at this time. The provider will need to make the determination if these medications may be used.
- Health Promotion and Disease Prevention
  - ○ Client education
    - Instruct the client to perform daily kick counts.
    - Educate the client about diet and exercise.
    - Instruct the client about self-administration of insulin.
    - Educate the client about the need for postpartum laboratory testing to include OGTT and blood glucose levels

98
RN MATERNAL NEWBORN NURSING

GESTATIONAL HYPERTENSION

Overview

- Hypertensive disease in pregnancy is divided into clinical subsets of the disease based on end-organ effects and progresses along a continuum from mild gestational hypertension, mild and severe preeclampsia, eclampsia, and hemolysis, elevated liver enzymes, and low platelets (HELLP) syndrome.

- Vasospasm contributing to poor tissue perfusion is the underlying mechanism for the manifestations of pregnancy hypertensive disorders.

- Gestational hypertension (GH), which begins after the 20th week of pregnancy, describes hypertensive disorders of pregnancy whereby the woman has an elevated blood pressure at 140/90 mm Hg or greater recorded at least twice, 4 to 6 hr apart, and within a 1-week period. There is no proteinuria. The presence of edema is no longer considered in the definition of hypertensive disease of pregnancy. The client's blood pressure returns to baseline by 6 weeks postpartum.

- Mild preeclampsia is GH with the addition of proteinuria of greater than 1+. Report of transient headaches may or may not occur along with episodes of irritability. Edema may be present.

- Severe preeclampsia consists of blood pressure that is 160/100 mm Hg or greater, proteinuria greater than 3+, oliguria, elevated serum creatinine greater than 1.2 mg/dL, cerebral or visual disturbances (headache and blurred vision), hyperreflexia with possible ankle clonus, pulmonary or cardiac involvement, extensive peripheral edema, hepatic dysfunction, epigastric and right upper-quadrant pain, and thrombocytopenia.

- Eclampsia is severe preeclampsia symptoms along with the onset of seizure activity or coma. Eclampsia is usually preceded by headache, severe epigastric pain, hyperreflexia, and hemoconcentrations, which are warning signs of probable convulsions.

- HELLP syndrome is a variant of GH in which hematologic conditions coexist with severe preeclampsia involving hepatic dysfunction. HELLP syndrome is diagnosed by laboratory tests, not clinically.

  - H – hemolysis resulting in anemia and jaundice

  - EL – elevated liver enzymes resulting in elevated alanine aminotransferase (ALT) or aspartate transaminase (AST), epigastric pain, and nausea and vomiting

  - LP – low platelets (less than 100,000/mm³), resulting in thrombocytopenia, abnormal bleeding and clotting time, bleeding gums, petechiae, and possibly disseminated intravascular coagulopathy (DIC)

- Gestational hypertensive disease and chronic hypertension may occur simultaneously.

- Gestational hypertensive diseases are associated with placental abruption, kidney failure, hepatic rupture, preterm birth, and fetal and maternal death.

Risk Factors

- No single profile identifies risks for gestational hypertensive disorders, but some high risks include the following:
  - Maternal age younger than 20 or older than 40
  - First pregnancy
  - Morbid obesity
  - Multifetal gestation
  - Chronic renal disease
  - Chronic hypertension
  - Familiar history of preeclampsia
  - Diabetes mellitus
  - Rh incompatibility
  - Molar pregnancy
  - Previous history of GH

Assessment

- Subjective Data
  - Severe continuous headache
  - Nausea
  - Blurring of vision
  - Flashes of lights or dots before the eyes
- Objective Data
  - Physical assessment findings
    - Hypertension
    - Proteinuria
    - Periorbital, facial, hand, and abdominal edema
    - Pitting edema of lower extremities
    - Vomiting
    - Oliguria
    - Hyperreflexia
    - Scotoma
    - Epigastric pain
    - Right upper quadrant pain
    - Dyspnea
    - Diminished breath sounds
    - Seizures
    - Jaundice
    - Signs of progression of hypertensive disease with indications of worsening liver involvement, renal failure, worsening hypertension, cerebral involvement, and developing coagulopathies

- Abnormal Laboratory Findings
  - Elevated liver enzymes (LDH, AST)
  - Increased creatinine
  - Increased plasma uric acid
  - Thrombocytopenia
  - Decreased Hgb
  - Hyperbilirubinemia
- Laboratory Tests
  - Liver enzymes
  - Serum creatinine, BUN, uric acid, and magnesium increase as renal function decreases
  - CBC
  - Clotting studies
  - Chemistry profile
- Diagnostic Procedures
  - Dipstick testing of urine for proteinuria
  - 24-hr urine collection for protein and creatinine clearance
  - Nonstress test, contraction stress test, biophysical profile, and serial ultrasounds to assess fetal status
  - Doppler blood flow analysis to assess fetal well-being

Patient-Centered Care

- Nursing Care
  - Assess the client's level of consciousness.
  - Obtain pulse oximetry.
  - Monitor the client's urine output and obtain a clean-catch urine sample to assess for proteinuria.
  - Obtain daily weights.
  - Monitor vital signs.
  - Encourage lateral positioning.
  - Perform NST and daily kick counts as prescribed.
  - Instruct the client to monitor I&O.
- Medications
  - Antihypertensive medications
    - Methyldopa (Aldomet).
    - Nifedipine (Adalat, Procardia).
    - Hydralazine (Apresoline, Neopresol).
    - Labetalol hydrochloride (Normodyne, Trandate).
    - Avoid ACE inhibitors and angiotensin II receptor blockers.

- ○ Anticonvulsant medications
  - ▪ Magnesium sulfate.
  - ▪ Medication of choice for prophylaxis or treatment to lower blood pressure and depress the CNS.
- ○ Nursing Considerations
  - ▪ Use an infusion control device to maintain a regular flow rate.
  - ▪ Inform the client that she may initially feel flushed, hot, and sedated with the magnesium sulfate bolus.
  - ▪ Monitor the client's blood pressure, pulse, respiratory rate, deep-tendon reflexes, level of consciousness, urinary output (indwelling urinary catheter for accuracy), presence of headache, visual disturbances, epigastric pain, uterine contractions, and FHR and activity.
  - ▪ Place the client on fluid restriction of 100 to 125 mL/hr, and maintain a urinary output of 30 mL/hr or greater.
  - ▪ Monitor the client for signs of magnesium sulfate toxicity.
    - □ Absence of patellar deep tendon reflexes
    - □ Urine output less than 30 mL/hr
    - □ Respirations less than 12/min
    - □ Decreased level of consciousness
    - □ Cardiac dysrhythmias
- ○ If magnesium toxicity is suspected:
  - ▪ Immediately discontinue infusion.
  - ▪ Administer antidote calcium gluconate.
  - ▪ Prepare for actions to prevent respiratory or cardiac arrest.
- • Health Promotion and Disease Prevention
  - ○ Discharge instructions
    - ▪ Maintain the client on bed rest, and encourage side-lying position.
    - ▪ Promote diversional activities.
    - ▪ Have the client avoid foods that are high in sodium.
    - ▪ Have the client avoid alcohol and limit caffeine.
    - ▪ Instruct the client to increase her fluid intake to 8 glasses/day.
    - ▪ Maintain a dark quiet environment to avoid stimuli that may precipitate a seizure.
    - ▪ Maintain a patent airway in the event of a seizure.
    - ▪ Administer antihypertensive medications as prescribed.

APPLICATION EXERCISES

1. A nurse is caring for a client at 14 weeks of gestation who has hyperemesis gravidarum. The nurse is aware that which of the following are risk factors for the client? (Select all that apply.)

X____ A. Obesity

X____ B. Multifetal pregnancy

____ C. Maternal age greater than 40

X____ D. Migraine headache

____ E. Oligohydramnios

2. A nurse is administering magnesium sulfate IV to a client who has severe preeclampsia for seizure prophylaxis. Which of the following indicates magnesium sulfate toxicity? (Select all that apply.)

X____ A. Respirations fewer than 12/min

X____ B. Urinary output less than 30 mL/hr

____ C. Hyperreflexic deep-tendon reflexes

X____ D. Decreased level of consciousness

____ E. Flushing and sweating

3. A nursing is caring for a client who is receiving IV magnesium sulfate. Which of the following medications should the nurse anticipate administering if magnesium sulfate toxicity is suspected?

A. Nifedipine (Adalat)

B. Pyridoxine (vitamin B$_6$)

C. Ferrous sulfate

(D) Calcium gluconate

4. A nurse is reviewing a new prescription for ferrous sulfate with a client who is at 12 weeks of gestation. Which of the following statements by the client indicates understanding of the teaching?

A. "I will take this pill with my breakfast."

B. "I will take this medication with a glass of milk."

(C.) "I plan to drink more orange juice while taking this pill."

D. "I plan to add more calcium-rich foods to my diet while taking this medication."

5. A nurse is caring for a client who has suspected hyperemesis gravidarum and is reviewing the client's laboratory reports. Which of the following findings is a clinical manifestation of this condition?

   A. Hgb 12.2 g/dL

   B. Urine ketones present

   C. Alanine aminotransferase (ALT) 20 IU/L

   D. Serum glucose 114 mg/dL

6. A nurse is preparing to teach a client who is at 20 weeks of gestation and is to undergo a prophylactic cervical cerclage. What should be included in the teaching? Use the ATI Active Learning Template: Therapeutic Procedure to complete this item to include:

   A. Description of the Procedure

   B. Potential Complications: Identify two.

   C. Client Education: Describe at least four instructions to be given to the client.

APPLICATION EXERCISES KEY

1. A. **CORRECT:** Obesity is a risk factor for hyperemesis gravidarum.

    B. **CORRECT:** Multifetal pregnancy is a risk factor for hyperemesis gravidarum.

    C. INCORRECT: Maternal age less than 20 is a risk factor for hyperemesis gravidarum.

    D. **CORRECT:** Migraine headache is a risk factor for hyperemesis gravidarum.

    E. INCORRECT: Oligohydramnios is not a risk factor for hyperemesis gravidarum.

    ℕ NCLEX® Connection: Physiological Adaptations, Alterations in Body Systems

2. A. **CORRECT:** A respiratory rate of less than 12/min is a sign of magnesium sulfate toxicity.

    B. **CORRECT:** Urinary output of less than 30 mL/hr is a sign of magnesium sulfate toxicity.

    C. INCORRECT: The absence of patellar deep-tendon reflexes is a sign of magnesium sulfate toxicity.

    D. **CORRECT:** Decreased level of consciousness is a sign of magnesium sulfate toxicity.

    E. INCORRECT: Flushing and sweating are adverse effects of magnesium sulfate but are not signs of toxicity.

    ℕ NCLEX® Connection: Pharmacological and Parenteral Therapies, Adverse Effects/Contraindications/ Side Effects/Interactions

3. A. INCORRECT: Nifedipine is an antihypertensive medication that may be administered to women who have gestational hypertension.

    B. INCORRECT: Pyridoxine (vitamin B_6) is a vitamin supplement prescribed for clients who have hyperemesis gravidarum.

    C. INCORRECT: Ferrous sulfate is a medication used in the treatment of iron deficiency anemia.

    D. **CORRECT:** Calcium gluconate is the antidote for magnesium sulfate.

    ℕ NCLEX® Connection: Physiological Adaptations, Unexpected Response to Therapies

4. A. INCORRECT: Ferrous sulfate should be taken on an empty stomach.

    B. INCORRECT: Ferrous sulfate is not compatible with dairy products or juices and should be taken with water.

    C. **CORRECT:** A diet with increased vitamin C improves the absorption of ferrous sulfate.

    D. INCORRECT: Although a diet of calcium-rich foods is appropriate for the client during pregnancy, it does not improve the effectiveness of ferrous sulfate.

     NCLEX® Connection: Pharmacological and Parenteral Therapies, Medication Administration

5. A. INCORRECT: Altered hematocrit is a clinical manifestation of hyperemesis gravidarum due to the hemoconcentration that occurs with dehydration.

    B. **CORRECT:** The presence of ketones in the urine is associated with the breakdown of proteins and fats that occurs in a client who has hyperemesis gravidarum.

    C. INCORRECT: Liver enzymes are elevated in a client who has hyperemesis gravidarum, and this finding is within the expected reference range.

    D. INCORRECT: Decreased serum glucose is anticipated in a client who has hyperemesis gravidarum, and this result is within the expected reference range.

    NCLEX® Connection: Reduction of Risk Potential, Laboratory Values

6. *Using the ATI Active Learning Template: Therapeutic Procedure*

    A. Description of the Procedure

    • Surgical reinforcement of the cervix with a heavy ligature (suture) that is placed submucosally around the cervix to strength it and prevent premature cervical dilation.

    B. Potential Complications

    • Uterine contractions
    • Rupture of membranes
    • Infection

    C. Client Education

    • Remain on activity restrictions/bed rest as prescribed.
    • Increase hydration to promote a relaxed uterus.
    • Refrain from sexual intercourse.
    • Signs and symptoms to report to the provider: preterm labor, rupture of membranes, signs of infection, strong contractions less than 5 min apart, perineal pressure, and the urge to push.
    • Use of home uterine activity monitor.
    • Home health agency to follow up.
    • Plan for removal of the cerclage at 37 weeks of gestation.

    NCLEX® Connection: Reduction of Risk Potential, Therapeutic Procedures

chapter 10

Overview

- Understanding the importance of identifying the onset of early labor in a client who is pregnant is crucial for maternal and fetal well-being.
- Preterm labor, premature rupture of membranes, and preterm premature rupture of membranes is covered in this chapter.

PRETERM LABOR

Overview

- Preterm labor is defined as uterine contractions and cervical changes that occur between 20 and 37 weeks of gestation.
- It is important for a nurse to have a thorough understanding of the risk factors, assessment findings, and nursing interventions to care for the client who has preterm labor.

Risk Factors

- Infections of the urinary tract, vagina, or chorioamnionitis (infection of the amniotic sac)
- Previous preterm birth
- Multifetal pregnancy
- Hydramnios (excessive amniotic fluid)
- Age below 17 or above 35
- Low socioeconomic status
- Smoking
- Substance use
- Domestic violence
- History of multiple miscarriages or abortions
- Diabetes mellitus or hypertension
- Lack of prenatal care
- Recurrent premature dilation of the cervix
- Placenta previa or abruptio placentae
- Preterm premature rupture of membranes
- Short interval between pregnancies
- Uterine abnormalities

Assessment

- Subjective Data
  - Persistent low backache
  - Pressure in the pelvis and cramping
  - Gastrointestinal cramping, sometimes with diarrhea
  - Urinary frequency
  - Vaginal discharge
- Objective Data
  - Physical assessment findings
    - Increase, change, or blood in vaginal discharge
    - Change in cervical dilation
    - Regular uterine contractions with a frequency of every 10 min or greater, lasting 1 hr or longer
    - Premature rupture of membranes
  - Laboratory Tests
    - Fetal fibronectin
    - Cervical cultures
    - CBC
    - Urinalysis
  - Diagnostic Procedures
    - Obtain swab of vaginal secretions for fetal fibronectin between 24 and 34 weeks of gestation. This protein can be found in the vaginal secretions when the fetal membrane integrity is lost. This test is used to determine preterm labor.
    - Measure endocervical length with an ultrasound to assess for a shortened cervix, which is suggested in certain studies to precede preterm labor.
    - Use home uterine activity monitoring (HUAM), which is a uterine contraction monitor that can be used by the client at home. HUAM is not considered to be effective in preventing preterm labor.
    - Obtain cervical cultures to detect if there is a presence of infectious organisms. Culture and sensitivity results guide prescription of an appropriate antibiotic, if indicated.
    - Perform a biophysical profile and/or a nonstress test to provide information about the fetal well-being.

Patient-Centered Care

- Nursing Care
  - Management of a client who is in preterm labor includes focusing on stopping uterine contractions.

    - Activity restriction
      - Instruct the client on ways to modify her environment to allow for modified bed rest, yet have the ability to fulfill role responsibilities. Strict bed rest has been found to have adverse effects.
      - Encourage the client to rest in the left lateral position to increase blood flow to the uterus and decrease uterine activity.
      - Tell the client to avoid sexual intercourse.
    - Ensuring hydration
      - Dehydration stimulates the pituitary gland to secrete an antidiuretic hormone and oxytocin. Preventing dehydration prevents the release of oxytocin, which stimulates uterine contractions.
    - Identifying and treating an infection
      - Have the client report any vaginal discharge, noting color, consistency, and odor.
      - Monitor vital signs and temperature.
    - Chorioamnionitis should be suspected with the occurrence of elevated temperature and tachycardia.
    - Monitor FHR and contraction pattern.
      - Fetal tachycardia, a prolonged increase in the FHR greater than 160/min may indicate infection, which is frequently associated with preterm labor.
- Medications
  - Nifedipine (Procardia, Adalat)
    - Classification and Therapeutic Intent
      - Nifedipine is a calcium channel blocker that is used to suppress contractions by inhibiting calcium from entering smooth muscles.
    - Nursing Considerations
      - Monitor for headache, flushing, dizziness, and nausea. These usually are related to orthostatic hypotension that occurs with administration.
      - Should not be administered concurrent with magnesium sulfate.
    - Client Education
      - Instruct the client to slowly change positions from supine to upright and to sit until dizziness disappears.
      - Inform the client to maintain adequate hydration to counter hypotension.
  - Magnesium sulfate
    - Classification and Therapeutic Intent
      - Magnesium sulfate is a commonly used tocolytic that relaxes the smooth muscle of the uterus and thus inhibits uterine activity by suppressing contractions.
    - Nursing Considerations
      - Monitor the client closely. Tocolytic therapy should be discontinued immediately if the client exhibits manifestations of pulmonary edema, which includes chest pain, shortness of breath, respiratory distress, audible wheezing and crackles, and/or a productive cough containing blood-tinged sputum.
      - Monitor for adverse effects.

Q̲
S̲

- □ Monitor for magnesium sulfate toxicity, and discontinue for any of the following adverse effects: loss of deep tendon reflexes, urinary output less than 30 mL/hr, respiratory depression less than 12/min, pulmonary edema, and/or chest pain.
- □ Administer calcium gluconate as an antidote for magnesium sulfate toxicity.
- □ Contraindications for tocolysis include active vaginal bleeding, dilation of the cervix greater than 6 cm, chorioamnionitis, greater than 34 weeks of gestation, and acute fetal distress.

- ■ Client Education
  - □ Instruct the client to notify the nurse of blurred vision, headache, nausea, vomiting, or difficulty breathing.

- ○ Indomethacin (Indocin)
  - ■ Classification and Therapeutic Intent
    - □ Indomethacin is a nonsteroidal anti-inflammatory drug (NSAID) that suppresses preterm labor by blocking the production of prostaglandins. This inhibition of prostaglandins suppresses uterine contractions.
  - ■ Nursing Considerations
    - □ Monitor the client closely. Tocolytic therapy should be discontinued immediately if the client exhibits manifestations of pulmonary edema, which includes chest pain, shortness of breath, respiratory distress, audible wheezing and crackles, and/or a productive cough containing blood-tinged sputum.
    - □ Indomethacin treatment should not exceed 48 hr.
    - □ Indomethacin should only be used if gestational age is less than 32 weeks of gestation.
    - □ Monitor for postpartum hemorrhage related to reduced platelet aggregation.
    - □ Administer indomethacin with food or rectally to decrease gastrointestinal distress.
    - □ Notify the provider if the client reports blurred vision, headache, nausea, vomiting, or difficulty breathing.
    - □ Monitor the neonate at birth.

- ○ Betamethasone (Celestone)
  - ■ Classification and Therapeutic Intent
    - □ Betamethasone is a glucocorticoid that is administered IM in two injections, 24 hr apart, and requires a 24-hr period to be effective. The therapeutic action is to enhance fetal lung maturity and surfactant production.
  - ■ Nursing Considerations
    - □ Administer the medication deep into the gluteal muscle 24 and 48 hr prior to birth of a preterm neonate.
    - □ Monitor the client and neonate for pulmonary edema by assessing lung sounds.
    - □ Monitor for maternal and neonate hyperglycemia.
    - □ Monitor the neonate for heart rate changes.
  - ■ Client Education
    - □ Educate the client regarding signs of pulmonary edema (chest pain, shortness of breath, and crackles).

PREMATURE RUPTURE OF MEMBRANES
AND PRETERM PREMATURE RUPTURE OF MEMBRANES

Overview

- Premature rupture of membranes (PROM) is the spontaneous rupture of the amniotic membranes 1 hr or more prior to the onset of true labor. For most women, PROM signifies the onset of true labor if gestational duration is at term.

- Preterm premature rupture of membranes (PPROM) is the premature spontaneous rupture of membranes after 20 weeks of gestation and prior to 37 weeks of gestation.

Risk Factors

- Infection is the major risk of PROM and PPROM for both the client and the fetus. Once the amniotic membranes have ruptured, micro-organisms can ascend from the vagina into the amniotic sac. PPROM is often preceded by infection.

- Chorioamnionitis is an infection of the amniotic membranes.

  ○ There is an increased risk of infection if there is a lag period over the 24-hr period from when the membranes rupture to delivery.

Assessment

- Subjective Data

  ○ Client reports a gush or leakage of clear fluid from the vagina.

- Objective Data

  ○ Physical assessment findings

    ▪ Temperature elevation

    ▪ Increased maternal heart rate or FHR

    ▪ Foul-smelling fluid or vaginal discharge

    ▪ Abdominal tenderness

  ○ Assess for a prolapsed umbilical cord.

    ▪ Abrupt FHR variable or prolonged deceleration

    ▪ Visible or palpable cord at the introitus

- Laboratory Tests

  ○ A positive Nitrazine paper test (blue, pH 6.5 to 7.5) or positive ferning test is conducted on amniotic fluid to verify rupture of membranes.

Patient-Centered Care

- Nursing Care
  - Prepare for birth if indicated.
  - Nursing management for PROM and PPROM is dependent on gestational duration, if there is evidence of infection, or an indication of fetal or maternal compromise.
  - Obtain vaginal cultures for streptococcus ß-hemolytic, chlamydia, and *Neisseria gonorrhoeae*.
  - Avoid vaginal exams.
  - Provide reassurance to reduce anxiety.
  - Assess vital signs every 2 hr. Notify the provider of a temperature greater than 38° C (100° F).
  - Assess FHR and uterine contractions.
  - Advise the client to adhere to bed rest with bathroom privileges.
  - Encourage hydration.
  - Obtain a CBC.
  - Instruct the client to perform daily fetal kick counts and to notify the nurse of uterine contractions.
- Medications
  - Ampicillin (Omnipen)
    - Classification and Therapeutic Intent
      - Ampicillin is an antibiotic that is used to treat infection.
  - Nursing Care
    - Obtain vaginal, urine, and blood cultures prior to administration of antibiotic.
  - Betamethasone (Celestone)
    - Classification and Therapeutic Intent
      - Betamethasone is a glucocorticoid that is administered IM in 2 injections, 24 hr apart, and requires a 24-hr period to be effective. The therapeutic action is to enhance fetal lung maturity and surfactant production.
      - A single dose is given with PROM at 24 to 31 weeks of gestation to reduce the risk of perinatal mortality, respiratory distress syndrome, and other morbidities.
  - Nursing Considerations
    - Administer the medication deep into the gluteal muscle 24 and 48 hr prior to birth of a preterm neonate.
    - Monitor the client and neonate for pulmonary edema by assessing lung sounds.
    - Monitor for maternal and neonate hyperglycemia.
    - Monitor the neonate for heart rate changes.
  - Client Education
    - Educate the client regarding signs of pulmonary edema (chest pain, shortness of breath, and crackles).

- Health Promotion and Disease Prevention
  - Discharge Instructions
    - Expect that the client will be discharged home if dilation is less than 3 cm, no evidence of infection, no contractions, and no malpresentation.
    - Advise the client to adhere to limited activity with bathroom privileges.
    - Encourage hydration.
  - Client Education for PROM and PPROM
    - The client should conduct a self-assessment for uterine contractions.
    - The client should record daily kick counts for fetal movement.
    - The client should monitor for foul-smelling vaginal discharge.
      - Refrain from inserting anything into the vagina.
    - The client should abstain from intercourse.
    - The client should avoid tub baths.
    - The client should wipe her perineal area from front to back after voiding and fecal elimination.
    - The client should take her temperature every 4 hr when awake and report a temperature that is greater than 38° C (100° F).

APPLICATION EXERCISES

1. A nurse is preparing to administer betamethasone acetate and betamethasone sodium phosphate (Celestone Soluspan) 6 mg IM to a client who will undergo a cesarean birth due to premature rupture of membranes. Available is betamethasone acetate 3 mg and betamethasone sodium phosphate 3 mg suspension per mL. How many mL should the nurse administer? (Round the answer to the nearest whole number.)

_____2_____ mL $\frac{6}{3} \times 1$

2. A nurse in labor and delivery is providing care for a client who is in preterm labor at 32 weeks of gestation. Which of the following medications should the nurse anticipate the provider will prescribe to hasten fetal lung maturity?

    A. Calcium gluconate

    B. Indomethacin (Indocin)

    C. Nifedipine (Procardia)

    D. Betamethasone (Celestone)

3. A nurse is caring for a client who is receiving nifedipine (Procardia) for prevention of preterm labor. The nurse should monitor the client for which of the following clinical manifestations?

    A. Blood-tinged sputum

    B. Dizziness

    C. Pallor

    D. Somnolence

4. A nurse is caring for a client who has a prescription for magnesium sulfate. The nurse should recognize that which of the following are contraindications for use of this medication. (Select all that apply.)

_____X_____ A. Acute fetal distress

_____ B. Preterm labor

_____X_____ C. Vaginal bleeding

_____X_____ D. Cervical dilation greater than 6 cm

_____ E. Severe gestational hypertension

5. A nurse is reviewing discharge teaching with a client who has premature rupture of membranes at 26 weeks of gestation. Which of the following should be included in the teaching?

    A. Use a condom with sexual intercourse.

    B. Avoid bubble bath solution when taking a tub bath.

    C. Wipe from the back to front when performing perineal hygiene.

    D. Keep a daily record of fetal kick counts.

6. A nurse in a prenatal clinic is reviewing preterm labor with a newly hired nurse. What should the nurse include in the discussion? Use the ATI Active Learning Template: Systems Disorder to complete this item to include the following:

    A. Description of the disorder.

    B. Subjective data: Describe at least three manifestations.

    C. Objective data: Describe at least three manifestations.

    D. Diagnostic procedures: Describe at least three.

APPLICATION EXERCISES KEY

1. **2** mL

Using Ratio and Proportion

STEP 1: *What is the unit of measurement to calculate?*
mL

STEP 2: *What is the dose needed? Dose needed = Desired*
6 mg

STEP 3: *What is the dose available? Dose available = Have*
3 mg

STEP 4: *Should the nurse convert the units of measurement?*
No

STEP 5: *What is the quantity of the dose available?*
1 mL

STEP 6: *Set up an equation and solve for X.*

$$\frac{\text{Have}}{\text{Quantity}} = \frac{\text{Desired}}{X}$$

$$\frac{3\ \text{mg}}{1\ \text{mL}} = \frac{6\ \text{mg}}{X\ \text{mL}}$$

X = 2

STEP 7: *Round if necessary.*

STEP 8: *Reassess to determine whether the amount to give makes sense.*
If there is 3 mg/mL and the prescribed amount is 6 mg, it makes sense to give 2 mL. The nurse should administer betamethasone acetate/ betamethasone sodium phosphate suspension 2 mL IM.

Using Desired Over Have

STEP 1: *What is the unit of measurement to calculate?*
mL

STEP 2: *What is the dose needed? Dose needed = Desired*
6 mg

STEP 3: *What is the dose available? Dose available = Have*
3 mg

STEP 4: *Should the nurse convert the units of measurement?*
No

STEP 5: *What is the quantity of the dose available?*
1 mL

STEP 6: *Set up an equation and solve for X.*

$$\frac{\text{Desired} \times \text{Quantity}}{\text{Have}} = X$$

$$\frac{6\ \text{mg} \times 1\ \text{mL}}{3\ \text{mg}} = X\ \text{mL}$$

X = 2

STEP 7: *Round if necessary.*

STEP 8: *Reassess to determine whether the amount to give makes sense.*
If there is 3 mg/mL and the prescribed amount is 6 mg, it makes sense to give 2 mL. The nurse should administer betamethasone acetate/ betamethasone sodium phosphate suspension 2 mL IM.

Using Dimensional Analysis

STEP 1: *What is the unit of measurement to calculate?*
mL

STEP 2: *What quantity of the dose is available?*
1 mL

STEP 3: *What is the dose available? Dose available = Have*
3 mg

STEP 4: *What is the dose needed? Dose needed = Desired*
6 mg

STEP 5: *Should the nurse convert the units of measurement?*
No

STEP 6: *Set up an equation of factors and solve for X.*

$$X = \frac{\text{Quantity}}{\text{Have}} \times \frac{\text{Conversion (Have)}}{\text{Conversion (Desired)}} \times \frac{\text{Desired}}{}$$

$$X\ \text{mL} = \frac{1\ \text{mL}}{3\ \text{mg}} \times \frac{6\ \text{mg}}{}$$

X = 2

STEP 7: *Round if necessary.*

STEP 8: *Reassess to determine whether the amount to give makes sense.*
If there is 3 mg/mL and the prescribed amount is 6 mg, it makes sense to give 2 mL. The nurse should administer betamethasone acetate/ betamethasone sodium phosphate suspension 2 mL IM.

Ⓝ NCLEX® Connection: Pharmacological and Parenteral Therapies, Dosage Calculation

2. A. INCORRECT: Calcium gluconate is administered as an antidote for magnesium sulfate toxicity.

    B. INCORRECT: Indomethacin is an NSAID used to suppress preterm labor by blocking prostaglandin production.

    C. INCORRECT: Nifedipine is a calcium channel blocker used to suppress uterine contractions.

    D. **CORRECT:** Betamethasone is a glucocorticoid that is given to clients in preterm labor to hasten surfactant production.

     NCLEX® Connection: Physiological Adaptations, Illness Management

3. A. INCORRECT: Blood-tinged sputum production is an adverse affect associated with indomethacin (Indocin).

    B. **CORRECT:** Dizziness and lightheadedness are associated with orthostatic hypotension, which occurs when taking nifedipine.

    C. INCORRECT: Facial flushing and heat sensation are adverse effects associated with nifedipine.

    D. INCORRECT: Nervousness, jitteriness, and sleep disturbances are adverse effects associated with nifedipine.

     NCLEX® Connection: Reduction of Risk Potential, Potential for Complications of Diagnostic Tests/ Treatments/Procedures

4. A. **CORRECT:** Acute fetal distress is a complication that is a contraindication for the use of magnesium sulfate therapy.

    B. INCORRECT: Preterm labor is an indication for the use of magnesium sulfate.

    C. **CORRECT:** Vaginal bleeding is a complication that is a contraindication for magnesium sulfate therapy.

    D. **CORRECT:** Cervical dilation greater than 6 cm is a complication that is a contraindication for magnesium sulfate therapy.

    E. INCORRECT: Severe gestational hypertension is an indiction for the use of magnesium sulfate.

     NCLEX® Connection: Pharmacological and Parenteral Therapies, Adverse Effects/Contraindications/ Side Effects/Interactions

5. A. INCORRECT: The client who has ruptured membranes should not insert anything into her vagina.

    B. INCORRECT: Showers should be taken, and tub baths should be avoided.

    C. INCORRECT: The client should be instructed that this is incorrect technique when performing perineal hygiene.

    D. **CORRECT:** The client should record daily fetal kick counts.

    (N) NCLEX® Connection: Health Promotion and Maintenance, Ante/Intra/Postpartum and Newborn Care

6. *Using the ATI Active Learning Template: Systems Disorder*

    A. Description of the Disorder
       • Uterine contractions and cervical changes that occur between 20 and 37 weeks of gestation.

    B. Subjective Data
       • Persistent low backache
       • Pressure in the pelvis and cramping
       • Gastrointestinal cramping, sometimes with diarrhea
       • Urinary frequency
       • Vaginal discharge

    C. Objective Data
       • Increase, change, or blood in vaginal discharge
       • Change in cervical dilation
       • Regular uterine contractions with a frequency of every 10 min or greater, lasting 1 hr or longer
       • Premature rupture of membranes

    D. Diagnostic Procedures
       • Test for fetal fibronectin
       • Ultrasound to measure endocervical length
       • Cervical culture to detect presence of infectious organisms
       • Biophysical profile
       • Nonstress test
       • Home uterine activity monitoring for uterine contractions

    (N) NCLEX® Connection: Health Promotion and Maintenance, Ante/Intra/Postpartum and Newborn Care

UNIT 2   Intrapartum Nursing Care

SECTIONS

› Labor and Delivery
› Complications of Labor and Delivery

NCLEX® CONNECTIONS

When reviewing the chapters in this unit, keep in mind the relevant sections of the NCLEX® outline, in particular:

Client Needs: Health Promotion and Maintenance

› Relevant topics/tasks include:
  » Ante/Intra/Postpartum and Newborn Care
    › Provide care to client in labor.

Client Needs: Physiological Adaptation

› Relevant topics/tasks include:
  » Alterations in Body Systems
    › Provide care for the client experiencing complications of pregnancy/labor and/or delivery.

Client Needs: Pharmacological and Parenteral Therapies

› Relevant topics/tasks include:
  » Adverse Effects/Contraindications/Side Effects/ Interactions
    › Identify contraindications to the administration of a medication to the client.
  » Dosage Calculation
    › Use clinical decision making/critical thinking when calculating dosages.
  » Medication Administration
    › Educate the client about medications.

Client Needs: Reduction of Risk Potential

› Relevant topics/tasks include:
  » Potential for Complications of Diagnostic Tests/ Treatments/Procedures
    › Evaluate responses to procedures and treatments.
  » Therapeutic Procedures
    › Assess the client's response to recovery from local, regional, or general anesthesia.

chapter 11

Overview

- An intrapartum nurse should care for three clients during each labor and delivery:
  - Fetus
  - Mother
  - Family unit
- Physiologic changes preceding labor (premonitory signs)
  - Backache – a constant low, dull backache, caused by pelvic muscle relaxation
  - Weight loss – a 0.5 to 1.4 kg (1 to 3 lb) weight loss
  - Lightening – fetal head descends into true pelvis about 14 days before labor; feeling that the fetus has "dropped;" easier breathing, but more pressure on bladder, resulting in urinary frequency; more pronounced in clients who are primigravida
  - Contractions – begin with irregular uterine contractions (Braxton Hicks) that eventually progress in strength and regularity
  - Bloody show – brownish or blood-tinged mucus discharge caused by expulsion of the cervical mucus plug resulting from the onset of cervical dilation and effacement
  - Energy burst – sometimes called "nesting" response
  - Gastrointestinal changes – less common, include nausea, vomiting, and indigestion
  - Rupture of membranes – spontaneous rupture of membranes can initiate labor or can occur anytime during labor, most commonly during the transition phase.
    - Labor usually occurs within 24 hr of the rupture of membranes.
    - Prolonged rupture of membranes greater than 24 hr before delivery of fetus may lead to an infection.
    - Immediately following the rupture of membranes, a nurse should assess the FHR for abrupt decelerations, which are indicative of fetal distress to rule out umbilical cord prolapse.
  - Assessment of amniotic fluid – completed once the membranes rupture
    - Should be watery, clear, and pale- to straw-yellow in color.
    - Odor should not be foul.
    - Volume is between 500 and 1,200 mL.
    - Nitrazine paper should be used by a nurse to confirm that amniotic fluid is present.
      - Amniotic fluid is alkaline: Nitrazine paper should be deep blue, indicating pH of 6.5 to 7.5. Urine is slightly acidic: Nitrazine paper remains yellow.
- An intrapartum nurse should collect assessment data on maternal and fetal well-being during labor, the progress of labor, and psychosocial and cultural factors that affect labor.

- There are five factors (the five "P's") that affect and define the labor and birth process: passenger, passageway, powers, position, and psychologic response.
  - Passenger – consists of the fetus and the placenta. The size of the fetal head, fetal presentation, lie, attitude, and position affect the ability of the fetus to navigate the birth canal. The placenta can be considered a passenger because it also must pass through the canal.
    - Presentation – the part of the fetus that is entering the pelvic inlet first. It can be the back of the head (occiput), chin (mentum), shoulder (scapula), or breech (sacrum or feet).
    - Lie – the relationship of the maternal longitudinal axis (spine) to the fetal longitudinal axis (spine).
      - Transverse – fetal long axis is horizontal and forms a right angle to maternal axis and will not accommodate vaginal birth. The shoulder is the presenting part and may require delivery by cesarean birth if the fetus does not rotate spontaneously.
      - Parallel or longitudinal – fetal long axis is parallel to maternal long axis, either a cephalic or breech presentation. Breech presentation may require a cesarean birth.
    - Attitude – relationship of fetal body parts to one another.
      - Fetal flexion – chin flexed to chest, extremities flexed into torso.
      - Fetal extension – chin extended away from chest, extremities extended.
    - Fetopelvic or fetal position – the relationship of the presenting part of the fetus (sacrum, mentum, or occiput), preferably the occiput, in reference to its directional position as it relates to one of the four maternal pelvic quadrants. It is labeled with three letters.
      - The first letter references either the right (R) or left (L) side of the maternal pelvis.
      - The second letter references the presenting part of the fetus, either occiput (O), sacrum (S), mentum (M), or scapula (Sc).
      - The third letter references either the anterior (A), posterior (P), or transverse (T) part of the maternal pelvis.
      - Station – measurement of fetal descent in centimeters with station 0 being at the level of an imaginary line at the level of the ischial spines, minus stations superior to the ischial spines, and plus stations inferior to the ischial spines.
  - Passageway – the birth canal that is composed of the bony pelvis, cervix, pelvic floor, vagina, and introitus (vaginal opening). The size and shape of the bony pelvis must be adequate to allow the fetus to pass through it. The cervix must dilate and efface in response to contractions and fetal descent.
  - Powers – uterine contractions cause effacement and dilation of the cervix and descent of the fetus. Involuntary urge to push and voluntary bearing down in the second stage of labor helps in the expulsion of the fetus.
  - Position – of the woman who is in labor. The client should engage in frequent position changes during labor to increase comfort, relieve fatigue, and promote circulation. Position during the second stage is determined by maternal preference, provider preference, and the condition of the mother and the fetus.
    - Gravity can aid in the fetal descent in upright, sitting, kneeling, and squatting positions.
  - Psychological response – maternal stress, tension, and anxiety can produce physiological changes that impair the progress of labor.

Nursing Interventions

- Preprocedure for Labor and Birth Process
  - ○ Nursing Actions
    - Leopold maneuvers – abdominal palpation of the number of fetuses, the fetal presenting part, lie, attitude, descent, and the probable location where fetal heart tones may be best auscultated on the woman's abdomen.
    - External electronic monitoring (tocotransducer) – separate transducer applied to the maternal abdomen over the fundus that measures uterine activity.
      - □ Displays uterine contraction patterns
      - □ Easily applied by the nurse but must be repositioned with maternal movement to ensure proper placement
    - External fetal monitoring (EFM) – transducer applied to the abdomen of the client to assess FHR patterns during labor and birth.
  - ○ Laboratory Analysis
    - Group B streptococcus – culture is obtained if results are not available from screening at 36 to 37 weeks.
      - □ If positive, intravenous prophylactic antibiotic is prescribed (exceptions are planned cesarean birth and membranes intact).
    - Urinalysis – clean-catch urine sample obtained to ascertain maternal:
      - □ Hydration status via specific gravity
      - □ Nutritional status via ketones
      - □ Proteinuria, which is indicative of gestational hypertension
      - □ Urinary tract infection via bacterial count
    - Blood Tests
      - □ Hct level
      - □ ABO typing and Rh-factor if not previously done
  - ○ Client Education
    - Provide the client and the client's partner with ongoing education regarding the labor and delivery process and procedures.
- Intraprocedure for Labor and Birth Process
  - ○ Nursing Actions
    - Assess maternal vital signs per agency protocol.
      - □ Check maternal temperature every 1 to 2 hr if membranes are ruptured.
    - Assess FHR to determine fetal well-being. This may be performed by use of EFM or spiral electrode that is applied to the fetal scalp.
      - □ Prior to electrode placement, cervical dilation and rupture of membranes must occur.
    - Assess uterine labor contraction characteristics by palpation (placing a hand over the fundus to assess contraction frequency, duration, and intensity) or by the use of external or internal monitoring.
      - □ Frequency – established from the beginning of one contraction to the beginning of the next.
      - □ Duration – the time between the beginning of a contraction to the end of that same contraction.

□ Intensity – strength of the contraction at its peak described as mild, moderate, or strong.

        □ Resting tone of uterine contractions – tone of the uterine muscle in between contractions.

            ► A prolonged contraction duration (greater than 90 seconds) or too frequent contractions (more than five in a 10-min period) without sufficient time for uterine relaxation (less than 30 seconds) in between can reduce blood flow to the placenta. This can result in fetal hypoxia and decreased FHR.

 View Image: Contraction Pattern

- Insert a solid, sterile, water-filled intrauterine pressure catheter inside the uterus to measure intrauterine pressure.

    □ Displays uterine contraction patterns on monitor.

    □ Requires the membranes to be ruptured and the cervix to be sufficiently dilated.

- Vaginal examination – performed digitally by the provider or qualified nurse to assess for the following:

    □ Cervical dilation (stretching of cervical os adequate to allow fetal passage) and effacement (cervical thinning and shortening)

    □ Descent of the fetus through the birth canal as measured by fetal station in centimeters

    □ Fetal position, presenting part, and lie

    □ Membranes that are intact or ruptured

CHARACTERISTICS OF TRUE VS. FALSE LABOR (BRAXTON HICKS CONTRACTIONS) TRUE LABOR LEADS TO CERVICAL DILATION AND EFFACEMENT	
True Labor	False Labor
› Contractions	› Contractions
» May begin irregularly, but become regular in frequency	» Painless, irregular frequency, and intermittent
» Stronger, last longer, and are more frequent	» Decrease in frequency, duration, and intensity with walking or position changes
» Felt in lower back, radiating to abdomen	» Felt in lower back or abdomen above umbilicus
» Walking can increase contraction intensity	» Often stop with sleep or comfort measures such as oral hydration or emptying of the bladder
» Continue despite comfort measures	› Cervix (assessed by vaginal exam)
› Cervix (assessed by vaginal exam)	» No significant change in dilation or effacement
» Progressive change in dilation and effacement	» Often remains in posterior position
» Moves to anterior position	» No significant bloody show
» Bloody show	› Fetus
› Fetus	» Presenting part is not engaged in pelvis
» Presenting part engages in pelvis	

- Mechanism of labor – the adaptations the fetus makes as it progresses through the birth canal during the birthing process.

  □ Engagement – occurs when the presenting part, usually biparietal (largest) diameter of the fetal head passes the pelvic inlet at the level of the ischial spines. Referred to as station 0.

  □ Descent – the progress of the presenting part (preferably the occiput) through the pelvis. Measured by station during a vaginal examination as either negative (-) station measured in centimeters if superior to station 0 and not yet engaged, or positive (+) station measured in centimeters if inferior to station 0.

  □ Flexion – when the fetal head meets resistance of the cervix, pelvic wall, or pelvic floor. The head flexes, bringing the chin close to the chest, presenting a smaller diameter to pass through the pelvis.

  □ Internal rotation – the fetal occiput ideally rotates to a lateral anterior position as it progresses from the ischial spines to the lower pelvis in a corkscrew motion to pass through the pelvis.

  □ Extension – the fetal occiput passes under the symphysis pubis, and then the head is deflected anteriorly and is born by extension of the chin away from the fetal chest.

  □ Restitution and external rotation – after the head is born, it rotates to the position it occupied as it entered the pelvic inlet (restitution) in alignment with the fetal body and completes a quarter turn to face transverse as the anterior shoulder passes under the symphysis.

  □ Expulsion – after birth of the head and shoulders, the trunk of the neonate is born by flexing it toward the symphysis pubis.

STAGES OF LABOR			
DURATION	BEGINS WITH	ENDS WITH	MATERNAL CHARACTERISTICS
FIRST STAGE			
› 12.5 hr	› Onset of labor	› Complete dilation	› Cervical dilation 1 cm/hr for clients who are primigravida, and 1.5 cm/hr for clients who are multigravida, on average
Latent Phase			
› Primigravida: 6 hr › Multigravida: 4 hr	› Cervix 0 cm › Irregular, mild to moderate contractions › Frequency 5 to 30 min › Duration 30 to 45 seconds	› Cervix 3 cm	› Some dilation and effacement › Talkative and eager
Active Phase			
› Primigravida: 3 hr › Multigravida: 2 hr	› Cervix 4 cm › More regular, moderate to strong contractions › Frequency 3 to 5 min › Duration 40 to 70 seconds	› Cervix 7 cm dilated	› Rapid dilation and effacement › Some fetal descent › Feelings of helplessness › Anxiety and restlessness increase as contractions become stronger
Transition			
› 20 to 40 min	› Cervix 8 cm › Strong to very strong contractions › Frequency 2 to 3 min › Duration 45 to 90 seconds	› Complete dilation at 10 cm	› Tired, restless, and irritable › Feeling out of control, client often states, "cannot continue" › May have nausea and vomiting › Urge to push › Increased rectal pressure and feelings of needing to have a bowel movement › Increased bloody show › Most difficult part of labor
SECOND STAGE			
› Primigravida: 30 min to 2 hr › Multigravida: 5 to 30 min	› Full dilation › Progresses to intense contractions every 1 to 2 min	› Birth	› Pushing results in birth of fetus
THIRD STAGE			
› 5 to 30 min	› Delivery of the neonate	› Delivery of placenta	› Placental separation and expulsion › Schultze presentation: shiny fetal surface of placenta emerges first › Duncan presentation: dull maternal surface of placenta emerges first
FOURTH STAGE			
› 1 to 4 hr	› Delivery of placenta	› Maternal stabilization of vital signs	› Achievement of vital sign homeostasis › Lochia scant to moderate rubra

M

View Media

› Stages of Labor (Video)   › Schultze and Dirty Duncan Placenta (Images)

- Postprocedure for Labor and Delivery Process
  - Nursing Assessments During the Fourth Stage
    - Maternal vital signs
    - Fundus
    - Lochia
    - Perineum
    - Urinary output
    - Maternal/newborn baby-friendly activities
  - Nursing Interventions During the Fourth Stage
    - Assess maternal vital signs every 15 min for the first hour and then according to facility protocol.
    - Assess fundus and lochia every 15 min for the first hour and then according to facility protocol.
    - Massage the uterine fundus and/or administer oxytocics as prescribed to maintain uterine tone to prevent hemorrhage.
    - Assess the client's perineum, and provide comfort measures as indicated.
    - Encourage voiding to prevent bladder distention.
    - Promote an opportunity for maternal/newborn bonding.
  - Client Education
    - Instruct the client to notify the nurse of increased vaginal bleeding or passage of blood clots. Offer assistance with breastfeeding, and provide reassurance.

APPLICATION EXERCISES

1. A nurse in the labor and delivery unit receives a phone call from a client who reports that her contractions started about 2 hr ago, did not go away when she had two glasses of water and rested, and became stronger since she started walking. Her contractions occur every 10 min and last about 30 seconds. She hasn't had any fluid leak from her vagina. However, she saw some blood when she wiped after voiding. Based on this report, the nurse should recognize that the client is experiencing

   A. Braxton Hicks contractions.

   B. rupture of membranes.

   C. fetal descent.

   D. true contractions.

2. A nurse in the labor and delivery unit is caring for a client in labor and applies an external fetal monitor and tocotransducer. The FHR is around 140/min. Contractions are every 8 min and 30 to 40 seconds in duration. The nurse performs a vaginal exam and finds the cervix is 2 cm dilated, 50% effaced, and the fetus is at a -2 station. Which of the following stages and phases of labor is this client experiencing?

   A. The first stage, latent phase

   B. The first stage, active phase

   C. The first stage, transition phase

   D. The second stage of labor

3. A client experiences a large gush of fluid from her vagina while walking in the hallway of the birthing unit. The nurse's first nursing action after establishing that the fluid is amniotic fluid should be to

   A. assess the amniotic fluid for meconium.

   B. monitor the FHR for distress.

   C. dry the client and make her comfortable.

   D. monitor the client's uterine contractions.

4. A nurse in labor and delivery is completing an admission history for a client who is at 39 weeks of gestation. The client reports that she has been leaking fluid from her vagina for 2 days. The nurse knows that this client is at risk for

   A. cord prolapse.

   B. infection.

   C. postpartum hemorrhage.

   D. hydramnios.

5. A nurse is caring for a client who is in active labor and becomes nauseous and vomits. The client is very irritable and feels the urge to have a bowel movement. She states, "I've had enough. I can't do this anymore. I want to go home right now." The nurse knows that these signs indicate the client is in the

    A. second stage of labor.

    B. fourth stage of labor.

    C. transition phase of labor.

    D. latent phase of labor.

6. The manager of a labor and delivery unit is reviewing the procedure for vaginal examination with a group of newly hired nurses. Which of the following interventions should be included in this discussion? Use the ATI Active Learning Template: Therapeutic Procedure to complete this item to include the following:

    A. Nursing Actions: Describe four actions that are preprocedure, intraprocedure, and postprocedure.

    B. Describe three assessment findings that can be determined by the procedure.

APPLICATION EXERCISES KEY

1. A. INCORRECT: Braxton Hicks contractions decrease with hydration and walking.

    B. INCORRECT: Rupture of membranes would be indicated by the presence of a gush of fluid that is unrelated to the client's activity.

    C. INCORRECT: Fetal descent is the downward movement of the fetus in the birth canal and cannot be evaluated based on the client's report.

    D. **CORRECT:** True contractions do not go away with hydration or walking. They are regular in frequency, duration, and intensity and become stronger with walking.

    Ⓝ NCLEX® Connection: Health Promotion and Maintenance, Ante/Intra/Postpartum and Newborn Care

2. A. **CORRECT:** In stage 1, latent phase, the cervix dilates from 0 to 3 cm, and contraction duration ranges from 30 to 45 seconds.

    B. INCORRECT: In stage 1, active phase, the cervix dilates from 4 to 7 cm, and contraction duration ranges from 40 to 70 seconds.

    C. INCORRECT: In stage 1, transition phase, the cervix dilates from 8 to 10 cm, and contraction duration ranges from 45 to 90 seconds.

    D. INCORRECT: The second stage of labor consists of the expulsion of the fetus.

    Ⓝ NCLEX® Connection: Health Promotion and Maintenance, Ante/Intra/Postpartum and Newborn Care

3. A. INCORRECT: The nurse assesses the color, clarity, odor, and amount of amniotic fluid, but this is not the first action the nurse should take.

    B. **CORRECT:** The greatest risk to the client and fetus is umbilical cord prolapse, leading to fetal distress following rupture of membranes. Therefore, the first action by the nurse is to monitor the FHR for signs of distress.

    C. INCORRECT: The nurse should provide comfort by drying the client following rupture of the membranes, but this is not the first action the nurse should take.

    D. INCORRECT: The nurse monitors the client's uterine contraction pattern after rupture of the membranes, but this is not the first action the nurse should take.

    Ⓝ NCLEX® Connection: Health Promotion and Maintenance, Ante/Intra/Postpartum and Newborn Care

4. A. INCORRECT: Although cord prolapse is a risk with rupture of membranes, it occurs when the fluid rushes out, rather than trickling or leaking out.

    B. **CORRECT:** Rupture of membranes for longer than 24 hr prior to delivery increases the risk that infectious organisms will enter the vagina and then eventually into the uterus.

    C. INCORRECT: The risk for postpartum hemorrhage by this client is not any greater than other clients who are pregnant.

    D. INCORRECT: This client is more likely to have oligohydramnios or insufficient amniotic fluid, rather than hydramnios, or excess amniotic fluid.

     NCLEX® Connection: Health Promotion and Maintenance, Ante/Intra/Postpartum and Newborn Care

5. A. INCORRECT: The second stage of labor occurs with the expulsion of the fetus.

    B. INCORRECT: The fourth stage of labor is the recovery period, following the delivery of the placenta.

    C. **CORRECT:** The transition phase of labor occurs when the client becomes irritable, feels rectal pressure similar to the need to have a bowel movement, and can become nauseous with emesis.

    D. INCORRECT: The latent phase of labor occurs in stage one, and coincides with mild contractions. The client is more relaxed, talkative, and eager for labor to progress.

     NCLEX® Connection: Health Promotion and Maintenance, Ante/Intra/Postpartum and Newborn Care

6. *Using the ATI Active Learning Template: Therapeutic Procedure*

    A. Nursing Actions
    - Explain procedure, and obtain client's permission for the examination.
    - Don sterile glove with antiseptic solution or soluble gel for lubrication.
    - Position the client to avoid supine hypotension.
    - Provide for privacy.
    - Cleanse the vulva or perineum if needed.
    - Insert index and middle finger into the client's vagina.
    - Explain findings to the client.
    - Document findings, and report to the provider.

    B. Assessment Findings
    - Cervical dilation, effacement, and position
    - Fetal presenting part, position, and station
    - Status of membranes
    - Characteristics of amniotic fluid if membranes ruptured

     NCLEX® Connection: Health Promotion and Maintenance, Ante/Intra/Postpartum and Newborn Care

chapter 12

Overview

- Pain is a subjective and individual experience, and each client's response to the pain of labor is unique.
- Sources of pain during the stages of labor
  - First stage – internal visceral pain that may be felt as back and leg pain, which is caused by
    - Dilation, effacement, and stretching of the cervix
    - Distention of the lower segment of the uterus
    - Contractions of the uterus with resultant uterine ischemia
  - Second stage – pain that is somatic and occurs with fetal descent and expulsion. Pain is caused by
    - Pressure and distention of the vagina and the perineum, described by the client as "burning, splitting, and tearing"
    - Pressure and pulling on the pelvic structures (ligaments, fallopian tubes, ovaries, bladder, and peritoneum)
    - Lacerations of soft tissues (cervix, vagina, and perineum)
  - Third stage – pain with the expulsion of the placenta is similar to the pain experienced during the first stage. Pain is caused by
    - Uterine contractions
    - Pressure and pulling of pelvic structures
  - Fourth stage – pain is caused by
    - Distention and stretching of the vagina and perineum incurred during the second stage with a splitting, burning, and tearing sensation
- Safety for the mother and fetus must be the first consideration of the nurse when planning pain management measures.

Pain Assessment

- Pain level cannot always be assessed by monitoring the outward expressions of a client. Client pain assessment may require persistent questioning and astute observation by the nurse. Cultural beliefs and behaviors of women during labor and delivery can affect the client's pain management.
  - Anxiety
    - Anxiety and fear are associated with pain. As fear and anxiety increase, muscle tension increases, and thus the experience of pain increases, becoming a cycle of pain. The fear, tension, and pain cycle is illustrated below.
      - Fear
      - Fatigue
      - Full bladder

◻ Individual pain tolerance

◻ Previous experiences with pain

◻ Fetal malposition

◻ Cephalopelvic disproportion

◻ Childbirth preparation

◻ Level of support during labor

- Assess the beliefs and expectations related to discomfort, pain relief, and birth plans regarding pain relief methods of the client who is in labor.

- Assess the client's level, quality, frequency, duration, intensity, and location of pain through verbal and nonverbal cues. Use an appropriate pain scale allowing the client to indicate the severity of her pain on a scale of 0 to 10, with 10 representing the most severe pain.

  ○ Indications of pain

    ▪ Behavioral manifestations such as crying, moaning, screaming, gesturing, writhing, avoidance or withdrawal, and inability to follow instructions

    ▪ Increasing blood pressure, tachycardia, and hyperventilation

- A nurse is responsible for helping the client maintain the proper position during administration of pharmacological interventions. The nurse is also responsible for assisting the client with positioning for comfort during labor and birth, and following pharmacological interventions.

- A nurse should provide client safety after any pharmacological intervention by putting the bed in a low position, maintaining side rails in the up position, placing the call light within the client's reach, and advising the client and her partner to call for assistance if she needs to leave the bed or ambulate.

- Evaluate the client's response to pain relief methods used (verbal report that pain is relieved or being relieved, appears relaxed between contractions).

TIMING AND EFFECTIVENESS OF PAIN RELIEF MEASURES DURING LABOR				
First Stage (Latent Phase)	First Stage (Active Phase)	Transition	Second Stage	Third Stage
Nonpharmacological methods ⟶				
Sedatives			Spinal block ⟶	
	Opioids			
	Epidural ⟶			
			Pudendal ⟶	
			Local infiltration ⟶	

Nonpharmacological Pain Management

- Nonpharmacological pain management measures reduce anxiety, fear, and tension, which are major contributing factors to pain in labor.

  ○ Gate-control theory of pain is based on the concept that the sensory nerve pathways that pain sensations use to travel to the brain will allow only a limited number of sensations to travel at any given time. By sending alternate signals through these pathways, the pain signals can be blocked from ascending the neurological pathway and inhibit the brain's perception and sensation of pain.

  ○ The gate-control theory of pain assists in the understanding of how nonpharmacological pain techniques can work to relieve pain.

- Interventions for nonpharmacological pain management

  ○ Childbirth preparation education, sensory and cutaneous strategies, and frequent maternal position changes

    ■ Childbirth preparation methods such as Lamaze and/or patterned breathing exercises are used to promote relaxation and pain management.

      □ Nursing implications include assessing for signs of hyperventilation (caused by low blood levels of PCO_2 from blowing off too much CO_2) such as light-headedness and tingling of the fingers. If this occurs, have the client breathe into a paper bag or her cupped hands.

    ■ Sensory stimulation strategies (based on the gate-control theory) to promote relaxation and pain relief

      □ Aromatherapy

      □ Breathing techniques

      □ Imagery

      □ Music

      □ Use of focal points

      □ Subdued lighting

    ■ Cutaneous strategies (based on the gate-control theory) to promote relaxation and pain relief

      □ Back rubs and massage

      □ Effleurage

        ▸ Light, gentle circular stroking of the client's abdomen with the fingertips in rhythm with breathing during contractions

      □ Sacral counterpressure

        ▸ Consistent pressure is applied by the support person using the heel of the hand or fist against the client's sacral area to counteract pain in the lower back

      □ Heat or cold therapy

      □ Hydrotherapy (whirlpool or shower) increases maternal endorphin levels

      □ Acupressure

- Frequent maternal position changes to promote relaxation and pain relief
  - □ Semi-sitting
  - □ Squatting
  - □ Kneeling
  - □ Kneeling and rocking back and forth
  - □ Supine position only with the placement of a wedge under one of the client's hips to tilt the uterus and avoid supine hypotension syndrome
  - ○ Client Education
    - Teach the client who is in labor about techniques to promote pain management, such as patterned breathing and progressive relaxation exercises.

Pharmacological Pain Management

- Pharmacological methods of pain management include analgesia and local/regional analgesics. To avoid slowing the progress of labor, prior to administering analgesic medications, the nurse should verify that labor is well established by performing a vaginal exam and evaluating uterine contraction pattern.

- Pharmacological Management
  - ○ Alleviates pain sensations or raises the threshold for pain perception
  - ○ Analgesia includes opioid analgesics.
    - Sedatives (barbiturates), such as secobarbital (Seconal), pentobarbital (Nembutal), and phenobarbital (Luminal), are not typically used during birth, but they can be used during the early or latent phase of labor to relieve anxiety and induce sleep.
      - □ Adverse effects of sedatives
        - ▸ Neonate respiratory depression secondary to the medication crossing the placenta and affecting the fetus. These medications should not be administered if birth is anticipated with 12 to 24 hr.
        - ▸ Unsteady ambulation of the client.
        - ▸ Inhibition of the mother's ability to cope with the pain of labor. Sedatives should not be given if the client is experiencing pain because apprehension can increase and cause the client to become hyperactive and disoriented.
      - □ Client Education
        - ▸ Explain to the client that the medication will cause drowsiness.
        - ▸ Instruct the client to request assistance with ambulation.
      - □ Nursing Actions
        - ▸ Dim the lights, and provide a quiet atmosphere.
        - ▸ Provide safety for the client by lowering the position of the bed and elevating the side rails.
        - ▸ Assist the mother to cope with labor.
        - ▸ Assess the neonate for respiratory depression.

- Opioid analgesics, such as meperidine hydrochloride (Demerol), fentanyl (Sublimaze), butorphanol (Stadol), and nalbuphine (Nubain), act in the CNS to decrease the perception of pain without the loss of consciousness. The client may be given opioid analgesics IM or IV, but the IV route is recommended during labor because the action is quicker.
  - □ Butorphanol (Stadol) and nalbuphine (Nubain) provide pain relief without causing significant respiratory depression in the mother or fetus. Both IM and IV routes are used.
  - □ Adverse effects of opioid analgesics
    - ▸ Crosses the placental barrier; if given to the mother too close to the time of delivery, opioid analgesics can cause respiratory depression in the neonate.
    - ▸ Reduces gastric emptying; increases the risk for nausea and emesis
    - ▸ Increases the risk for aspiration of food or fluids in the stomach
    - ▸ Sedation
    - ▸ Tachycardia
    - ▸ Hypotension
    - ▸ Decreased FHR variability
    - ▸ Allergic reaction
  - □ Client Education
    - ▸ Explain to the client that the medication will cause drowsiness.
    - ▸ Instruct the client to request assistance with ambulation.
  - □ Nursing Actions
    - ▸ Prior to administering analgesic medication, the nurse should verify that labor is well established by performing a vaginal exam that reveals cervical dilation of at least 4 cm with a fetus that is engaged.
    - ▸ Administer antiemetics as prescribed.
    - ▸ Monitor maternal vital signs, uterine contraction pattern, continuous FHR monitoring.
- Naloxone (Narcan), an opioid antagonist, should be readily available for reversal of opioid-induced respiratory depression.
- Ondansetron (Zofran) and metoclopramide (Reglan) can control nausea and anxiety. They do not relieve pain and are used as an adjunct with opioids.
  - □ Adverse effects include dry mouth and sedation.
  - □ Nursing Actions
    - ▸ Provide ice chips or mouth swabs.
    - ▸ Provide safety measures for the client.
- Epidural and spinal regional analgesia consists of using analgesics such as fentanyl (Sublimaze) and sufentanil (Sufenta), which are short-acting opioids that are administered as a motor block into the epidural or intrathecal space without anesthesia. These opioids produce regional analgesia providing rapid pain relief while still allowing the client to sense contractions and maintain the ability to bear down.
  - □ Adverse effects of epidural and spinal analgesia
    - ▸ Decreased gastric emptying resulting in nausea and vomiting
    - ▸ Inhibition of bowel and bladder elimination sensations
    - ▸ Bradycardia or tachycardia
    - ▸ Hypotension

- ▸ Respiratory depression
- ▸ Allergic reaction and pruritus
- ▸ Elevated temperature
  - ▫ Client Education
    - ▸ Provide the client with ongoing education related to expectations for procedure.
  - ▫ Nursing Actions
    - ▸ Institute safety precautions, such as putting side rails up on the client's bed. The client may experience dizziness and sedation, which increases maternal risk for injury.
    - ▸ Assess the client for nausea and emesis, and administer antiemetics as prescribed.
    - ▸ Monitor maternal vital signs per facility protocol.
    - ▸ Monitor for allergic reaction.
    - ▸ Continue FHR pattern monitoring.
- Pharmacological Anesthesia
  - ○ Pharmacological anesthesia eliminates pain perceptions by interrupting the nerve impulses to the brain.
  - ○ Anesthesia used in childbirth includes regional blocks and general anesthesia.
    - ▪ Regional blocks are most commonly used and consist of pudendal block, epidural block, spinal block, and paracervical nerve block.
      - ▫ Pudendal block consists of a local anesthetic, such as lidocaine (Xylocaine) or bupivacaine (Marcaine), being administered transvaginally into the space in front of the pudendal nerve. This type of block has no maternal or fetal systemic effects, but it does provide local anesthesia to the perineum, vulva, and rectal areas during delivery, episiotomy, and episiotomy repair. It is administered during the second stage of labor 10 to 20 min before delivery providing analgesia prior to spontaneous expulsion of the fetus or forceps-assisted or vacuum-assisted birth.
      - ▫ Adverse effects of Pudendal Block
        - ▸ Broad ligament hematoma
        - ▸ Compromise of maternal bearing down reflex
      - ▫ Nursing Actions
        - ▸ Instruct the client about the method.
        - ▸ Coach the client about when to bear down.
        - ▸ Assess the perineal and vulvar area postpartum for hematoma.
    - ▪ An epidural block consists of a local anesthetic, bupivacaine (Marcaine), along with an analgesic, morphine (Duramorph) or fentanyl (Sublimaze), injected into the epidural space at the level of the fourth or fifth vertebrae. This eliminates all sensation from the level of the umbilicus to the thighs, relieving the discomfort of uterine contractions, fetal descent, and pressure and stretching of the perineum. It is administered when the client is in active labor and dilated to at least 4 cm. Continuous infusion or intermittent injections may be administered through an indwelling epidural catheter. Patient-controlled epidural analgesia is a technique for labor analgesia and is a favored method of pain management for labor and birth.
      - ▫ Adverse effects of an epidural block
        - ▸ Maternal hypotension
        - ▸ Fetal bradycardia
        - ▸ Inability to feel the urge to void
        - ▸ Loss of the bearing down reflex

- ☐ Nursing Actions
  - ▸ Administer a bolus of IV fluids to help offset maternal hypotension as prescribed.
  - ▸ Help to position and steady the client into either a sitting or side-lying modified Sims' position with her back curved to widen the intervertebral space for insertion of the epidural catheter.
  - ▸ Encourage the client to remain in the side-lying position after insertion of the epidural catheter to avoid supine hypotension syndrome with compression of the vena cava.
  - ▸ Coach the client in pushing efforts, and request an evaluation of epidural pain management by anesthesia personnel if pushing efforts are ineffective.
  - ▸ Monitor maternal blood pressure and pulse, and observe for hypotension, respiratory depression, and decreased oxygen saturation.
  - ▸ Assess FHR patterns continuously.
  - ▸ Maintain the IV line, and have oxygen and suction available.
  - ▸ Assess for orthostatic hypotension. If present, be prepared to administer an IV vasopressor such as ephedrine, position the client laterally, increase rate of IV fluid administration, and initiate oxygen.
  - ▸ Provide client safety such as raising the side rails of the bed. Do not allow the client to ambulate unassisted.
  - ▸ Assess the client's bladder for distention at frequent intervals, and catheterize if necessary to prevent discomfort and interference with uterine contractions.
  - ▸ Monitor for the return of sensation and motor control in the client's legs after delivery but prior to standing. Assist the client with standing and walking for the first time after a delivery that included epidural anesthesia.

  > **M⬗** View Video: Epidural Catheter Placement

- ☐ Client Education
  - ▸ Provide ongoing instructions related to the procedure and nursing actions.
- ▪ Spinal block consists of a local anesthetic that is injected into the subarachnoid space into the spinal fluid at the third, fourth, or fifth lumbar interspace. This can be done alone or in combination with an analgesic such as fentanyl (Sublimaze). The spinal block eliminates all sensations from the level of the nipples to the feet. It is commonly used for cesarean births. A low spinal block may be used for a vaginal birth, but it is not used for labor. A spinal block is administered in the late second stage or before cesarean birth.
  - ☐ Adverse Effects of a Spinal Block
    - ▸ Maternal hypotension
    - ▸ Fetal bradycardia
    - ▸ Loss of the bearing down reflex in the mother with a higher incidence of operative births
    - ▸ Potential headache from leakage of cerebrospinal fluid at the puncture site
    - ▸ Higher incidence of maternal bladder and uterine atony following birth

◽ Nursing Actions

▸ Assess maternal vital signs every 10 min.

▸ Manage maternal hypotension by administering an IV fluid bolus as prescribed, positioning the mother laterally, increasing the rate of IV fluid administration, and initiating oxygen.

▸ Assess the client's uterine contractions.

▸ Assess level of anesthesia.

▸ Assess FHR patterns.

▸ Provide client safety to prevent injury by raising the side rails of the bed, and assisting the client with repositioning.

▸ Recognize signs of impending birth including sitting on one buttock, making grunting sounds, and bulging of the perineum.

▸ Encourage interventions to relieve a postpartum headache resulting from a cerebrospinal fluid leak. Interventions include placing the client in a supine position, promoting bed rest in a dark room, administering oral analgesics, caffeine, and fluids. An autologous blood patch is the most beneficial and reliable relief measure for cerebrospinal fluid leaks.

◽ Client Education

▸ Instruct the client about the method.

▸ Instruct the client to bear down for expulsion of the fetus because during a vaginal birth, the mother will not feel her contractions.

▪ General anesthesia is rarely used for vaginal or cesarean births when there are no complications present. It is used only in the event of a delivery complication or emergency when there is a contraindication to nerve block analgesia or anesthesia. General anesthesia produces unconsciousness.

◽ Nursing Actions

▸ Monitor maternal vital signs.

▸ Monitor FHR patterns.

▸ Ensure that the client has had nothing by mouth.

▸ Ensure that the IV infusion is in place.

▸ Apply antiemboli stockings and/or sequential compression devices.

▸ Premedicate the client with oral antacid to neutralize acidic stomach contents.

▸ Administer a histamine$_2$ receptor antagonist such as ranitidine (Zantac) to decrease gastric acid production.

▸ Administer metoclopramide (Reglan) to increase gastric emptying as prescribed.

▸ Place a wedge under one of the client's hips to displace the uterus.

▸ Maintain an open airway and cardiopulmonary function.

▸ Assess the client postpartum for decreased uterine tone, which can lead to hemorrhage and be produced by pharmacological agents used in general anesthesia.

◽ Client Education

▸ Facilitate parent-newborn attachment as soon as possible.

APPLICATION EXERCISES

1. A nurse is caring for a client at 40 weeks of gestation who is experiencing contractions every 3 to 5 min and becoming stronger. A vaginal exam reveals that the client's cervix is 3 cm dilated, 80% effaced, and -1 station. The client asks for pain medication. Which of the following actions should the nurse take at this time? (Select all that apply.)

_____X_____ A. Encourage the use of patterned breathing techniques.

_____ B. Insert an indwelling urinary catheter.

_____✓_____ C. Administer opioid analgesic medication as prescribed.

_____X_____ D. Suggest application of cold.

_____ E. Provide ice chips.

2. A nurse is caring for a client who is in active labor. The client reports lower back pain. The nurse suspects that this pain is related to a persistent occiput posterior fetal position. Which of the following nonpharmacological nursing interventions is appropriate?

A. Abdominal effleurage

B. Sacral counterpressure

C. Showering if not contraindicated

D. Back rub and massage

3. A nurse is caring for a client following the administration of an epidural block and is preparing to administer a prescribed IV fluid bolus. The client's partner asks about the purpose of the IV fluids. Which of the following is an appropriate response by the nurse?

A. "It is needed to promote increased urine output."

B. "It is needed to counteract respiratory depression."

C. "It is needed to counteract hypotension."

D. "It is needed to prevent oligohydramnios."

4. A nurse in the labor and delivery unit is caring for a client who is in the second stage of labor. The client's labor has been progressing, and she is expected to deliver vaginally in 20 min. The provider is preparing to administer lidocaine (Xylocaine) for pain relief and perform an episiotomy. The nurse should know that the type of regional anesthetic block that is to be administered is which of the following?

A. Pudendal block

B. Epidural block

C. Spinal block

D. Paracervical block

5. A nurse in the labor and delivery unit is caring for a client who is using patterned breathing during labor. The client reports numbness and tingling of the fingers. Which of the following actions should the nurse take?

A. Administer oxygen via nasal cannula at 2 L/min.

B. Apply a warm blanket.

C. Assist the client to a side-lying position.

D. Place an oxygen mask over the client's nose and mouth.

6. A nurse in a prenatal clinic is teaching a childbirth education class on methods to promote relaxation and pain management to a group of women in the third trimester. Which nonpharmacological pain management strategies should be included in the discussion? Use the ATI Active Learning Template: Basic Concept to complete this item to include the following:

A. Describe the underlying principle for the use of sensory stimulation and cutaneous strategies.

B. Describe three sensory stimulation strategies.

C. Describe three cutaneous strategies.

APPLICATION EXERCISES KEY

1. A. **CORRECT:** Encouraging the use of patterned breathing techniques can assist with pain management at this time.

    B. INCORRECT: There is no indication for the insertion of an indwelling urinary catheter at this time.

    C. **CORRECT:** An opioid analgesic can be safely administered at this time.

    D. **CORRECT:** The use of a nonpharmacological approach, such as the application of cold, is an appropriate intervention at this time.

    E. INCORRECT: This action does not address the client's request for assistance with pain management.

    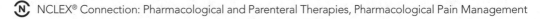 NCLEX® Connection: Pharmacological and Parenteral Therapies, Pharmacological Pain Management

2. A. INCORRECT: Abdominal effleurage is an appropriate pain management technique but does not address the pressure on the pelvis due to the fetal position.

    B. **CORRECT:** Sacral counterpressure to the lower back relieves the pressure exerted on the pelvis and spinal nerves by the fetus.

    C. INCORRECT: A shower is an appropriate pain management strategy but does not address the pressure on the pelvis due to the fetal position.

    D. INCORRECT: A back rub with massage is an appropriate pain management strategy but does not address the pressure on the pelvis due to the fetal position.

    NCLEX® Connection: Basic Care and Comfort, Non-Pharmacological Comfort Interventions

3. A. INCORRECT: Urinary output is not affected by an epidural block.

    B. INCORRECT: Oxygen is administered to counteract respiratory depression that can occur following an epidural block.

    C. **CORRECT:** Maternal hypotension can occur following an epidural block and can be offset by administering an IV fluid bolus.

    D. INCORRECT: Oligohydramnios does not occur as a result of an epidural block.

    NCLEX® Connection: Pharmacological and Parenteral Therapies, Medication Administration

4. A. **CORRECT:** A pudendal block is a transvaginal injection of local anesthetic that anesthetizes the perineal area for the episiotomy and repair, and the expulsion of the fetus.

    B. INCORRECT: Epidural blocks are administered during labor and allow the client to participate in the second stage while remaining comfortable.

    C. INCORRECT: Spinal blocks are administered in the late second stage but most commonly preceding a cesarean birth.

    D. INCORRECT: Paracervical blocks are used early in labor to block pain of uterine contractions but are rarely used today.

     NCLEX® Connection: Health Promotion and Maintenance, Ante/Intra/Postpartum and Newborn Care

5. A. INCORRECT: The client is experiencing hyperventilation caused by low levels of serum PCO_2. Supplying additional oxygen will not resolve this issue.

    B. INCORRECT: The client is experiencing hyperventilation caused by low levels of serum PCO_2. Applying a warm blanket will not resolve this issue.

    C. INCORRECT: The client is experiencing hyperventilation caused by low serum levels of PCO_2. Assisting the client to a side-lying position will not resolve this issue.

    D. **CORRECT:** The client is experiencing hyperventilation caused by low serum levels of PCO_2. Placing an oxygen mask over the client's nose and mouth or having the client breathe into a paper bag will reduce the intake of oxygen, allowing the PCO_2 to rise and alleviate the numbness and tingling.

    NCLEX® Connection: Health Promotion and Maintenance, Ante/Intra/Postpartum and Newborn Care

6. *Using the ATI Active Learning Template: Basic Concept*

    A. Underlying Principle
    - Gate control theory of pain is based on the concept that the sensory nerve pathways that pain sensations use to travel to the brain will allow only a limited number of sensations to travel at any given time. By sending alternate signals through these pathways, the pain signals can be blocked from ascending the neurological pathway and inhibit the brain's perception and sensation of pain.

    B. Sensory Stimulation Strategies
    - Aromatherapy
    - Breathing techniques
    - Imagery
    - Music
    - Use of focal points

    C. Cutaneous Strategies
    - Back rubs and massage
    - Effleurage
    - Sacral counterpressure
    - Heat or cold therapy
    - Hydrotherapy
    - Acupressure

    NCLEX® Connection: Basic Care and Comfort, Non-Pharmacological Comfort Interventions

UNIT 2   **INTRAPARTUM NURSING CARE**
               SECTION: LABOR AND DELIVERY

CHAPTER 13   Fetal Assessment During Labor

Overview

- Describe fetal assessment during labor.

- The diagnostic procedures mentioned in this chapter include Leopold maneuvers, and FHR pattern and uterine contraction monitoring.

LEOPOLD MANEUVERS

- Description of Procedure

   View Video: Leopold Maneuvers

  ○ Leopold maneuvers consist of performing external palpations of the maternal uterus through the abdominal wall to determine the following:

    ▪ Number of fetuses

    ▪ Presenting part, fetal lie, and fetal attitude

    ▪ Degree of descent of the presenting part into the pelvis

    ▪ Expected location of the point of maximal impulse (PMI)

      □ PMI is the optimal location where the fetal heart tones are auscultated the loudest on the woman's abdomen. These tones are best heard directly over the fetal back.

      □ In vertex presentation, PMI is either in the right- or left-lower quadrant or below the maternal umbilicus.

      □ In breech presentation, PMI is either in the right- or left-upper quadrant above the maternal umbilicus.

- Nursing Actions

  ○ Preparation of the Client

    ▪ Ask the client to empty her bladder before beginning the assessment.

    ▪ Place the client in the supine position with a pillow under her head, and have her flex her knees slightly.

    ▪ Place a wedge under her right hip to displace the uterus to the left and prevent supine hypotension syndrome.

○ Ongoing care

- Identify the fetal part occupying the fundus. The head should feel round, firm, and move freely. The breech should feel irregular and soft. This maneuver identifies the fetal lie (longitudinal or transverse) and presenting part (cephalic or breech).

- Locate and palpate the smooth contour of the fetal back using the palm of one hand and the irregular small parts of the hands, feet, and elbows using the palm of the other hand. This maneuver validates the presenting part.

- Determine the part that is presenting over the true pelvis inlet by gently grasping the lower segment of the uterus between the thumb and fingers. If the head is presenting and not engaged, determine whether the head is flexed or extended. This maneuver assists in identifying the descent of the presenting part into the pelvis.

- Face the client's feet and outline the fetal head using the palmar surface of the fingertips on both hands to palpate the cephalic prominence. If the cephalic prominence is on the same side as the small parts, the head is flexed with vertex presentation. If the cephalic prominence is on the same side as the back, the head is extended with a face presentation. This maneuver identifies the fetal attitude.

○ Interventions

- Auscultate the FHR postmaneuvers to assess the fetal tolerance to the procedure.

- Document the findings from the maneuvers.

FHR PATTERN AND UTERINE CONTRACTION MONITORING

- Description of Procedure

  ○ Intermittent auscultation and uterine contraction palpation

  - Intermittent auscultation of the FHR is a low-technology method that can be performed during labor using a hand-held Doppler ultrasound device, an ultrasound stethoscope, or fetoscope to assess FHR. In conjunction, palpation of contractions at the fundus for frequency, duration, and intensity is used to evaluate fetal well-being. During labor, uterine contractions compress the uteroplacental arteries, temporarily stopping maternal blood flow into the uterus and intervillous spaces of the placenta, decreasing fetal circulation and oxygenation. Circulation to the uterus and placenta resumes during uterine relaxation between contractions. For low-risk labor and delivery, this procedure allows the woman freedom of movement and can be done at home or a birthing center.

  - Guidelines for intermittent auscultation or continuous electronic fetal monitoring

    □ Low-risk women

    ▸ During latent phase, every 60 min

    ▸ During active phase, every 30 min

    ▸ During second stage, every 15 min

    □ High-risk women

    ▸ During latent phase, every 30 min

    ▸ During active phase, every 15 min

    ▸ During second stage, every 5 min

- Indications
  - Potential diagnoses
    - Rule out labor
    - Active labor
  - Guidelines for intermittent auscultation following routine procedures
    - Rupture of membranes, either spontaneously or artificially
    - Preceding and subsequent to ambulation
    - Prior to and following administration of or a change in medication analgesia
    - At peak action of anesthesia
    - Following vaginal examination
    - Following expulsion of an enema
    - After urinary catheterization
    - In the event of abnormal or excessive uterine contractions
- Interpretation of Findings
  - A normal, reassuring FHR is 110 to 160/min with increases and decreases from baseline.
- Nursing Actions
  - Preparation of the client
    - Based on findings obtained using Leopold maneuvers, auscultate at PMI using listening device.
    - Palpate the uterine fundus to assess uterine activity.
    - Count FHR for 30 to 60 seconds to determine baseline rate.
    - Auscultate FHR during a contraction and for 30 seconds following the completion of the contraction.
  - Ongoing care
    - Identify FHR patterns and characteristics of uterine contractions.
  - Interventions
    - It is the responsibility of the nurse to assess FHR patterns and characteristics of uterine contractions, implement nursing interventions, and report nonreassuring patterns or abnormal uterine contractions to the provider.

    - Cultural considerations, as well as the emotional, educational, and comfort needs of the mother and the family, must be incorporated into the plan of care while continuing to assess the FHR pattern's response to uterine contractions during the labor process.
  - The method and frequency of fetal surveillance during labor will vary and depend on maternal-fetal risk factors as well as the preference of the facility, provider, and client.

- Description of Procedure
  - Continuous electronic fetal monitoring
    - Continuous external fetal monitoring is accomplished by securing an ultrasound transducer over the client's abdomen to determine PMI, which records the FHR pattern, and a tocotransducer on the fundus that records the uterine contractions.
    - Advantages of external fetal monitoring
      - Noninvasive and reduces risk for infection
      - Membranes do not have to be ruptured
      - Cervix does not have to be dilated
      - Placement of transducers can be performed by the nurse
      - Provides permanent record of FHR and uterine contraction tracing
    - Disadvantages of external fetal monitoring
      - Contraction intensity is not measurable
      - Movement of the client requires frequent repositioning of transducers
      - Quality of recording is affected by client obesity and fetal position
- Indications for Monitoring
  - Potential diagnoses
    - Multiple gestations, oxytocin (Pitocin) infusion (augmentation or induction of labor)
    - Placenta previa
    - Fetal bradycardia
    - Maternal complications (diabetes mellitus, gestational hypertension, kidney disease)
    - Intrauterine growth restriction
    - Postdate
    - Active labor
    - Meconium-stained amniotic fluid
    - Abruption placenta – suspected or actual
    - Abnormal nonstress test or contraction stress test
    - Abnormal uterine contractions
    - Fetal distress
  - Interpretation of Findings
    - A normal fetal heart rate baseline at term is 110 to 160/min excluding accelerations, decelerations, and periods of marked variability within a 10 min window. At least 2 min of baseline segments in a 10 min window should be present. A single number should be documented instead of a baseline range.
    - Fetal heart rate baseline variability is described as fluctuations in the FHR baseline that are irregular in frequency and amplitude. Classification of variability is as follows:
      - Absent or undetectable variability (considered nonreassuring)
      - Minimal variability (greater than undetectable but less than 5/min)
      - Moderate variability (6 to 25/min)
      - Marked variability (greater than 25/min)

- Changes in fetal heart rate patterns are categorized as episodic or periodic changes. Episodic changes are not associated with uterine contractions, and periodic changes occur with uterine contractions. These changes include accelerations and decelerations.

- Current recommendations for fetal monitoring include a three-tier fetal heart rate interpretation system.

  □ Category I: All of the following are included in the fetal heart rate tracing:

    ‣ Baseline fetal heart rate of 110 to 160/min

    ‣ Baseline fetal heart rate variability: moderate

    ‣ Accelerations: present or absent

    ‣ Early decelerations: present or absent

    ‣ Variable or late decelerations: absent

  □ Category II: Category II tracings include all fetal heart rate tracings not categorized as Category I or Category III. Examples of Category II fetal heart rate tracings contain any of the following:

    ‣ Baseline rate

      ▷ Tachycardia

      ▷ Bradycardia not accompanied by absent baseline variability

    ‣ Baseline FHR variability

      ▷ Minimal baseline variability

      ▷ Absent baseline variability not accompanied by recurrent decelerations

      ▷ Marked baseline variability

    ‣ Episodic or periodic decelerations

      ▷ Prolonged fetal heart rate deceleration greater than 2 min but less than 10 min

      ▷ Recurrent late decelerations with moderate baseline variability

      ▷ Recurrent variable decelerations with minimal or moderate baseline variability

      ▷ Variable decelerations with additional characteristics, including "overshoots," "shoulders," or slow return to baseline fetal heart rate

    ‣ Accelerations

      ▷ Absence of induced accelerations after fetal stimulation

  □ Category III: Category III fetal heart rate tracings include either:

    ‣ Sinusoidal pattern

    ‣ Absent baseline fetal heart rate variability and any of the following:

      ▷ Recurrent variable decelerations

      ▷ Recurrent late decelerations

      ▷ Bradycardia

- Each uterine contraction is comprised of the following:
  - Increment – the beginning of the contraction as intensity is increasing
  - Acme – the peak intensity of the contraction
  - Decrement – the decline of the contraction intensity as the contraction is ending
- Nonreassuring FHR patterns are associated with fetal hypoxia and include the following:
  - Fetal bradycardia
  - Fetal tachycardia
  - Absence of FHR variability
  - Late decelerations
  - Variable decelerations

FHR PATTERNS	
CAUSES/COMPLICATIONS	NURSING INTERVENTIONS
Accelerations (variable transitory increase in the FHR above baseline)	
› Healthy fetal/placental exchange › Intact fetal central nervous system (CNS) response to fetal movement › Vaginal exam › Fundal pressure	› Reassuring. › No interventions required. › Indicate reactive nonstress test.
Fetal bradycardia (FHR less than 110/min for 10 min or more)	
› Uteroplacental insufficiency › Umbilical cord prolapse › Maternal hypotension › Prolonged umbilical cord compression › Fetal congenital heart block › Anesthetic medications	› Discontinue oxytocin (Pitocin) if being administered. › Assist the client to a side-lying position. › Administer oxygen by mask at 8 to 10 L/min. › Insert an IV catheter if one is not in place. › Administer a tocolytic medication as prescribed. › Notify the provider.
Fetal tachycardia (FHR greater than 160 beats/min for 10 min or more)	
› Maternal infection, chorioamnionitis › Fetal anemia › Fetal heart failure › Fetal cardiac dysrhythmias › Maternal use of cocaine or methamphetamines › Maternal dehydration	› Administer prescribed antipyretics for maternal fever, if present. › Administer oxygen by mask at 8 to 10 L/min. › Administer IV fluid bolus.

FHR PATTERNS	
CAUSES/COMPLICATIONS	**NURSING INTERVENTIONS**
Decrease or loss of FHR variability (decrease or loss of irregular fluctuations in the baseline of the FHR)	
› Medications that depress the CNS, such as narcotics, barbiturates, tranquilizers, or general anesthetics › Fetal hypoxemia with resulting acidosis › Fetal sleep cycle › Congenital abnormalities	› Stimulate the fetal scalp. › Assist provider with application of scalp electrode. › Place client in left-lateral position.
Early deceleration of FHR (slowing of FHR with start of contraction with return of FHR to baseline at end of contraction)	
› Compression of the fetal head resulting from uterine contraction › Vaginal exam › Fundal pressure	› No intervention required.
Late deceleration of FHR (slowing of FHR after contraction has started with return of FHR to baseline well after contraction has ended)	
› Uteroplacental insufficiency causing inadequate fetal oxygenation › Maternal hypotension, abruptio placentae, uterine hyperstimulation with oxytocin (Pitocin)	› Place client in side-lying position. › Insert an IV catheter if not in place, and increase rate of IV fluid administration. › Discontinue oxytocin (Pitocin) if being infused. › Administer oxygen by mask at 8 to 10 L/min. › Notify the provider. › Prepare for an assisted vaginal birth or cesarean birth.
Variable deceleration of FHR (transitory, abrupt slowing of FHR less than 110 beats/min, variable in duration, intensity, and timing in relation to uterine contraction)	
› Umbilical cord compression › Short cord › Prolapsed cord › Nuchal cord (around fetal neck) › Oligohydramnios	› Reposition client from side to side or into knee-chest. › Discontinue oxytocin (Pitocin) if being infused. › Administer oxygen by mask at 8 to 10 L/min. › Perform or assist with a vaginal examination. › Assist with an amnioinfusion if prescribed.

View Images

› Early Decelerations

› Variable Decelerations

› Late Decelerations

› Minimal Variability

- Nursing Actions
  - Preparation of the Client
    - Based on findings obtained using Leopold maneuvers, auscultate at PMI using listening device.
    - Palpate the fundus to identify uterine activity for proper placement of the tocotransducer to monitor uterine contractions.
  - Ongoing Care
    - Provide education regarding the procedure to the client and the client's partner during placement and adjustments of the fetal monitor equipment.
    - Encourage frequent maternal position changes, which may require adjustments of the transducers with position changes.
    - If the client needs to void and can ambulate, and it is not contraindicated, the nurse can disconnect the external monitor for the client to use the bathroom.
    - If disconnecting the FHR monitor is contraindicated or an internal FHR monitor is being used, the nurse can bring the client a bedpan.
- Description of Procedure
  - Continuous internal fetal monitoring
    - Continuous internal fetal monitoring with a scalp electrode is performed by attaching a small spiral electrode to the presenting part of the fetus to monitor the FHR. The electrode wires are then attached to a leg plate that is placed on the client's thigh and then attached to the fetal monitor.
    - Continuous internal fetal monitoring may be used in conjunction with an intrauterine pressure catheter (IUPC), which is a solid or fluid-filled transducer placed inside the client's uterine cavity to monitor the frequency, duration, and intensity of contractions. The average pressure is usually 50 to 85 mm Hg.
      - Advantages of internal fetal monitoring
        - Early detection of abnormal FHR patterns suggestive of fetal distress.
        - Accurate assessment of FHR variability.
        - Accurate measurement of uterine contraction intensity.
        - Allows greater maternal freedom of movement because tracing is not affected by fetal activity, maternal position changes, or obesity.
      - Disadvantages of internal fetal monitoring
        - Membranes must have ruptured to use internal monitoring.
        - Cervix must be adequately dilated to a minimum of 2 to 3 cm.
        - Presenting part must have descended to place electrode.
        - Potential risk of injury to fetus if electrode is not properly applied.
        - A provider, nurse practitioner/midwife, or specially trained registered nurse must perform this procedure.
        - Contraindicated with vaginal bleeding.
        - Potential risk of infection to the client and the fetus.

- Nursing Actions
  - Preparation of the Client
    - Ensure electronic fetal monitoring equipment is functioning properly.
    - Use aseptic techniques when assisting with procedures.
  - Ongoing Care
    - Monitor maternal vital signs, and obtain maternal temperature every 1 to 2 hr.
    - Encourage frequent repositioning of the client. If the client is lying supine, place a wedge under one of the client's hips to tilt her uterus.
- Complications
  - Misinterpretation of FHR patterns
  - Maternal or fetal infection
  - Fetal trauma if fetal monitoring electrode or IUPC are inserted into the vagina improperly
  - Supine hypotension secondary to internal monitor placement

APPLICATION EXERCISES

1. A nurse is providing care for a client who is in active labor. Her cervix is dilated to 5 cm, and her membranes are intact. Based on the use of external electronic fetal monitoring, the nurse notes a FHR of 115 to 125/min with occasional increases up to 150 to 155/min that last for 25 seconds, and have beat-to-beat variability of 20/min. There is no slowing of FHR from the baseline. The nurse should recognize that this client is exhibiting signs of which of the following? (Select all that apply.)

_____ A. Moderate variability

_____ B. FHR accelerations

_____ C. FHR decelerations

_____ D. Normal baseline FHR

_____ E. Fetal tachycardia

2. A nurse is caring for a client who is having an induction of labor. Based on the use of external electronic fetal monitoring, the nurse notes that the FHR variability is decreased and resembles a straight line. The client has not received pain medication. Which of the following should occur first before the nurse can apply an internal scalp electrode?

A. Dilation

B. Rupture of the membranes

C. Effacement

D. Engagement

3. A nurse is reviewing the electronic monitor tracing of a client who is in active labor. The nurse knows that a fetus receives more oxygen when which of the following appears on the tracing?

A. Peak of the uterine contraction

B. Moderate variability

C. FHR acceleration

D. Relaxation between uterine contractions

4. A nurse is caring for a client who is in labor and observes late decelerations on the electronic fetal monitor. Which of the following is the first action the nurse should take?

A. Assist the client into the left-lateral position.

B. Apply a fetal scalp electrode.

C. Insert an IV catheter.

D. Perform a vaginal exam.

5. A nurse is performing Leopold maneuvers on a client who is in labor. Which of the following techniques should the nurse use to identify the fetal lie?

   A. Apply palms of both hands to sides of uterus.

   B. Palpate the fundus of the uterus.

   C. Grasp lower uterine segment between thumb and fingers.

   D. Stand facing client's feet with fingertips outlining cephalic prominence.

6. A nurse in labor and delivery is reviewing intermittent fetal auscultation and uterine contraction palpation with a recently hired nurse. What should be included in the review? Use the ATI Active Learning Template: Therapeutic Procedure to complete this item to include the following sections:

   A. Indications: Describe four situations when this procedure should be performed.

   B. Interpretation of Findings: Describe normal expected FHR findings.

   C. Nursing Actions:
   - Preprocedure: Describe the three types of devices that are used to auscultate FHR.
   - Intraprocedure: Identify the time frame for counting FHR to determine the baseline rate and when auscultation should take place.

APPLICATION EXERCISES KEY

1. A. **CORRECT:** There is moderate variability of 20 beats/min (6 to 25/min is expected).

   B. **CORRECT:** FHR accelerations are present with increases up to 150 to 155/min lasting for 25 seconds.

   C. INCORRECT: There are no FHR decelerations because the FHR does not slow down.

   D. **CORRECT:** There is a normal baseline FHR of 115 to 125/min (110 to 160/min is expected).

   E. INCORRECT: There is no evidence of fetal tachycardia because there is a normal baseline FHR of 115 to 125/min.

    NCLEX® Connection: Health Promotion and Maintenance, Ante/Intra/Postpartum and Newborn Care

2. A. INCORRECT: The cervix must be dilated 2 to 3 cm before internal monitoring can be used, but this is not the first criterion to consider.

   B. **CORRECT:** The membranes must be ruptured prior to the insertion of an internal electrode or intrauterine pressure catheter.

   C. INCORRECT: Effacement of the cervix must occur before internal monitoring can be used, but this is not the first criterion to consider.

   D. INCORRECT: Engagement of the presenting part must occur before internal monitoring can be used, but this is not the first criterion to consider.

    NCLEX® Connection: Reduction of Risk Potential, Diagnostic Tests

3. A. INCORRECT: Compression of the arteries to the uteroplacental intervillous spaces is most acute at the peak (acme) of the uterine contraction, resulting in a decrease in fetal circulation and oxygenation.

   B. INCORRECT: Moderate variability indicates fluctuations in the fetal heart and is not an indication the fetus is receiving more oxygen.

   C. INCORRECT: FHR accelerations indicate an intact fetal CNS and is not an indication the fetus is receiving more oxygen.

   D. **CORRECT:** A fetus is most oxygenated during the relaxation period between contractions. During contractions, the arteries to the uteroplacental intervillous spaces are compressed, resulting in a decrease in fetal circulation and oxygenation.

    NCLEX® Connection: Health Promotion and Maintenance, Ante/Intra/Postpartum and Newborn Care

4. A. **CORRECT:** The greatest risk to the fetus during late decelerations is uteroplacental insufficiency. The initial nursing action should be to place the client into the left-lateral position to increase uteroplacental perfusion.

   B. INCORRECT: The application of a fetal scalp electrode will assist in the assessment of fetal well-being, but this is not the first action the nurse should take.

   C. INCORRECT: Inserting an IV catheter is an intervention for late decelerations, but this is not the first action the nurse should take.

   D. INCORRECT: The nurse may perform a vaginal exam to assess dilation, but this is not the first action the nurse should take.

    NCLEX® Connection: Management of Care, Establishing Priorities

5. A. INCORRECT: Using the palms of the hands on the sides of the uterus to identify the fetal back and small body parts verifies the presenting part.

   B. **CORRECT:** Palpating the fundus of the uterus identifies the fetal part that is present, indicating the fetal lie (longitudinal or transverse).

   C. INCORRECT: The descent of the presenting part into the pelvis is determined by gently grasping the lower uterine segment between the thumb and fingers.

   D. INCORRECT: Fetal attitude is identified by facing the client's feet and outlining the cephalic prominence (fetal head) using the fingertips of both hands.

    NCLEX® Connection: Health Promotion and Maintenance, Ante/Intra/Postpartum and Newborn Care

6. *Using the ATI Active Learning Template: Therapeutic Procedure*

   A. Indications
   - Rupture of membranes, spontaneously or artificially
   - Preceding and subsequent to ambulation
   - Prior to and following administration of or a change in medication analgesia
   - At the peak action of anesthesia
   - Following vaginal examination
   - Following expulsion of an enema
   - After urinary catheterization
   - In the event of abnormal or excessive uterine contractions

   B. Interpretation of Findings
   - A normal, reassuring FHR is 110 to 160/min with increases and deceases from baseline.

   C. Nursing Actions
   - Preprocedure
     ○ Hand-held Doppler ultrasound
     ○ Ultrasound stethoscope
     ○ Fetoscope
   - Intraprocedure
     ○ Count FHR for 30 to 60 seconds to determine the baseline rate.
     ○ Auscultate during and for 30 seconds following the completion of a contraction.

    NCLEX® Connection: Health Promotion and Maintenance, Ante/Intra/Postpartum and Newborn Care

chapter 14

Overview

- Labor occurs in four stages.
- It is the responsibility of a nurse to care, monitor, and provide interventions during each stage.
- Nursing responsibilities
  - Assess the client
    - Orient her and her partner to the unit during admission.
    - Assess the client prior to admission to the birthing facility.

      - Provide culturally competent care that respects and is compatible with the client's culture.
        - Hispanic – Prefer mother to be present rather than partner
        - African American – Prefer female family members for support
        - Asian American –May prefer mother to be present; partner not an active participant; labor in silence; caesarean birth undesirable
        - Native American – Prefer female nursing personnel; family involved in birth; use of herbs during labor; squatting position for birth
        - European American – Birth is public concern; focus on technology; partner expected to be involved; provider seen as head of health care team
      - Conduct an admission history, review of antepartum care, and review of the birth plan.
      - Obtain laboratory reports.
      - Monitor baseline fetal heart tones and uterine contraction patterns for 20 to 30 min.
      - Obtain maternal vital signs.
      - Check the status of the amniotic membranes.
  - Perform maternal and fetal assessments continuously throughout the labor process and immediately after birth.
  - Avoid vaginal examinations in the presence of vaginal bleeding or until placenta previa or placenta abruptio is ruled out. If necessary, vaginal examinations should be done by the provider.
  - Cervical dilation is the single most important indicator of the progress of labor.
  - The progress of labor is affected by fetal lie, presentation, attitude, and fetal size in relationship to the mother's pelvis.
  - The frequency, duration, and strength (intensity) of the uterine contractions cause fetal descent and cervical dilation.

First Stage

- Nursing Assessments During the First Stage
  - ○ Leopold maneuvers performed
  - ○ Perform a vaginal examination as indicated (if no evidence of progress) to allow the examiner to assess whether client is in true labor and whether membranes have ruptured.
    - ▪ Encourage the client to take slow, deep breaths prior to the vaginal exam.
    - ▪ Monitor the cervical dilation and effacement.
    - ▪ Monitor the station and fetal presentation.
    - ▪ Prepare for an impending delivery as the presenting part moves into positive stations and begins to push against the pelvic floor (crowning).
  - ○ Assessments related to possible rupture of membranes
    - ▪ When there is suspected rupture of membranes, the nurse should first assess the FHR to ensure there is no fetal distress from possible umbilical cord prolapse, which can occur with the gush of amniotic fluid.
    - ▪ Verify presence of alkaline amniotic fluid using nitrazine paper (turns blue, pH 6.5 to 7.5).
    - ▪ A sample of the fluid may be obtained and viewed on a slide under a microscope. Amniotic fluid will exhibit a frondlike ferning pattern. Assess the amniotic fluid for color and odor: clear, straw color, and free of odor. Abnormal findings include the presence of meconium, abnormal color (yellow or port wine), a foul odor.
  - ○ Perform bladder palpation on a regular basis to prevent bladder distention, which can impede fetal descent through the birth canal and cause trauma to the bladder.
    - ▪ Clients may not feel the urge to void secondary to the labor process or anesthesia.
    - ▪ Encourage the client to void frequently.
  - ○ Blood pressure, pulse, and respiration measurements
    - ▪ Latent phase every 30 to 60 min
    - ▪ Active phase every 30 min
    - ▪ Transition phase every 15 to 30 min
  - ○ Temperature assessment every 4 hr (every 1 to 2 hr if membranes have ruptured)
  - ○ Contraction monitoring
    - ▪ Latent phase every 30 to 60 min
    - ▪ Active phase every 15 to 30 min
    - ▪ Transition phase every 10 to 15 min
  - ○ FHR monitoring (normal range 110 to 160/min)
    - ▪ Latent phase every 30 to 60 min
    - ▪ Active phase every 15 to 30 min
    - ▪ Transitional phase every 15 to 30 min

- Nursing Interventions During the First Stage of Labor
  - Provide teaching to the client and her partner about what to expect during labor and on implementing relaxation measures: breathing (deep cleansing breaths help divert focus away from contractions), effleurage (gentle circular stroking of the abdomen in rhythm with breathing during contractions), diversional activities (distraction, concentration on a focal point, or imagery).
  - Encourage upright positions, application of warm/cold packs, ambulation, or hydrotherapy if not contraindicated to promote comfort.
  - Encourage voiding every 2 hr.
    - During first stage, active phase of labor
      - Provide client/fetal monitoring.
      - Encourage frequent position changes.
      - Encourage voiding at least every 2 hr.
      - Encourage deep cleansing breaths before and after modified paced breathing.
      - Encourage relaxation.
      - Provide nonpharmacological comfort measures.
      - Provide pharmacological pain relief as prescribed.
    - During first stage, transition phase of labor
      - Continue to encourage voiding every 2 hr.
      - Continue to monitor and support the client and fetus.
      - Encourage a rapid pant-pant-blow breathing pattern if the client has not learned a particular breathing pattern.
      - Discourage pushing efforts until the cervix is fully dilated.
      - Listen for client statements expressing the need to have a bowel movement. This sensation is a sign of complete dilation and fetal descent.
      - Prepare the client for the birth.
      - Observe for perineal bulging or crowning (appearance of the fetal head at the perineum).
      - Encourage the client to begin bearing down with contractions once the cervix is fully dilated.

Second Stage

- Nursing Assessments During the Second Stage (begins with complete dilation and effacement)
  - Blood pressure, pulse, and respiration measurements every 5 to 30 min
  - Uterine contractions
  - Pushing efforts by client
  - Increase in bloody show
  - FHR every 15 min and immediately following birth

- ○ Assessment for perineal lacerations, which usually occur as the fetal head is expulsed. Perineal lacerations are defined in terms of depth.
  - First degree – Laceration extends through the skin of the perineum and does not involve the muscles.
  - Second degree – Laceration extends through the skin and muscles into the perineum.
  - Third degree – Laceration extends through the skin, muscles, perineum, and anal sphincter muscle.
  - Fourth degree – Laceration extends through skin, muscles, anal sphincter, and the anterior rectal wall.
- • Nursing Interventions During the Second Stage
  - ○ Continue to monitor the client/fetus.
  - ○ Assist in positioning the client for effective pushing.
  - ○ Assist in partner involvement with pushing efforts and in encouraging bearing down efforts during contractions.
  - ○ Promote rest between contractions.
  - ○ Provide comfort measures such as cold compresses.
  - ○ Cleanse the client's perineum as needed if fecal material is expelled during pushing.
  - ○ Prepare for episiotomy, if needed.
  - ○ Provide feedback on labor progress to the client.
  - ○ Prepare for care of neonate. A nurse trained in neonatal resuscitation should be present at delivery.
    - Check oxygen flow and tank on warmer.
    - Preheat radiant warmer.
    - Lay out newborn stethoscope and bulb syringe.
    - Have resuscitation equipment in working order (resuscitation bag, laryngoscope) and emergency medications available.
    - Check suction apparatus.

Third Stage

- • Nursing Assessments During the Third Stage
  - ○ Blood pressure, pulse, and respiration measurements every 15 min
  - ○ Signs of placental separation from the uterus as indicated by
    - Fundus firmly contracting
    - Swift gush of dark blood from introitus
    - Umbilical cord appears to lengthen as placenta descends
    - Vaginal fullness on exam
  - ○ Assignment of 1 and 5 min Apgar scores to the neonate

- Nursing Interventions During the Third Stage
  - Instruct the client to push once signs of placental separation are indicated.
  - Promote baby-friendly activities between the family and the newborn, which facilitates the release of endogenous maternal oxytocin.
  - Administer analgesics as prescribed.
  - Administer oxytocics once the placenta is expulsed to stimulate the uterus to contract and thus prevent hemorrhage.
  - Gently cleanse the perineal area with warm water or 0.9% sodium chloride, and apply a perineal pad or ice pack to the perineum.

Fourth Stage

- Nursing Assessments During the Fourth Stage
  - Maternal vital signs
  - Fundus
  - Lochia
  - Urinary output
  - Baby-friendly activities of the family
- Nursing Interventions During the Fourth Stage

  - Assess maternal vital signs every 15 min for the first hour and then according to facility protocol.
  - Assess fundus and lochia every 15 min for the first hour and then according to facility protocol.
  - Massage the uterine fundus and/or administer oxytocics as prescribed to maintain uterine tone and to prevent hemorrhage.
  - Encourage voiding to prevent bladder distention.
  - Promote an opportunity for parental-newborn bonding.

APPLICATION EXERCISES

1. A nurse is caring for a client and her partner during the second stage of labor. The client's partner asks the nurse to explain how he will know when crowning occurs. Which of the following is an appropriate response by the nurse?

    A. "The placenta will protrude from the vagina."

    B. "Your partner will report a decrease in the intensity of contractions."

    C. "The vaginal area will bulge as the baby's head appears."

    D. "Your partner will report less rectal pressure."

2. A nurse is caring for a client in the third stage of labor. Which of the following findings indicate that placental separation has occurred? (Select all that apply.)

    X   A. Lengthening of the umbilical cord.

    _____ B. Swift gush of clear amniotic fluid.

    _____ C. Softening of the lower uterine segment.

    X   D. Appearance of dark blood from the vagina.

    X   E. Fundus is firm upon palpation.

3. A nurse is caring for a client who is in the transition phase of labor and reports that she needs to have a bowel movement with the peak of contractions. Which of the following is an appropriate nursing intervention?

    A. Assist the client to the bathroom.

    B. Prepare for an impending delivery.

    C. Prepare to remove a fecal impaction.

    D. Encourage the client to take deep, cleansing breaths.

4. A nurse in labor and delivery is planning care for a newly admitted client who reports she is in labor and has been having vaginal bleeding for 2 weeks. Which of the following should the nurse include in the plan of care?

    A. Inspect the introitus for a prolapsed cord.

    B. Perform a test to identify the ferning pattern.

    C. Monitor station of the presenting part.

    D. Defer vaginal examinations.

5. A nurse is caring for a client who is in the first stage of labor and encourages the client to void every 2 hr. The nurse explains that a

    A. full bladder increases the risk for fetal trauma.

    B. full bladder increases the risk for bladder infections.

    C. distended bladder will be traumatized by frequent pelvic exams.

    D. distended bladder reduces pelvic space needed for birth.

6. A nurse is caring for a client in the fourth stage of labor. What actions should the nurse take? Use the ATI Active Learning Template: Basic Concept to complete this item to include the following:

    A. Underlying Principle: Describe.

    B. Nursing Interventions: Describe four.

APPLICATION EXERCISES KEY

1. A. INCORRECT: The appearance of the placenta occurs after crowning and the birth of the neonate.

    B. INCORRECT: Crowning occurs with an increase in the intensity of contractions and the urge to push.

    C. **CORRECT:** Crowning is bulging of the perineum and the appearance of the fetal head.

    D. INCORRECT: Crowning occurs with an increase in rectal pressure as the fetal head descends onto the perineum.

    Ⓝ NCLEX® Connection: Health Promotion and Maintenance, Ante/Intra/Postpartum and Newborn Care

2. A. **CORRECT:** The umbilical cord lengthens as the placenta is being expulsed.

    B. INCORRECT: A sudden gush of clear amniotic fluid occurs when membranes rupture.

    C. INCORRECT: Softening of the lower uterine segment is not an indication of placental separation.

    D. **CORRECT:** A gush of dark blood from the introitus is an indication of placental separation.

    E. **CORRECT:** The uterus contracts firmly with placental separation.

    Ⓝ NCLEX® Connection: Health Promotion and Maintenance, Ante/Intra/Postpartum and Newborn Care

3. A. INCORRECT: The urge to have a bowel movement indicates fetal descent and complete dilation. Assisting the client to the bathroom is not an appropriate action in view of the impending delivery.

    B. **CORRECT:** The urge to have a bowel movement indicates fetal descent and complete dilation. Preparing for an imminent delivery is appropriate.

    C. INCORRECT: The nurse cleanses the perineal area to remove fecal matter that can be expelled due to the descent of the fetus. The nurse does not prepare to remove an impaction.

    D. INCORRECT: Deep cleansing breaths are encouraged between contractions. The client will be encouraged to push because the sensation of a bowel movement indicates complete dilation and fetal descent.

    Ⓝ NCLEX® Connection: Health Promotion and Maintenance, Ante/Intra/Postpartum and Newborn Care

4. A INCORRECT: Active vaginal bleeding is not an indication of ruptured membranes. Therefore, the nurse should not anticipate cord prolapse.

   B. INCORRECT: A test for ferning is performed if there is suspected amniotic fluid and there is no indication of ruptured membranes.

   C. INCORRECT: Station is monitored by vaginal examination, which should not be performed if there is vaginal bleeding, which may be related to placenta previa or placenta abruptio.

   D. **CORRECT:** Vaginal examinations should not be performed until placenta previa or placenta abruptio has been ruled out as the cause of vaginal bleeding.

    NCLEX® Connection: Physiological Adaptations, Alterations in Body Systems

5. A. INCORRECT: A full bladder does not place the fetus at risk for trauma.

   B. INCORRECT: Urinary stasis, which occurs due to long periods between voiding, increases the risk for bladder infections.

   C. INCORRECT: The urethra may be traumatized by frequent pelvic exams.

   D. **CORRECT:** A distended bladder reduces pelvic space, impedes fetal descent, and places the bladder at risk for trauma during the labor process.

    NCLEX® Connection: Health Promotion and Maintenance, Ante/Intra/Postpartum and Newborn Care

6. *Using the ATI Active Learning Template: Basic Concept*

   A. Underlying Principle
   - The focus of care in the fourth stage is to maintain uterine tone and to prevent hemorrhage.

   B. Nursing Interventions
   - Assess vital signs, fundus, and lochia every 15 min for the first hour, then according to facility protocol.
   - Massage the uterus.
   - Encourage voiding to prevent bladder distention.
   - Promote parental-newborn bonding.

    NCLEX® Connection: Health Promotion and Maintenance, Ante/Intra/Postpartum and Newborn Care

chapter 15

Overview

- In this chapter, the various therapeutic procedures to assist with labor and delivery will be discussed.

- The therapeutic procedures that will be reviewed include external cephalic version, Bishop score, cervical ripening, induction/augmentation of labor, amniotomy, amnioinfusion, episiotomy, vacuum-assisted delivery, forceps-assisted delivery, cesarean birth, and vaginal delivery after cesarean birth.

EXTERNAL CEPHALIC VERSION

Overview

- Description of Procedure

  - External cephalic version (ECV) is the attempt to manipulate the abdominal wall to direct a malpositioned fetus into a normal vertex presentation after 37 weeks of gestation. There is a high risk of prolapse of the umbilical cord with this procedure. Contraindications to performing a version include uterine anomalies, previous cesarean birth, cephalopelvic disproportion, placenta previa, multifetal gestation, and/or oligohydramnios.

- Indications

  - Potential diagnoses

    - A malpositioned fetus in a breech or transverse position after 37 weeks of gestation.

- Nursing Actions

  - Preparation of the client

    - Obtain an informed consent form from the client.

    - The provider will perform ultrasound screening prior to the procedure to evaluate fetal position, locate the umbilical cord, assess placental placement to rule out placenta previa, determine the amount of amniotic fluid, determine fetal age, assess for the presence of anomalies, evaluate pelvic adequacy for delivery, and/or guide the direction of the fetus during the procedure.

    - Perform a nonstress test to evaluate fetal well-being.

    - Ensure that $RH_o(D)$ immune globulin (RhoGAM) was administered at 28 weeks of gestation if the mother is Rh-negative.

    - Administer IV fluid and tocolytics to relax uterus to permit easier manipulation.

○ Ongoing care

- Continuous monitoring of FHR patterns to assess for bradycardia and variable decelerations during the version and for 1 hr following the procedure.

- Monitor vital signs.

- Assess for hypotension to determine whether vena cava compression is occurring.

- Monitor for client report of pain.

- Rh-negative clients require a Kleihauer-Betke test to detect for the presence and amount of fetal blood in the maternal circulation because a version can cause fetomaternal bleeding. If more than 15 mL of fetal blood is present, $Rh_o(D)$ immune globulin (RhoGAM) must be administered to suppress the maternal immune response to fetal Rh-positive blood.

○ Interventions

- Monitor uterine activity, contraction frequency, duration, and intensity.

- Monitor for rupture of membranes.

- Monitor for bleeding until maternal condition is stable.

- Monitor for a decrease in fetal activity.

BISHOP SCORE

Overview

- Description of Procedure

    ○ A Bishop score is used to determine maternal readiness for labor by evaluating whether the cervix is favorable by rating the following:

      - Cervical dilation

      - Cervical effacement

      - Cervical consistency (firm, medium, or soft)

      - Cervical position (posterior, midposition, or anterior)

      - Station of presenting part

    ○ The five factors are assigned a numerical value of 0 to 3, and the total score is calculated.

- Client Readiness

    ○ A 2012 American Congress of Obstetricians and Gynecologists (ACOG) update states that a Bishop score for a client at 39 weeks of gestation should be greater than 8 for a multiparous client and greater than 10 for a nulliparous client as an indicator of readiness for labor induction.

- Indications

    ○ Potential diagnoses

      - Any condition in which augmentation or induction of labor is indicated.

CERVICAL RIPENING

Overview

- Description of Procedure
  - Cervical ripening by various methods increases cervical readiness for labor through promotion of cervical softening, dilation, and effacement.
    - Cervical ripening can eliminate the need for oxytocin (Pitocin) administration to induce labor, lower the dosage of oxytocin needed and promote a more successful induction.
    - Administration of a low-dose infusion of oxytocin is used for cervical priming.
  - Mechanical and physical methods
    - A balloon catheter is inserted into the intracervical canal to dilate the cervix.
    - Membrane stripping and an amniotomy may be performed.
    - Hygroscopic dilators and sponges may be inserted to absorb fluid from surrounding tissues and then enlarge. Fresh dilators may be inserted if further dilation is required.
      - ☐ Laminaria tents are made from desiccated seaweed.
      - ☐ Synthetic dilators contain magnesium sulfate (Lamicel).
  - Chemical agents based on prostaglandins are used to soften and thin the cervix. They can be in the form of oral medication or vaginal suppositories/gels.
    - Misoprostol (Cytotec) – prostaglandin E_1
    - Dinoprostone (Cervidil, Prostin E_2, Prepidil) – prostaglandin E_2
- Potential Diagnoses
  - Any condition in which augmentation or induction of labor is indicated.
- Client Presentation
  - Failure of the cervix to dilate and efface
  - Failure of labor to progress
- Nursing Actions
  - Ongoing care includes the nurse assessing for
    - Urinary retention
    - Rupture of membranes
    - Uterine tenderness or pain
    - Contractions
    - Vaginal bleeding
    - Fetal distress

- ○ Interventions
  - ▪ Document the number of dilators and/or sponges inserted during the procedure.
  - ▪ The client should remain in a side-lying position.
  - ▪ Assist with augmentation or induction of labor as prescribed.
  - ▪ Monitor the client for potential side effects such as, hypertension, diarrhea, and vomiting.
  - ▪ The nurse should proceed with caution in clients who have glaucoma, asthma, and cardiovascular or renal disorders.
- • Complications
  - ○ Hyperstimulation
    - ▪ Nursing actions
      - ▫ Administer subcutaneous injection of terbutaline (Brethine).
  - ○ Fetal distress
    - ▪ Nursing actions
      - ▫ Apply O_2 via face mask at 10 L/min.
      - ▫ Position the client on her left side.
      - ▫ Increase rate of IV fluid administration.
      - ▫ Notify the provider.

INDUCTION OF LABOR

Overview

- • Description of Procedure
  - ○ Induction of labor is the deliberate initiation of uterine contractions to stimulate labor before spontaneous onset to bring about the birth either by chemical or mechanical means.
  - ○ Methods
    - ▪ Mechanical or chemical approaches
    - ▪ Administration of IV oxytocin (Pitocin)
    - ▪ Nipple stimulation to trigger the release of endogenous oxytocin
- • Indications
  - ○ Any condition in which augmentation or induction of labor is indicated. Elective induction for nonmedical indications must meet the criteria of at least 39 weeks of gestation and a Bishop score of greater than 8 for a multiparous client and greater than 10 for a nulliparous (ACOG, 2012). Elective inductions that do not meet recommended criteria can result in increased risk for infection, premature delivery, longer labor, and need for cesarean birth.
- • Client Presentation
  - ○ Postterm pregnancy (beyond 42 weeks of gestation)
  - ○ Dystocia (prolonged, difficult labor) due to inadequate uterine contractions.
  - ○ Prolonged rupture of membranes predisposes the client and fetus to risk of infection.

- ○ Maternal medical complications
    - ▪ Rh-isoimmunization
    - ▪ Diabetes mellitus
    - ▪ Pulmonary disease
    - ▪ Gestational hypertension
  - ○ Fetal demise
  - ○ Chorioamnionitis
- • Nursing Actions
  - ○ Prepare the client for cervical ripening.
    - ▪ Obtain the client's informed consent form.
    - ▪ If cervical-ripening agents are used, baseline data on fetal and maternal well-being should be obtained.
    - ▪ The nurse may initiate oxytocin (Pitocin) 6 to 12 hr after administration of the prostaglandin.
    - ▪ The nurse should monitor FHR and uterine activity after administration of cervical-ripening agents.
    - ▪ The nurse should notify the provider if uterine hyperstimulation or fetal distress is noted.
  - ○ Prepare the client for an amniotomy or amniotic membrane stripping.
  - ○ Prepare of the client for oxytocin (Pitocin).
    - ▪ Prior to the administration of oxytocin, it is essential that the nurse confirm that the fetus is engaged in the birth canal at a minimum of station 0.
    - ▪ Use the infusion port closest to the client for administration. Oxytocin should be connected "piggyback" to the main IV line and administered via an infusion pump.
    - ▪ An intrauterine pressure catheter (IUPC) may be used to monitor frequency, duration, and intensity of contractions.
    - ▪ When oxytocin is administered, assessments include maternal blood pressure, pulse, and respirations every 30 min and with every change in dose.
    - ▪ Monitor FHR and contraction pattern every 15 min and with every change in dose.
    - ▪ Assess fluid intake and urinary output.
    - ▪ A Bishop score rating should be obtained prior to starting any labor induction protocol.
  - ○ Ongoing care
    - ▪ Assist with or perform administration of labor induction agents as prescribed.
      - □ Increase oxytocin as prescribed until desired contraction pattern is obtained and then maintain the dose if there is a:
        - ▸ Contraction frequency of 2 to 3 min.
        - ▸ Contraction duration of 60 to 90 seconds.
        - ▸ Contraction intensity of 40 to 90 mm Hg on IUPC.
        - ▸ Uterine resting tone of 10 to 15 mm Hg.
        - ▸ Cervical dilation of 1 cm/hr.
        - ▸ Reassuring FHR between 110 to 160/min.

- Discontinue oxytocin if uterine hyperstimulation occurs. Symptoms of uterine hyperstimulation include the following:
  - □ Contraction frequency more often than every 2 min.
  - □ Contraction duration longer than 90 seconds.
  - □ Contraction intensity that results in pressures greater than 90 mm Hg as shown by IUPC.
  - □ Uterine resting tone greater than 20 mm Hg between contractions.
  - □ No relaxation of uterus between contractions
- Complications
  - A nonreassuring FHR is noted.
    - □ An abnormal baseline less than 110 or greater than 160/min
    - □ Loss of variability
    - □ Late or prolonged decelerations
- Interventions
  - Notify the provider.
  - Position the client in a side-lying position to increase uteroplacental perfusion.
  - Keep the IV line open and increase the rate of IV fluid administration to 200 mL/hr unless contraindicated.
  - Administer O_2 by a face mask at 8 to 10 L/min as prescribed.
  - Administer the tocolytic terbutaline (Brethine) 0.25 mg subcutaneously as prescribed to diminish uterine activity.
  - Monitor FHR and patterns in conjunction with uterine activity.
  - Document responses to interventions.
  - If unable to restore reassuring FHR, prepare for an emergency cesarean birth.

AUGMENTATION OF LABOR

Overview

- Description of Procedure
  - Augmentation of labor is the stimulation of hypotonic contractions once labor has spontaneously begun, but progress is inadequate.
  - Certain providers favor active management of labor to establish effective labor with the aggressive use of oxytocin (Pitocin) or rupture of membranes. This ensures that the client delivers within 12 hr of admission to the labor unit so that the risk of cesarean birth will be decreased.
- Risk factors requiring augmentation of labor, administration procedures, nursing assessments and interventions, and possible procedure complications are the same for labor induction.

AMNIOTOMY

Overview

- Description of Procedure
  - An amniotomy is the artificial rupture of the amniotic membranes (AROM) by the provider using an Amnihook or other sharp instrument.
  - Labor typically begins within 12 hr after the membranes rupture.
  - The client is at an increased risk for cord prolapse or infection.
- Indications
  - Labor progression is too slow and augmentation or induction of labor is indicated.
  - An amnioinfusion is indicated for cord compression.
- Nursing Actions
  - Ongoing care
    - Ensure that the presenting part of the fetus is engaged prior to an amniotomy to prevent cord prolapse.
    - Monitor FHR prior to and following AROM to assess for cord prolapse as evidenced by variable or late decelerations.
    - Assess and document characteristics of amniotic fluid including color, odor, and consistency.
  - Interventions
    - Document the time of rupture.
    - Obtain temperature every 2 hr.

AMNIOINFUSION

Overview

- Description of Procedure
  - An amnioinfusion of 0.9% sodium chloride or lactated Ringer's solution, as prescribed, is instilled into the amniotic cavity through a transcervical catheter introduced into the uterus to supplement the amount of amniotic fluid. The instillation will reduce the severity of variable decelerations caused by cord compression.
- Indications
  - Potential diagnoses
    - Oligohydramnios (scant amount or absence of amniotic fluid) caused by any of the following:
      - Uteroplacental insufficiency
      - Premature rupture of membranes
      - Postmaturity of the fetus
    - Fetal cord compression secondary to:
      - Postmaturity of fetus (macrosomic, large body), which places the fetus at risk for variable deceleration from cord compression

- Nursing Actions
  - Interventions
    - Assist with the amniotomy if membranes have not already ruptured. Membranes must have ruptured to perform an amnioinfusion.
    - Warm fluid using a blood warmer prior to infusion.
    - Perform nursing measures to maintain comfort and dryness because the infused fluid will leak continuously.
    - Monitor the client to prevent uterine overdistention and increased uterine tone, which can initiate, accelerate, or intensify uterine contractions and cause nonreassuring FHR changes.
    - Continually assess intensity and frequency of the client's uterine contractions.
    - Continually monitor FHR.
    - Monitor fluid output from vagina to prevent uterine overdistention.

VACUUM-ASSISTED DELIVERY

Overview

- Description of Procedure
  - A vacuum-assisted birth involves the use of a cuplike suction device that is attached to the fetal head. Traction is applied during contractions to assist in the descent and birth of the head, after which, the vacuum cup is released and removed preceding delivery of the fetal body.
  - Recommendations by the manufacturer should be followed for product use to ensure safety.
  - Conditions for use of a vacuum-assisted birth
    - Vertex presentation
    - Absence of cephalopelvic disproportion
    - Ruptured membranes
  - Risks associated with vacuum-assisted births
    - Scalp lacerations
    - Subdural hematoma of the neonate
    - Cephalohematoma
    - Maternal lacerations to the cervix, vagina, or perineum
- Indications
  - Maternal exhaustion and ineffective pushing efforts
  - Fetal distress during second stage of labor

- Nursing Actions
  - Preparation of the client
    - Provide the client and her partner with support and education regarding the procedure.
    - Assist the client into the lithotomy position to allow for sufficient traction of the vacuum cup when it is applied to the fetal head.
    - Assess and record FHR before and during vacuum assistance.
    - Assess for bladder distention, and catheterize if necessary.
  - Ongoing care
    - Prepare for a forceps-assisted birth if a vacuum-assisted birth is not successful.
  - Interventions
    - Alert postpartum care providers that vacuum assistance was used.
    - Observe the neonate for lacerations, cephalohematomas, or subdural hematomas after delivery.
    - Check the neonate for caput succedaneum. Caput succedaneum is a normal occurrence and should resolve within 24 hr.

FORCEPS-ASSISTED BIRTH

Overview

- Description of Procedure
  - A forceps-assisted birth consists of using an instrument with two curved spoon-like blades to assist in the delivery of the fetal head. Traction is applied during contractions.
- Indications
  - Client presentation
    - Fetal distress during labor
    - Abnormal presentation or a breech position requiring delivery of the head
    - Arrest of rotation
- Nursing Actions
  - Preparation of the client
    - Explain the procedure to the client and her partner.
    - Assist the client into the lithotomy position.
    - Assess to ensure that the client's bladder is empty, and catheterize if necessary.
    - Assess to ensure that the fetus is engaged and that membranes have ruptured.
    - Assess and record FHR before, during, and after forceps assistance.
  - Ongoing care
    - Assist with the procedure as necessary.

- ○ Interventions
  - Assess and record FHR before, during, and after forceps assistance.
    - □ Compression of the cord between the fetal head and forceps will cause a decrease in the FHR.
    - □ If a FHR decrease occurs, the forceps are removed and reapplied.
  - Observe the neonate for bruising and abrasions at the site of forceps application after delivery.
  - Check the client for any possible injuries after birth.
    - □ Vaginal or cervical lacerations indicated by bleeding in spite of contracted uterus
    - □ Urine retention resulting from bladder or urethral injuries
    - □ Hematoma formation in the pelvic soft tissues resulting from blood vessel damage
  - Report to the postpartum nursing caregivers that forceps or vacuum-assisted delivery methods were used.
- • Complications
  - ○ Lacerations of the cervix
  - ○ Lacerations of the vagina and perineum
  - ○ Injury to the bladder
  - ○ Facial nerve palsy of the neonate
  - ○ Facial bruising on the neonate

EPISIOTOMY

Overview

- • Description of Procedure
  - ○ An episiotomy is an incision made into the perineum to enlarge the vaginal opening to facilitate delivery and minimize soft tissue damage.
- • Indications for an episiotomy
  - ○ Shorten the second stage of labor
  - ○ Facilitate forceps-assisted or vacuum-assisted delivery
  - ○ Prevent cerebral hemorrhage in a fragile preterm fetus
  - ○ Facilitate birth of a macrosomic (large) infant
- • The site and direction of the incision designates the type of episiotomy.
  - ○ A median (midline) episiotomy extends from the vaginal outlet toward the rectum, and is the most commonly used.
    - Easier to repair
    - Less blood loss
    - Associated with a higher incidence of third- and fourth-degree lacerations

- A mediolateral episiotomy extends from the vaginal outlet posterolateral, either to the left or right of the midline, and is used when posterior extension is likely.
  - Third-degree laceration may occur.
  - Blood loss is greater, and the repair is more difficult.
  - Local anesthetic is administered to the perineum prior to the incision.
- Nursing Actions
  - Ongoing care
    - Encourage alternate labor positions to reduce pressure on the perineum and promote perineal stretching to reduce the necessity for an episiotomy.

CESAREAN BIRTH

Overview

- Description of Procedure
  - A cesarean birth is the delivery of the fetus through a transabdominal incision of the uterus to preserve the life or health of the client and fetus when there is evidence of complications.
    - Incisions are made horizontally into the lower segment of the uterus.
- Indications
  - Potential diagnoses
    - Malpresentation, particularly breech presentation
    - Cephalopelvic disproportion
    - Fetal distress
    - Placental abnormalities
      - Placenta previa
      - Abruptio placenta
    - High-risk pregnancy
      - Positive HIV status
      - Hypertensive disorders such as preeclampsia and eclampsia
      - Diabetes mellitus
      - Active genital herpes lesions
    - Previous cesarean birth
    - Dystocia
    - Multiple gestations
    - Umbilical cord prolapse

- Preprocedure
  - Nursing actions
    - Assess and record FHR and vital signs.
    - Assist with obtaining an ultrasound to determine whether a cesarean birth is indicated.
    - Position the client in a supine position with a wedge under one hip to prevent compression of the vena cava.
    - Insert an indwelling urinary catheter.
    - Apply anti-embolism stockings and sequential compression device.
    - Administer preoperative medications as prescribed.
    - Prepare the surgical site.
    - Insert an IV catheter, and initiate administration of IV fluids as prescribed.
    - Obtain an informed consent form from the client.
    - Determine whether the client has had nothing by mouth since midnight before the procedure. If the client has, notify the anesthesiologist.
    - Ensure that preoperative diagnostic tests are complete, including an Rh-factor test.
  - Client education
    - Explain the procedure to the client and her partner.
    - Provide emotional support.
- Intraprocedure
  - Nursing actions
    - Assist in positioning the client on the operating table.
    - Continue to monitor FHR.
    - Continue to monitor vital signs, IV fluids, and urinary output.
- Postprocedure
  - Nursing actions
    - Monitor for evidence of infection and excessive bleeding at the incision site.
    - Assess the uterine fundus for firmness or tenderness.
    - Assess the lochia for amount and characteristics.
      - A tender uterus and foul-smelling lochia may indicate endometritis.
    - Assess for productive cough or chills, which could be a manifestation of pneumonia.
    - Assess for indications of thrombophlebitis, which include tenderness, pain, and heat on palpation.
    - Monitor I&O.
    - Monitor vital signs per protocol.
    - Provide pain relief and antiemetics as prescribed.
    - Encourage the client to turn, cough, and deep breathe to prevent pulmonary complications.
    - Encourage splinting of the incision with pillows.
    - Encourage ambulation to prevent thrombus formation.
    - Assess the client for burning and pain on urination, which could be suggestive of a urinary tract infection.

- Complications
  - Maternal
    - Aspiration
    - Amniotic fluid pulmonary embolism
    - Wound infection
    - Wound dehiscence
    - Severe abdominal pain
    - Thrombophlebitis
    - Hemorrhage
    - Urinary tract infection
    - Injuries to the bladder or bowel
    - Anesthesia associated complications
  - Fetal
    - Premature birth of fetus if gestational age is inaccurate
    - Fetal injuries during surgery

VAGINAL DELIVERY AFTER CESAREAN BIRTH

Overview

- A vaginal birth after cesarean birth is when the client delivers vaginally after having had a previous cesarean birth.
- Indications
  - Client presentation
    - Previous documented low-segment transverse incision
    - No current contraindications
      - Large for gestational age newborn
      - Malpresentation
      - Cephalopelvic disproportion
      - Previous classical vertical uterine incision
- Nursing Actions
  - Preprocedure
    - Nursing actions
      - Review medical records for evidence of a previous low-segment transverse cesarean incision.
    - Client education
      - Explain the procedure to the client and her partner.

- ○ Intraprocedure
  - ▪ Nursing actions
    - ▫ Assess and record FHR during the labor.
    - ▫ Assess and record contraction patterns for strength, duration, and frequency of contractions.
    - ▫ Assess for evidence of uterine rupture.
    - ▫ Promote relaxation and breathing techniques during labor.
    - ▫ Provide analgesia as prescribed and requested.
- ○ Postprocedure
  - ▪ Nursing actions
    - ▫ Nursing interventions for a vaginal delivery after a cesarean birth are the same as for a vaginal delivery.

APPLICATION EXERCISES

1. A nurse is caring for a client who is at 42 weeks of gestation and is admitted to the labor and delivery unit. During an ultrasound, it is noted that the fetus is large for gestational age. The nurse reviews the prescription from the provider to begin an amnioinfusion. The nurse should know that an amnioinfusion is indicated for which of the following reasons? (Select all that apply.)

_____X_____ A. Oligohydramnios

_____ B. Hydramnios

_____X_____ C. Fetal cord compression

_____ D. Hydration

_____ E. Fetal immaturity

2. A nurse is caring for a client who has been in labor for 12 hr, and her membranes are intact. The provider has decided to perform an amniotomy in an effort to facilitate the progress of labor. The nurse performs a vaginal examination to ensure which of the following prior to the performance of the amniotomy?

A. Fetal engagement

B. Fetal lie

C. Fetal attitude

D. Fetal position

3. A nurse is caring for client who had no prenatal care, is Rh-negative and will undergo an external version at 37 weeks of gestation. The nurse anticipates a prescription for which of the following medications to be administered prior to the version?

A. Prostaglandin gel (Cervidil)

B. Magnesium sulfate

C. $Rh_o(D)$ immune globulin (RhoGAM)

D. Oxytocin (Pitocin)

4. A nurse is caring for a client who is receiving oxytocin (Pitocin) for induction of labor and has an intrauterine pressure catheter (IUPC) placed to monitor uterine contractions. For which of the following contraction patterns should the nurse discontinue the infusion of oxytocin?

A. Frequency of every 2 min

B. Duration of 90 to 120 seconds

C. Intensity of 60 to 90 mm Hg

D. Resting tone of 15 mm Hg

5. A nurse educator in the labor and delivery unit is reviewing the use of chemical agents to promote cervical ripening with a group of newly hired nurses. Which of the following statements by a nurse indicates understanding of the teaching?

A. "They are administered in an oral form."

B. "They act by absorbing fluid from tissues."

C. "They promote dilation of the os."

D. "They include an amniotomy."

6. A nurse is planning care for a client who experienced a cesarean birth. What should be included in the plan of care? Use the ATI Active Learning Template: Therapeutic Procedure to complete this item to include the following:

A. Procedure: Describe.

B. Indications: Describe at least four.

C. Nursing Actions: Describe four that are preprocedure.

D. Complications: Describe two that are maternal and two that are fetal.

APPLICATION EXERCISES KEY

1. A. **CORRECT:** Oligohydramnios is an indication for an amnioinfusion because inadequate amniotic fluid can contribute to intrauterine growth restriction of the fetus, restrict fetal movement, and cause fetal distress during labor.

   B. INCORRECT: Hydramnios is excessive amniotic fluid.

   C. **CORRECT:** Oligohydramnios results in fetal cord compression, which decreases fetal oxygenation. Amnioinfusion prevents cord compression.

   D. INCORRECT: Amnioinfusion does not increase hydration. IV fluids or oral intake would provide this.

   E. INCORRECT: Fetal immaturity is not a reason for performing an amnioinfusion.

   Ⓝ NCLEX® Connection: Physiological Adaptations, Alterations in Body Systems

2. A. **CORRECT:** Prior to the performance of an amniotomy, the amniotic membranes should have ruptured. It is also imperative that the fetus is engaged at 0 station and at the level of the maternal ischial spines to prevent prolapse of the umbilical cord.

   B. INCORRECT: Fetal lie pertains to the axis of the maternal spine in relation to the fetal spine and is determined by Leopold maneuvers.

   C. INCORRECT: Fetal attitude is the relationship of the fetal extremities and chin to the fetal torso. It is determined by Leopold maneuvers.

   D. INCORRECT: Fetal position refers to the direction of a reference point in the fetal presenting part to the maternal pelvis. It is not a criterion when performing an amniotomy.

   Ⓝ NCLEX® Connection: Health Promotion and Maintenance, Ante/Intra/Postpartum and Newborn Care

3. A. INCORRECT: Prostaglandin gel is a cervical ripening agent and is not administered prior to an external version.

    B. INCORRECT: Magnesium sulfate is a tocolytic, which may be administered prior to the version. But because the client had no prenatal care and is Rh-negative, there is another medication the nurse should anticipate administering.

    C. **CORRECT:** $Rh_o(D)$ immune globulin (RhoGAM) is administered to a Rh-negative client at 28 weeks of gestation. Because this client had no prenatal care, it should be given prior to the version to prevent isoimmunization.

    D. INCORRECT: Oxytocin is administered to increase contraction frequency, intensity and duration. It is not administered prior to an external version.

     NCLEX® Connection: Health Promotion and Maintenance, Ante/Intra/Postpartum and Newborn Care

4. A. INCORRECT: This contraction pattern does not require discontinuing the infusion of oxytocin.

    B. **CORRECT:** Oxytocin is discontinued if uterine hyperstimulation occurs with contraction duration longer than 90 seconds.

    C. INCORRECT: This contraction pattern does not require discontinuing the infusion of oxytocin.

    D. INCORRECT: This contraction pattern does not require discontinuing the infusion of oxytocin.

     NCLEX® Connection: Pharmacological and Parenteral Therapies, Adverse Effects/Contraindications/ Side Effects/Interactions

5. A. **CORRECT:** Chemical agents that promote cervical ripening include medications administered in oral form.

    B. INCORRECT: Hygroscopic sponges, which are a mechanical method to promote cervical ripening, act by absorbing fluid from surrounding tissues to enlarge the cervical opening.

    C. INCORRECT: Mechanical and physical methods promote cervical ripening by dilation.

    D. INCORRECT: An amniotomy is a mechanical method to promote cervical ripening.

     NCLEX® Connection: Pharmacological and Parenteral Therapies, Expected Actions/Outcomes

6. *Using the ATI Active Learning Template: Therapeutic Procedure*

   A. Procedure
      - Delivery of the fetus through a transabdominal incision of the uterus to preserve the life or health of the client and fetus when there is evidence of complications; incisions are made horizontally into the lower uterine segment.

   B. Indications
      - Malpresentation, breech
      - Cephalopelvic disproportion
      - Fetal distress
      - Placenta previa
      - Abruptio placenta
      - HIV-positive status
      - Dystocia
      - Multiple gestations
      - Umbilical cord prolapse
      - Preeclampsia
      - Eclampsia
      - Active herpes lesions
      - Previous cesarean birth

   C. Nursing Actions
      - Assess and record FHR, vital signs.
      - Assist with ultrasound.
      - Position client in a supine position with a wedge under one hip.
      - Insert an indwelling urinary catheter.
      - Administer preoperative medications as prescribed.
      - Prepare the surgical site.
      - Insert an IV catheter, and administer IV fluids as prescribed.
      - Obtain signed informed consent form.
      - Determine client's NPO status.
      - Verify preoperative testing results.
      - Provide emotional support.

   D. Complications
      - Maternal
        - Aspiration
        - Amniotic fluid pulmonary embolism
        - Wound infection
        - Wound dehiscence
        - Severe abdominal pain
        - Thrombophlebitis
        - Hemorrhage
        - Urinary tract infection
        - Injury to bladder or bowel
        - Anesthesia-associated complications
      - Fetal
        - Premature birth
        - Fetal injury during surgery

   Ⓝ NCLEX® Connection: Reduction of Risk Potential, Therapeutic Procedures

chapter 16

Overview

- Complications occurring during the labor process are emergent and require immediate intervention in order to improve maternal fetal outcomes. This chapter explores prolapsed umbilical cord, meconium-stained amniotic fluid, fetal distress, dystocia (dysfunctional labor), precipitous labor, uterine rupture, and anaphylactoid syndrome of pregnancy (amniotic fluid embolism). Assessment findings, interventions, and therapeutic outcomes are discussed.

PROLAPSED UMBILICAL CORD

Overview

- A prolapsed umbilical cord occurs when the umbilical cord is displaced, preceding the presenting part of the fetus, or protruding through the cervix. This results in cord compression and compromised fetal circulation.

 View Image: Prolapsed Cord

Risk Factors

- Rupture of amniotic membranes
- Abnormal fetal presentation (any presentation other than vertex [occiput as presenting part])
- Transverse lie – Presenting part is not engaged, which leaves room for the cord to descend.
- Small-for-gestational-age fetus
- Unusually long umbilical cord
- Multifetal pregnancy
- Cephalopelvic disproportion – due to unusual space between maternal pelvis and presenting part, which allows for cord descent
- Placenta previa
- Intrauterine tumor – prevents engagement of presenting part
- Hydramnios or polyhydramnios

Assessment

- Subjective Data
  - Client reports that she feels something coming through her vagina.
- Objective Data
  - Physical assessment findings
    - Visualization or palpation of the umbilical cord protruding from the introitus
    - FHR monitoring shows variable or prolonged deceleration
    - Excessive fetal activity followed by cessation of movement; suggestive of severe fetal hypoxia

Patient-Centered Care

- Nursing Care
  - Call for assistance immediately.
  - Notify the provider.
  - Use a sterile-gloved hand, insert two fingers into the vagina, and apply finger pressure on either side of the cord to the fetal presenting part to elevate it off of the cord.
  - Reposition the client in a knee-chest, Trendelenburg, or a side-lying position with a rolled towel under the client's right or left hip to relieve pressure on the cord.
  - Apply a warm, sterile, saline-soaked towel to the visible cord to prevent drying and to maintain blood flow.
  - Provide continuous electronic monitoring of FHR for variable decelerations, which indicate fetal asphyxia and hypoxia.
  - Administer oxygen at 8 to 10 L/min via a face mask to improve fetal oxygenation.
  - Initiate IV access, and administer IV fluid bolus.
  - Prepare for a cesarean birth if other measures fail.
  - Inform and educate the client and her partner about the interventions.

MECONIUM-STAINED AMNIOTIC FLUID

Overview

- Meconium passage in the amniotic fluid during the antepartum period prior to the start of labor is typically not associated with an unfavorable fetal outcome.
- The fetus has had an episode of loss of sphincter control, allowing meconium to pass into amniotic fluid.

Risk Factors

- There is an increased incidence for meconium in the amniotic fluid after 38 weeks of gestation due to fetal maturity of normal physiological functions.
- Umbilical cord compression results in fetal hypoxia that stimulates the vagal nerve in mature fetuses.
- Hypoxia stimulates the vagal nerve, which induces peristalsis of the fetal gastrointestinal tract and relaxation of the anal sphincter.

Assessment

- Objective Data
  - Physical assessment findings
    - Amniotic fluid may vary in color – black to greenish, yellow, or brown. Consistency may be thin or heavy.
    - Criteria for evaluation of meconium-stained amniotic fluid
      - Often present in breech presentation, and may not indicate fetal hypoxia
      - Present with no changes in FHR
      - Stained fluid accompanied by variable or late decelerations in FHR (ominous sign)
  - Diagnostic Procedures – electronic fetal monitoring

Patient-Centered Care

- Nursing Care
  - Document color and consistency of stained amniotic fluid.
  - Notify neonatal resuscitation team to be present at birth.
  - Gather equipment needed for neonatal resuscitation.
  - Follow designated suction protocol.
    - Assess neonate's respiratory efforts, muscle tone, and heart rate.
    - Suction mouth and nose using bulb syringe if respiratory efforts strong, muscle tone good, and heart rate greater than 100/min.
    - Suction below the vocal cords using an endotracheal tube before spontaneous breaths occur if respirations are depressed, muscle tone decreased, and heart rate less than 100/min.

FETAL DISTRESS

Overview

- Fetal distress is present when
  - The FHR is below 110/min or above 160/min.
  - The FHR shows decreased or no variability.
  - There is fetal hyperactivity or no fetal activity.

Risk Factors

- Fetal anomalies
- Uterine anomalies
- Complications of labor and birth

Assessment

- Objective Data
  - Nonreassuring FHR pattern with decreased or no variability
  - Diagnostic procedures
    - Monitor uterine contractions.
    - Monitor FHR.
    - Monitor findings of ultrasound and any other prescribed diagnostics.

Patient-Centered Care

- Nursing Care
  - Monitor vital signs and FHR.
  - Position the client in a left side-lying reclining position with legs elevated.
  - Administer 8 to 10 L/min of oxygen via a face mask.
  - Discontinue oxytocin (Pitocin) if being administered.
  - Increase IV fluid rate to treat hypotension if indicated.
  - Prepare the client for an emergency cesarean birth.

DYSTOCIA (DYSFUNCTIONAL LABOR)

Overview

- Dystocia, or dysfunctional labor, is a difficult or abnormal labor related to the five powers of labor (passenger, passageway, powers, position, and psychologic response).
- Atypical uterine contraction patterns prevent the normal process of labor and its progression. Contractions can be hypotonic (weak, inefficient, or completely absent) or hypertonic (excessively frequent, uncoordinated, and of strong intensity with inadequate uterine relaxation) with failure to efface and dilate the cervix.
- Risk factors
  - Short stature, overweight status
  - Age greater than 40 years
  - Uterine abnormalities
  - Pelvic soft tissue obstructions or pelvic contracture
  - Cephalopelvic disproportion (fetal head is larger than maternal pelvis)
  - Fetal macrosomia
  - Fetal malpresentation, malposition
  - Multifetal pregnancy
  - Hypertonic or hypotonic uterus
  - Maternal fatigue, fear, or dehydration
  - Inappropriate timing of anesthesia or analgesics

Assessment

- Objective Data
  - Physical assessment findings
    - Lack of progress in dilatation, effacement, or fetal descent during labor.
      - A hypotonic uterus is easily indentable, even at peak of contractions.
      - A hypertonic uterus cannot be indented, even between contractions.
    - Client is ineffective in pushing with no voluntary urge to bear down.
      - Persistent occiput posterior presentation is when the fetal occiput is directed toward the posterior maternal pelvis rather than the anterior pelvis.
      - Persistent occiput posterior position prolongs labor and the client reports greater back pain as the fetus presses against the maternal sacrum.
  - Diagnostic/Therapeutic Procedures
    - Ultrasound
    - Amniotomy or stripping of membranes if not ruptured
    - Oxytocin (Pitocin) infusion
    - Vacuum-assisted birth
    - Cesarean birth

Patient-Centered Care

- Nursing Care
  - Dysfunctional Labor
    - Assist with application of fetal scalp electrode and/or intrauterine pressure catheter.
    - Assist with amniotomy (artificial rupture of membranes).
    - Encourage client to engage in regular voiding to empty her bladder.
    - Encourage position changes to aid in fetal descent or to open up the pelvic outlet.
      - Assist client to a position on her hands and knees to help the fetus to rotate from a posterior to anterior position.
    - Encourage ambulation to enhance the progression of labor.
    - Encourage hydrotherapy and other relaxation techniques to aid in the progression of labor.
    - Apply counterpressure using fist or heel of hand to sacral area to alleviate discomfort.
    - Assist the client into a beneficial position for pushing and coach her about how to bear down with contractions.
    - Prepare for a possible forceps-assisted, vacuum-assisted, or cesarean birth.
    - Continue monitoring FHR in response to labor.

- ○ Hypertonic Contractions
    - ▪ Maintain hydration.
    - ▪ Promote rest and relaxation, and provide comfort measures between contractions.
    - ▪ Place the client in a lateral position, and provide oxygen by mask.
- • Medications
    - ○ Oxytocin (Pitocin)
        - ▪ Therapeutic intent
            - ▫ Used to augment labor and strengthen uterine contractions
        - ▪ Nursing considerations
            - ▫ Administer oxytocin if prescribed to augment labor. Oxytocin is not administered for hypertonic contractions.
    - ○ Administer analgesics if prescribed (for rest from hypertonic contractions).

PRECIPITOUS LABOR

Overview

- • Precipitous labor is defined as labor that lasts 3 hr or less from the onset of contractions to the time of delivery.

Risk Factors

- ○ Hypertonic uterine dysfunction
    - ▪ Nonproductive, uncoordinated, painful, uterine contractions during labor that are too frequent and too long in duration and do not allow for relaxation of the uterine muscle between contractions (uterine tetany).
    - ▪ Hypertonic contractions do not contribute to the progression of labor (cervical effacement, dilation, and fetal descent).
    - ▪ Hypertonic contractions can result in uteroplacental insufficiency leading to fetal hypoxia.
- ○ Oxytocin (Pitocin) stimulation
    - ▪ Administered to augment or induce labor by increasing intensity and duration of contractions.
    - ▪ Oxytocin stimulation can lead to hypertonic uterine contractions.
- ○ Multiparous client
    - ▪ May move through the stages of labor more rapidly.

Assessment

- Subjective Data (during labor)
  - Low backache
  - Abdominal pressure and cramping
- Objective Data
  - Increased or bloody vaginal discharge
  - Palpable uterine contractions
  - Progress of cervical dilation and effacement
  - Diarrhea
  - Fetal presentation, station, and position
  - Status of amniotic membranes (membranes can be intact or ruptured)
- Physical Assessment Findings (postbirth)
  - Assess maternal perineal area for signs of trauma or lacerations.
  - Assess neonate's color and for signs of hypoxia.
  - Assess for signs of trauma to presenting part of neonate, especially on cephalic presentation.

Patient-Centered Care

- Nursing Care
  - Do not leave the client unattended.
    - Provide reassurance and emotional support to help the client remain calm.
    - Prepare for emergency delivery of the neonate.
  - Encourage the client to pant with an open mouth between contractions to control the urge to push.

Q
EBP

  - Encourage the client to maintain a side-lying position to optimize uteroplacental perfusion and fetal oxygenation.
  - Prepare for rupturing of membranes upon crowning (fetal head visible at perineum) if not already ruptured.
  - Do not attempt to stop delivery.
  - Control rapid delivery by applying light pressure to the perineal area and fetal head, gently pressing upward toward the vagina. This eases the rapid expulsion of the fetus and prevents cerebral damage to the newborn and perineal lacerations to the client.
    - Deliver the fetus between contractions assuring the cord is not around the fetal neck.
    - If the cord is around the fetal neck, attempt to gently slip it over the head. If not possible, clamp the cord with two clamps and cut between the clamps.
  - Suction mucus from the fetal mouth and nose with a bulb syringe when the head appears.

○ Next, deliver the anterior shoulder located under the maternal symphysis pubis: next, the posterior shoulder; and then allow the rest of the fetal body to slip out.

○ Assess for complications of precipitous labor.

- Maternal

  □ Cervical, vaginal, and/or perineal lacerations

  □ Resultant tissue trauma secondary to rapid birth

  □ Uterine rupture

  □ Amniotic fluid embolism

  □ Postpartum hemorrhage

- Fetal/neonate

  □ Fetal hypoxia due to hypertonic contractions or umbilical cord around fetal neck

  □ Fetal intracranial hemorrhage due to head trauma from rapid birth

RUPTURE OF THE UTERUS

Overview

- Complete rupture involves the uterine wall, peritoneal cavity, and/or broad ligament. Internal bleeding is present.

- Incomplete rupture occurs with dehiscence at the site of a prior scar (cesarean birth, surgical intervention). Internal bleeding may not be present.

Risk Factors

○ Congenital uterine abnormality

○ Uterine trauma due to accident or surgery (previous multiple cesarean births)

○ Overdistention of the uterus from a fetus who is large for gestational age, a multifetal gestation, or polyhydramnios

○ Hyperstimulation of the uterus, either spontaneous or from oxytocin (Pitocin) administration

○ External or internal fetal version done to correct malposition of the fetus

○ Forceps-assisted birth

○ Multigravida clients

Assessment

- Subjective Data

  ○ Client reports sensation of "ripping," "tearing," or sharp pain.

  ○ Client reports abdominal pain, uterine tenderness.

- Objective Data
  - Physical assessment findings
    - Nonreassuring FHR with signs of distress, bradycardia, variable and late decelerations, and absent or minimal variability
    - Change in uterine shape and fetal parts palpable
    - Cessation of contractions and loss of fetal station
    - Manifestations of hypovolemic shock: tachypnea, hypotension, pallor, and cool, clammy skin

Patient-Centered Care

- Nursing Care
  - Administer IV fluids.
  - Administer blood product transfusions if prescribed.
  - Prepare the client for an immediate cesarean birth, which may involve a laparotomy and/or hysterectomy.
  - Inform the client and her partner about the treatment.

ANAPHYLACTOID SYNDROME OF PREGNANCY (AMNIOTIC FLUID EMBOLISM)

Overview

- An amniotic fluid embolism occurs when there is a rupture in the amniotic sac or maternal uterine veins accompanied by high intrauterine pressure that causes infiltration of the amniotic fluid into the maternal circulation. The amniotic fluid then travels to and obstructs pulmonary vessels and causes respiratory distress and circulatory collapse.

- Meconium-stained amniotic fluid or fluid containing particulate matter can cause devastating maternal damage because it readily clogs the pulmonary veins completely.

- Serious coagulation problems, such as disseminated intravascular coagulopathy (DIC), can occur.

- Risk factors
  - Multiparity and advanced maternal age
  - Tumultuous labor
  - Placenta previa or abruptio placentae
  - Preeclampsia
  - Oxytocin (Pitocin) administration
  - Fetal macrosomia
  - Hydramnios
  - Fetal demise
  - Meconium-stained amniotic fluid

Assessment

- Subjective Data
  - ○ Report of sudden chest pain
- Objective Data
  - ○ Physical assessment findings
    - Indications of respiratory distress
      - □ Restlessness
      - □ Cyanosis
      - □ Dyspnea
      - □ Pulmonary edema
      - □ Respiratory arrest
    - Indications of coagulation failure
      - □ Bleeding from incisions and venipuncture sites
      - □ Petechiae and ecchymosis
      - □ Uterine atony
    - Indications of circulatory collapse
      - □ Tachycardia
      - □ Hypotension
      - □ Shock
      - □ Cardiac arrest

Patient-Centered Care

- Nursing Care
  - ○ Administer oxygen via a mask at 8 to 10 L/min.
  - ○ Assist with intubation and mechanical ventilation as indicated.
  - ○ Perform cardiopulmonary resuscitation if necessary.
  - ○ Administer IV fluids.
  - ○ Position the client on her side with her pelvis tilted at a 30° angle to displace the uterus.
  - ○ Administer blood products as prescribed to correct coagulation failure.
  - ○ Insert an indwelling urinary catheter, and measure hourly urine output.
  - ○ Monitor maternal and fetal status.
  - ○ Prepare the client for an emergency cesarean birth if the fetus is not yet delivered.

APPLICATION EXERCISES

1. A nurse is caring for a client who is in labor and experiencing incomplete uterine relaxation between hypertonic contractions. The nurse recognizes the adverse effect of this contraction pattern is

    A. prolonged labor.

    B. reduced fetal oxygen supply.

    C. delayed cervical dilation.

    D. increased maternal stress.

2. A nurse is caring for a client who is in active labor and reports severe back pain. During assessment, the fetus is noted to be in the occiput posterior position. Which of the following maternal positions should the nurse suggest to the client to facilitate normal labor progress?

    A. Hands and knees

    B. Lithotomy

    C. Trendelenburg

    D. Supine with a rolled towel under one hip

3. A nurse is caring for a client who is admitted to the labor and delivery unit. With the use of Leopold maneuvers, it is noted that the fetus is in a breech presentation. For which of the following possible complications should the nurse observe?

    A. Precipitous labor

    B. Premature rupture of membranes

    C. Postmaturity syndrome

    D. Prolapsed umbilical cord

4. A nurse is caring for a client who is at 42 weeks of gestation and in active labor. The nurse should understand that the fetus is at risk for which of the following?

    A. Intrauterine growth restriction

    B. Hyperglycemia

    C. Meconium aspiration

    D. Polyhydramnios

5. A nurse is caring for a client in active labor. When last examined 2 hr ago, the client's cervix was 3 cm dilated, 100% effaced, membranes intact, and the fetus was at a -2 station. The client suddenly states "my water broke." The monitor reveals a FHR of 80 to 85/min, and the nurse performs a vaginal examination, noticing clear fluid and a pulsing loop of umbilical cord in the client's vagina. Which of the following actions should the nurse perform first?

 A. Place the client in the Trendelenburg position.

 B. Apply pressure to the presenting part with her fingers.

 C. Administer oxygen at 10 L/min via a face mask.

 D. Call for assistance.

6. A nurse is caring for a client and observes meconium-stained amniotic fluid upon rupture of the client's membranes. What actions should the nurse take? Use the ATI Active Learning Template: Systems Disorder to complete this item to include the following sections:

 A. Assessment: Describe at least two observations the nurse should make.

 B. Risk Factors: Describe two.

 C. Nursing Care: Describe three actions the nurse should take.

APPLICATION EXERCISES KEY

1. A. INCORRECT: Precipitous labor, not prolonged labor, is often the result of hypertonic contractions and inadequate uterine relaxation between contractions.

    B. **CORRECT:** Inadequate uterine relaxation results in reduced oxygen supply to the fetus.

    C. INCORRECT: Hypertonic contractions and inadequate relaxation of the uterus between contractions does not delay cervical dilation.

    D. INCORRECT: A contraction pattern of hypertonic contractions and inadequate relaxation between contractions will increase maternal distress, but this is not an adverse effect.

     NCLEX® Connection: Health Promotion and Maintenance, Ante/Intra/Postpartum and Newborn Care

2. A. **CORRECT:** Having the client assume a position on her hands and knees may help the fetus rotate from a posterior to an anterior position.

    B. INCORRECT: The lithotomy position is when the client lies on her back with her knees elevated and is not used to facilitate labor progress.

    C. INCORRECT: The Trendelenburg position requires the client to lie on her back and does not assist in the rotation of the fetus.

    D. INCORRECT: The supine position with a rolled towel under one hip can assist in preventing vena cava syndrome but does not assist in the rotation of the fetus.

    NCLEX® Connection: Basic Care and Comfort, Non-Pharmacological Comfort Interventions

3. A. INCORRECT: Breech presentation would most likely cause dystocia (prolonged, difficult labor) rather than a precipitous labor.

    B. INCORRECT: Breech presentation has no effect on rupture of the membranes.

    C. INCORRECT: Breech presentation is not associated with postmaturity syndrome.

    D. **CORRECT:** A prolapsed umbilical cord is a potential complication for a fetus in a breech presentation.

    NCLEX® Connection: Health Promotion and Maintenance, Ante/Intra/Postpartum and Newborn Care

4.   A. INCORRECT: Intrauterine growth restriction occurs earlier in the pregnancy and not at this point.

  B. INCORRECT: A postterm neonate is at risk for hypoglycemia, not hyperglycemia.

  C. **CORRECT:** Postterm neonates are at risk for aspiration of meconium.

  D. INCORRECT: Postterm pregnancies result in oligohydramnios, not polyhydramnios.

  (N) NCLEX® Connection: Physiological Adaptations, Alterations in Body Systems

5.   A. INCORRECT: This is not the first action the nurse should take. There is another action the nurse should perform first.

  B. INCORRECT: This is not the first action the nurse should take. There is another action the nurse should perform first.

  C. INCORRECT: This is not the first action the nurse should take. There is another action the nurse should perform first.

  D. **CORRECT:** Calling for assistance is the first action the nurse should take.

  (N) NCLEX® Connection: Physiological Adaptations, Medical Emergencies

6.   *Using ATI Active Learning Template: Systems Disorder*

  A. Assessment
    • Color and consistency
    • FHR pattern (presence of decelerations)

  B. Risk Factors
    • 38 weeks or later in gestation
    • Episodes of fetal hypoxia due to cord compression

  C. Nursing Care
    • Document color and consistency of amniotic fluid.
    • Notify neonatal resuscitation team to be present at birth.
    • Gather equipment needed for neonatal resuscitation and make available.
    • Follow designated suction protocol.
    • Assess neonate's respiratory efforts, muscle tone, and heart rate.
      ○ If respiratory efforts are strong, muscle tone good, and heart rate greater than 100/min, suction mouth and nose using bulb syringe.
      ○ If respirations are depressed, muscle tone decreased, and heart rate less than 100/min, suction below the vocal cords using an endotracheal tube before spontaneous breaths occur.

  (N) NCLEX® Connection: Physiological Adaptations, Alterations in Body Systems

UNIT 3 ## Postpartum Nursing Care

SECTIONS

› Routine Postpartum Care
› Complications of the Postpartum Period

NCLEX® CONNECTIONS

When reviewing the chapters in this unit, keep in mind the relevant sections of the NCLEX® outline, in particular:

Client Needs: Health Promotion and Maintenance	Client Needs: Pharmacological and Parenteral Therapies	Client Needs: Reduction of Risk Potential

› Relevant topics/tasks include:
» Ante/Intra/Postpartum and Newborn Care
  › Provide postpartum care and education.
» Developmental Stages and Transitions
  › Assist the client to cope with life transitions.
» Health Promotion/Disease Prevention
  › Provide information about health promotion and maintenance recommendations (e.g., physician visits, immunizations).
	› Relevant topics/tasks include:
	» Adverse Effects/ Contraindications/Side Effects/Interactions
	  › Notify the provider of side effects, adverse effects, and contraindications of medications and parenteral therapy.
	» Expected Actions/Outcomes
	  › Evaluate client response to medication (e.g., therapeutic effects, side effects, adverse reactions).
	» Medication Administration
	  › Review pertinent data prior to medication administration (e.g., contraindications, lab results, allergies, potential interactions).
		› Relevant topics/tasks include:
		» Changes/Abnormalities in Vital Signs
		  › Assess and respond to changes in the client's vital signs.
		» Laboratory Values
		  › Educate the client about the purpose and procedure of prescribed laboratory tests.
		» Potential for Complications from Surgical Procedures and Health Alterations
		  › Apply knowledge of pathophysiology to monitoring for complications.

chapter 17

Overview

- It is important for a nurse to provide comfort measures for the client during the fourth stage of labor. This maternal recovery period starts with the delivery of the placenta and lasts from 1 to 4 hr. Also during this stage, parent-newborn bonding should begin to occur.

- The main goal during the immediate postpartum period is to prevent postpartum hemorrhage. Other goals include assisting in a client's recovery, identifying deviations in the expected recovery process, providing comfort measures and pharmacologic pain relief as prescribed, providing client education about newborn and self-care, and providing baby-friendly activities to promote infant/family bonding.

- The postpartum period, also known as the puerperium, includes physiological and psychological adjustments. This period begins after the delivery of the placenta and ends when the body returns to the prepregnant state. This process takes approximately 6 weeks.

  ○ Physiological maternal changes consist of uterine involution; lochia flow; cervical involution; decrease in vaginal distention; alteration in ovarian function and menstruation; and cardiovascular, urinary tract, breast, and gastrointestinal tract changes.

  ○ The greatest risks during the postpartum period are hemorrhage, shock, and infection.

  ○ Oxytocin, a hormone released from the pituitary gland, coordinates and strengthens uterine contractions.

    ▪ Breastfeeding stimulates the release of endogenous oxytocin from the pituitary gland.

    ▪ Pitocin (exogenous oxytocin) may be administered postpartum to improve the quality of the uterine contractions. A firm and contracted uterus prevents excessive bleeding and hemorrhage.

    ▪ Uncomfortable uterine cramping is referred to as afterpains.

  ○ After delivery of the placenta, hormones (estrogen, progesterone, and placental enzyme insulinase) decrease, thus resulting in decreased blood glucose, estrogen, and progesterone levels.

    ▪ Decreased estrogen is associated with breast engorgement, diaphoresis (profuse perspiration), and diuresis (increased formation and excretion of urine) of excess extracellular fluid accumulated during pregnancy.

    ▪ Decreased estrogen diminishes vaginal lubrication. Local dryness and intercourse discomfort may persist until ovarian function returns and menstruation resumes.

    ▪ Decreased progesterone results in an increase in muscle tone throughout the body.

    ▪ Decreased placental enzyme insulinase results in reversal of the diabetogenic effects of pregnancy, which lowers blood glucose levels immediately in the puerperium.

- ○ Lactating and nonlactating women differ in the timing of the first ovulation and the resumption of menstruation.

    - ▪ In lactating women, the serum prolactin levels remain elevated and suppress ovulation.

        - □ The return of ovulation is influenced by breastfeeding frequency, the length of each feeding, and the use of supplementation.

        - □ The infant's suck is also believed to affect prolactin levels.

        - □ Length of time to the first postpartum ovulation is approximately 6 months.

    - ▪ In nonlactating women, prolactin declines and reaches the prepregnant level by the third week postpartum.

        - □ Ovulation occurs 27 to 75 days after birth.

        - □ Menses resume by 4 to 6 weeks postpartum.

- ○ Therapeutic and diagnostic procedures and nursing considerations

    - ▪ Rh-negative mothers

        - □ $RH_O(D)$ immune globulin (RhoGAM) is administered within 72 hr to women who are Rh-negative and gave birth to infants who are Rh-positive to prevent sensitization in future pregnancies.

        - □ The Kleihauer-Betke test determines the amount of fetal blood in maternal circulation if a large fetomaternal transfusion is suspected. If 15 mL or more of fetal blood is detected, the mother should receive an increased RhoGAM dose.

        - □ Laboratory tests may include CBC with monitoring of Hgb, Hct, and WBC and platelet counts.

- ○ Nursing assessments and interventions

    - ▪ Postpartum assessments immediately following delivery include monitoring vital signs, uterine firmness and its location in relation to the umbilicus, uterine position in relation to the midline of the abdomen, and amount of vaginal bleeding.

        - □ If the client is stable, vital signs will be monitored every 15 min x 4 for the first hour, every 30 min x 2 for the second hr, hourly x 2 for at least 2 hr, then every 4 to 8 hr depending on the prescriptions set forth by the provider.

M View Video: Postpartum Assessment

    - ▪ A focused postpartum physical assessment should include assessing the client's

        - □ B – Breasts

        - □ U – Uterus (fundal height, uterine placement, and consistency)

        - □ B – Bowel and GI function

        - □ B – Bladder function

        - □ L – Lochia (color, odor, consistency, and amount [COCA])

        - □ E – Episiotomy (edema, ecchymosis, approximation)

        - □ Vital signs, to include pain assessment

        - □ Teaching needs

Thermoregulation

- Postpartum chill, which occurs in the first 2 hr puerperium, is an uncontrollable shaking chill immediately following birth. Postpartum chill is possibly related to a nervous system response, vasomotor changes, a shift in fluids, and/or the work of labor. This is a normal occurrence unless accompanied by an elevated temperature.
  - ○ Provide warm blankets and fluids.
  - ○ Assure client that these chills are a self-limiting, common occurrence that will last only a short while.

Fundus

- Physical changes of the uterus include involution of the uterus. Involution occurs with contractions of the uterine smooth muscle, whereby the uterus returns to its prepregnant state. The uterus also rapidly decreases in size from approximately 1,000 g (2.2 lb) to 50 to 60 g over a period of 6 weeks with the fundal height steadily descending into the pelvis approximately one fingerbreadth (1 cm) per day.

 View Image: Fundal Height

  - ○ Immediately after delivery, the fundus should be firm, midline with the umbilicus, and approximately at the level of the umbilicus. At 12 hr postpartum, the fundus may be palpated at 1 cm above the umbilicus.
  - ○ Every 24 hr, the fundus should descend approximately 1 to 2 cm. It should be halfway between the symphysis pubis and the umbilicus by the sixth postpartum day.
  - ○ By day 10, the uterus should lie within the true pelvis and should not be palpable.
- The nurse should assess the fundal height, uterine placement, and uterine consistency at least every 8 hr after the recovery period has ended.
  - ○ Explain the procedure to the client.
  - ○ Apply clean gloves, a lower perineal pad, and observe lochia flow as the fundus is palpated.
  - ○ Cup one hand just above the symphysis pubis to support the lower segment of the uterus, and with the other hand, palpate the client's abdomen to locate the fundus.
  - ○ Document the fundal height, location, and uterine consistency.
    - Determine the fundal height by placing fingers on the abdomen and measuring how many fingerbreadths (centimeters) fit between the fundus and the umbilicus above, below, or at the umbilical level.
    - Determine whether the fundus is midline in the pelvis or displaced laterally (caused by a full bladder).
    - Determine whether the fundus is firm or boggy. If the fundus is boggy (not firm), lightly massage the fundus in a circular motion.

- Nursing interventions related to uterine involution
  - Administer oxytocics intramuscularly or IV as prescribed after the placenta is delivered to promote uterine contractions and to prevent hemorrhage.
    - Oxytocics include oxytocin (Pitocin), methylergonovine maleate (Methergine), and carboprost tromethamine (Hemabate). Misoprostol (Cytotec), a prostaglandin, also may be administered.
  - Monitor for adverse affects of medications.
    - Oxytocin and misoprostol may cause hypotension.
    - Methylergonovine maleate, ergonovine maleate, and carboprost tromethamine may cause hypertension.
  - Encourage early breastfeeding for a client who is lactating. This will stimulate the production of natural oxytocin and prevent hemorrhage.
  - Encourage emptying of the bladder every 2 to 3 hr to prevent possible uterine displacement and atony.

Lochia

- Physical changes in vaginal discharge include lochia, which is the blood flow from the uterus during puerperium.
  - Three stages of lochia
    - Lochia rubra – bright red color, bloody consistency, fleshy odor, may contain small clots, transient flow increases during breastfeeding and upon rising. Lasts 1 to 3 days after delivery.
    - Lochia serosa – pinkish brown color and serosanguineous consistency. Lasts from approximately day 4 to day 10 after delivery.
    - Lochia alba – yellowish, white creamy color, fleshy odor. Lasts from approximately day 11 up to and beyond 6 weeks postpartum.
  - Lochia amount is assessed by the quantity of saturation on the perineal pad as being either:
    - Scant (less than 2.5 cm)
    - Light (less than 10 cm)
    - Moderate (more than 10 cm)
    - Heavy (one pad saturated within 2 hr)
    - Excessive blood loss (one pad saturated in 15 min or less, or pooling of blood under buttocks)

M   View Image: Vaginal Bleeding

- The nurse should assess the lochia flow for normal color, amount, and consistency.
  - Lochia typically trickles from the vaginal opening but flows more steadily during uterine contractions.
  - Assess for pooled lochia on the pad under the client, which may not be felt by the client. Massaging the uterus or ambulation may result in a gush of lochia with the expression of clots and dark blood that has pooled in the vagina, but should soon decrease back to a trickle of bright red lochia when in the early puerperium.

- Nursing interventions for abnormal lochia include notifying the provider and performing prescribed interventions based on the cause of the abnormality.

  ○ Abnormal lochia is evidenced by

    ▪ Excessive spurting of bright red blood from the vagina, possibly indicating a cervical or vaginal tear.

    ▪ Numerous large clots and excessive blood loss (saturation of one pad in 15 min or less), which may indicate hemorrhage.

    ▪ Foul odor, which is suggestive of infection.

    ▪ Persistent lochia rubra in the early postpartum period beyond day 3, which may indicate retained placental fragments.

    ▪ Continued flow of lochia serosa or alba beyond the normal length of time may indicate endometritis, especially if it is accompanied by fever, pain, or abdominal tenderness.

Cervix, Vagina, and Perineum

- Physical changes of the cervix, vagina, and perineum are as follows:

  ○ The cervix is soft directly after birth and may be edematous, bruised, and have small lacerations. Within 2 to 3 days postpartum, it shortens, regains its form, and becomes firm, with the os gradually closing.

    ▪ Lacerations can delay the production of estrogen-influenced cervical mucus and are a predisposing factor to infection.

  ○ The vagina, which has distended, gradually returns to its prepregnancy size with the reappearance of rugae and a thickening of the vaginal mucosa. However, muscle tone is never restored completely.

  ○ The soft tissues of the perineum may be erythematous and edematous, especially in areas of an episiotomy or lacerations. Hematomas or hemorrhoids may be present. The pelvic floor muscles may be overstretched and weak.

- The nurse should assess for cervical, vaginal, and perineal healing.

  ○ Observe the perineum for erythema, edema, and hematoma.

  ○ Assess episiotomy and lacerations for approximation, drainage, quantity, and quality.

    ▪ A bright red trickle of blood from the episiotomy site in the early postpartum period is a normal finding.

- Nursing interventions for perineal tenderness, laceration, and episiotomy

  ○ Promote measures for the client to help soften her stools.

  ○ Educate the client about proper cleansing to prevent infection.

    ▪ The client should wash her hands thoroughly before and after voiding.

    ▪ The client should use a squeeze bottle filled with warm water or antiseptic solution after each voiding to cleanse the perineal area.

    ▪ The client should clean her perineal area from front to back (urethra to anus).

- The client should blot dry, not wipe.

- The client should sparingly use a topical application of antiseptic cream or spray.

- The client's perineal pad should be changed from front to back after voiding or defecating.

○ Promote comfort measures.

- Apply ice packs to the client's perineum for the first 24 to 48 hr to reduce edema and provide anesthetic effect.

- Encourage sitz baths at a temperature of 38° to 40° C (100° to 104° F) or cooler at least twice a day.

- Administer analgesia, such as nonopioids (acetaminophen [Tylenol]), nonsteroidal anti-inflammatories (ibuprofen [Advil]), and opioids (codeine, hydrocodone), as prescribed for pain and discomfort.

- Opioid analgesia may be administered via a PCA (patient-controlled analgesia) pump after cesarean birth. Continuous epidural infusions may also be used for pain control after cesarean birth.

- Apply topical anesthetics (Americaine spray or Dermoplast) to the client's perineal area as needed or witch hazel compresses (Tuck's Pads) to the rectal area for hemorrhoids.

Breasts

- Physical changes of the breasts include the secretion of colostrum, which occurs during pregnancy and 2 to 3 days immediately after birth. Milk is produced 2 to 3 days after the delivery of the newborn.

- The nurse should assess the client's breasts as well as her ability to assist the newborn with latching on if breastfeeding.

○ Colostrum secretion in lactating and nonlactating clients.

○ Engorgement of the breast tissue as a result of lymphatic circulation, milk production, and temporary vein congestion.

○ Redness and tenderness of the breast.

○ Cracked nipples and indications of mastitis (infection in a milk duct of the breast with concurrent flulike symptoms).

○ Ascertain that the newborn who is breastfeeding has latched on correctly to prevent sore nipples.

○ Ineffective newborn feeding patterns related to maternal dehydration, maternal discomfort, newborn positioning, or difficulty with the newborn latching onto the breast.

- Nursing interventions pertaining to the client's breasts and breastfeeding

○ Encourage early demand breastfeeding for the client who is lactating, which will also stimulate the production of natural oxytocin and help prevent uterine hemorrhage.

○ Assist the client into a comfortable position, and have her try various positions during breastfeeding (cradle hold, side-lying, and football hold) Explain how varying positions can prevent nipple soreness.

○ Teach the client the importance of proper latch techniques (the newborn takes in part of the areola and nipple, not just the tip of the nipple) to prevent nipple soreness.

○ Inform the client that breastfeeding causes the release of oxytocin, which stimulates uterine contractions. This is a normal occurrence and beneficial to uterine tone.

Cardiovascular System and Fluid and Hematologic Status

- Physical changes in the cardiovascular system during the postpartum period
  - The cardiovascular system undergoes a decrease in blood volume during the postpartum period related to:
    - Blood loss during childbirth (average blood loss is 500 mL in an uncomplicated vaginal delivery and 1,000 mL for a cesarean birth).
    - Diaphoresis and diuresis of the excess fluid accumulated during the last part of the pregnancy. Loss occurs within the first 2 to 3 days postdelivery.
  - Hypovolemic shock does not usually occur in response to the normal blood loss of labor and birth because of the expanded blood volume of pregnancy and the readjustment in the maternal vasculature, which occurs in response to the following:
    - Elimination of the placenta, diverting 500 to 750 mL of blood into the maternal systemic circulation.
    - Rapid reduction in the size of the uterus, putting more blood into the maternal systemic circulation.
- Physical changes in blood values, coagulation factors, and fibrinogen levels during the puerperium
  - Increased Hct and Hgb values are present immediately after delivery for up to 72 hr. Leukocytosis (white blood cell count elevation) of up to 20,000 to 25,000/mm³ occurs for the first 10 to 14 days without the presence of infection and then returns to normal.
  - Coagulation factors and fibrinogen levels increase during pregnancy and remain elevated for 2 to 3 weeks postpartum. Hypercoagulability predisposes the postpartum client to thrombus formation and thromboembolism.
- Vital sign changes
  - Blood pressure is usually unchanged with an uncomplicated pregnancy but may have an insignificant, slight transient increase.
  - Possible orthostatic hypotension within the first 48 hr postpartum may occur immediately after standing up with feelings of faintness or dizziness resulting from splanchnic (viscera/internal organs) engorgement that can occur after birth.
  - Elevation of pulse, stroke volume, and cardiac output for the first hour postpartum occurs and then gradually decreases to a prepregnant state baseline by 8 to 10 weeks.
  - Elevation of temperature to 38° C (100° F) resulting from dehydration after labor during the first 24 hr may occur, but should return to normal after 24 hr postpartum.
- The nurse should assess for cardiovascular and vital sign changes and monitor blood component changes.
  - The nurse should also inspect the client's legs for redness, swelling, and warmth, which are additional signs of venous thrombosis.
- Nursing interventions for alterations in findings include notifying the provider and performing prescribed interventions based on the cause of the alteration.
  - Encourage early ambulation to prevent venous stasis and thrombosis.
  - Apply antiembolism hose to the client's lower extremities if she is at high risk for developing venous stasis and thrombosis. The hose should be removed as soon as the client is ambulating.
  - Administer medications as prescribed.

Gastrointestinal System and Bowel Function

- Physical changes in the gastrointestinal system
  - An increased appetite following delivery
  - Constipation with bowel evacuation delayed until 2 to 3 days after birth
  - Hemorrhoids
- The nurse should assess the gastrointestinal system including bowel function.
  - Assess the client for reports of hunger. The nurse should expect the client to have a good appetite.
  - Assess the client for bowel sounds and the return of normal bowel function.
    - Spontaneous bowel movement may not occur for 2 to 3 days after delivery secondary to decreased intestinal muscle tone during labor and puerperium and prelabor diarrhea and dehydration. The client may also anticipate discomfort with defecation because of perineal tenderness, episiotomy, lacerations, or hemorrhoids.
  - Assess the client's rectal area for varicosities (hemorrhoids).
  - Operative vaginal birth (forceps-assisted and vacuum-assisted) and anal sphincter lacerations increase the risk of temporary postpartum anal incontinence that usually resolves within 6 months.
- Nursing interventions for gastrointestinal and bowel function
  - Encourage the client to take measures to soften her stools and promote bowel function (early ambulation, increased fluids, and high-fiber food sources).
  - Administer stool softeners (docusate sodium) as prescribed to prevent constipation.
    - Enemas and suppositories are contraindicated.

Urinary System and Bladder Function

- The urinary system may show evidence of:
  - Urinary retention secondary to loss of bladder elasticity and tone and/or loss of bladder sensation resulting from trauma, medications, or anesthesia.
    - A distended bladder as a result of urinary retention can cause uterine atony and displacement to one side, usually to the right. The ability of the uterus to contract is also lessened.
  - Postpartal diuresis with increased urinary output begins within 12 hr of delivery.
- The nurse should assess the urinary system and bladder function.
  - Assess the client's ability to void every 2 to 3 hr (perineal/urethral edema may cause pain and difficulty in voiding during the first 24 to 48 hr).
  - Assess the client's bladder elimination pattern (client should be voiding every 2 to 3 hr). Excessive urine diuresis (1,500 to 3,000 mL/day) is normal within the first 2 to 3 days after delivery.

- ○ Assess for evidence of a distended bladder.
  - ▪ Fundal height above the umbilicus or baseline level
  - ▪ Fundus displaced from the midline over to the side
  - ▪ Bladder bulges above the symphysis pubis
  - ▪ Excessive lochia
  - ▪ Tenderness over the bladder area
  - ▪ Frequent voiding of less than 150 mL of urine is indicative of urinary retention with overflow
- • Nursing interventions for the urinary system and bladder function
  - ○ Encourage the client to empty her bladder frequently (every 2 to 3 hr) to prevent possible displacement of the uterus and atony.
  - ○ Measure the client's first few voidings after delivery to assess for bladder emptying.
  - ○ Encourage the client to increase her oral fluid intake to replace fluids lost at delivery and to prevent or correct dehydration.
  - ○ Catheterize if necessary for bladder distention if the client is unable to void to ensure complete emptying of the bladder and allow uterine involution.

Musculoskeletal System

- • Physical changes of the musculoskeletal system involve a reversal of the musculoskeletal adaptations that occurred during pregnancy. By 6 to 8 weeks after birth:
  - ○ The joints return to their prepregnant state and are completely restabilized. The feet, however, may remain permanently increased in size.
  - ○ Muscle tone begins to be restored throughout the body with the removal of progesterone's effect following delivery of the placenta.
    - ▪ The rectus abdominis muscles of the abdomen and the pubococcygeal muscle tone are restored following placental expulsion and return to the prepregnant state within 2 to 6 weeks postpartum.
- • The nurse should assess the musculoskeletal system for changes.
  - ○ Assess the client's abdominal wall for diastasis recti (a separation of the rectus muscle) anywhere from 2 to 4 cm. It usually resolves within 6 weeks.
- • Nursing interventions pertaining to the musculoskeletal system
  - ○ Teach the client postpartum strengthening exercises, advising her to start with simple exercises, and then gradually progressing to more strenuous ones.
  - ○ Instruct clients who have had a cesarean birth to postpone abdominal exercises until about 4 weeks after delivery, or follow recommendations of her health care provider.
  - ○ Advise the client on good body mechanics and proper posture.

Immune System

- Review rubella status – A client who has a titer of less than 1:8 is administered a subcutaneous injection of rubella vaccine or a measles, mumps, and rubella vaccine during the postpartum period to protect a subsequent fetus from malformations. The client should not get pregnant for 1 month following the immunization.

- Review hepatitis B status – Newborns born to infected mothers should receive the hepatitis B vaccine and the hepatitis B immune globulin within 12 hr of birth.

- Review the Rh status – All Rh-negative mothers who have newborns who are Rh-positive must be given $RH_O(D)$ immune globulin (RhoGAM) administered IM within 72 hr of the newborn being born to suppress antibody formation in the mother.

- Test the client who receives both the rubella vaccine and RhoGAM after 3 months to determine whether immunity to rubella has been developed.

- Review varicella status – If the client has no immunity, varicella vaccine is administered before discharge. The client should not get pregnant for 1 month following the immunization. A second dose of vaccine is given at 4 to 8 weeks.

- Review tetanus-diphtheria-acellular pertussis vaccine status – The vaccine is recommended for women who have not previously received the vaccine. Administer prior to discharge or as soon as possible in the postpartum period.

Comfort Level

- Nursing assessments and interventions for the client's comfort level
  - Assess pain related to episiotomy, lacerations, incisions, afterpains, and sore nipples.
  - Assess location, type, and quality of the pain to guide nursing interventions and client education.
  - Administer pain medications as prescribed.

APPLICATION EXERCISES

1. A nurse is performing a fundal assessment for a client in her second postpartum day and observes the client's perineal pad for lochia. She notes the pad to be saturated approximately 12 cm with lochia that is bright red in color and contains small clots. The nurse knows that this finding is

    A. moderate lochia rubra.

    B. excessive lochia rubra.

    C. light lochia rubra.

    D. scant lochia serosa.

2. During ambulation to the bathroom, a postpartum client experiences a gush of dark red blood that soon stops. On assessment, a nurse finds the client's uterus to be firm and midline and at the level of the umbilicus. The nurse interprets this finding as

    A. evidence of a possible vaginal hematoma.

    B. an indication of a cervical or perineal laceration.

    C. a normal postural discharge of lochia.

    D. abnormally excessive lochia rubra flow.

3. A nurse is assessing a postpartum client for fundal height, location, and consistency. The fundus is found to be displaced laterally to the right, and there is uterine atony. Which of the following is the cause of the uterine atony?

    A. Poor involution

    B. Urinary retention

    C. Hemorrhage

    D. Infection

4. A nurse is completing postpartum discharge teaching to a client who had no immunity to varicella and was given varicella vaccine. Which of the following statements by the client indicates understanding of the teaching?

    A. "I will need to use contraception for 3 months before considering pregnancy."

    B. "I need a second vaccination at my postpartum visit."

    C. "I was given the vaccine because my baby is O-positive."

    D. "I will be tested in 3 months to see if I have developed immunity."

5. A nurse is caring for a client who is 1 hr following a vaginal birth and experiencing uncontrollable shaking. The nurse should understand that the shaking is due to which of the following? (Select all that apply.)

_____ A. A change in body fluids

_____ B. The metabolic effort of labor

_____ C. Diaphoresis

_____ D. A decrease in body temperature

_____ E. A decrease in prolactin levels

6. A nurse on the postpartum unit is leading a discussion with a group of clients about perineal care after delivery. What should be included in the discussion? Use the ATI Active Learning Template: Basic Concept to complete this item to include the following sections:

A. Underlying Principles: Describe three concepts that are the basis for perineal hygiene.

B. Nursing Interventions:
- Describe four actions the client should take to prevent infection.
- Describe four actions the nurse can take to promote client comfort.

APPLICATION EXERCISES KEY

1. A. **CORRECT:** The client has moderate lochia rubra containing small clots, which is an expected finding for the second day postpartum.

    B. INCORRECT: Excessive lochia rubra is saturation of a perineal pad in 15 min or less or pooling of blood under the client's buttocks.

    C. INCORRECT: Light lochia rubra is a perineal pad that is saturated less than 10 cm with lochia.

    D. INCORRECT: Scant lochia serosa (less than 2.5 cm area on perineal pad) is pinkish brown in color and serosanguineous in consistency. It occurs on day 4 to 12 following delivery.

    Ⓝ NCLEX® Connection: Health Promotion and Maintenance, Ante/Intra/Postpartum and Newborn Care

2. A. INCORRECT: A client who has a vaginal hematoma may report excessive pain or vaginal pressure.

    B. INCORRECT: Excessive spurting of bright red blood from the vagina indicates a possible cervical or perineal laceration.

    C. **CORRECT:** Lochia typically trickles from the vaginal opening but flows more steadily during uterine contractions. Massaging the uterus or ambulation may result in a gush of lochia with the expression of clots and dark blood that has been pooled in the vagina, but it should soon decrease back to a trickle of bright red lochia in the early puerperium.

    D. INCORRECT: Excessive blood loss consists of one pad saturated in 15 min or less or the pooling of blood under the buttocks, which is not affected by the client's postural changes.

    Ⓝ NCLEX® Connection: Health Promotion and Maintenance, Ante/Intra/Postpartum and Newborn Care

3. A. INCORRECT: Poor involution is the result of uterine atony and does not cause it.

    B. **CORRECT:** Urinary retention can result in a distention of the bladder. A distended bladder can cause uterine atony and lateral displacement from the midline, usually to the right.

    C. INCORRECT: Hemorrhage is the result of uterine atony and does not cause it.

    D. INCORRECT: Infection does not cause uterine displacement or atony and would be characterized by foul-smelling vaginal discharge and elevated temperature.

    Ⓝ NCLEX® Connection: Health Promotion and Maintenance, Ante/Intra/Postpartum and Newborn Care

4. A. INCORRECT: A client is instructed to not get pregnant for 1 month following administration of varicella vaccine.

    B. **CORRECT:** A second varicella immunization is needed at 4 to 8 weeks following delivery by clients who had no history of immunity.

    C. INCORRECT: $RH_o(D)$ immune globulin is administered to a Rh-negative mother who has a Rh-positive newborn.

    D. INCORRECT: A client requires testing for immunity at 3 months following administration of rubella vaccine and RhoGAM.

    Ⓝ NCLEX® Connection: Health Promotion and Maintenance, Health Promotion/Disease Prevention

5. A. **CORRECT:** A shift in body fluids during the first 2 hr puerperium can cause a postpartum chill.

    B. **CORRECT:** The work of labor can cause a postpartum chill during the first 2 hr puerperium.

    C. INCORRECT: Diaphoresis is the mechanism by which the excess fluid of pregnancy is removed from the body. It usually occurs within the first 2 to 3 days following delivery.

    D. INCORRECT: An increase in body temperature is associated with a postpartum chill, but it is not the cause of it.

    E. INCORRECT: Changes in prolactin levels affect ovulation and menses and are not the cause of a postpartum chill.

    Ⓝ NCLEX® Connection: Health Promotion and Maintenance, Ante/Intra/Postpartum and Newborn Care

6. *Using the ATI Active Learning Template: Basic Concept*

    A. Underlying Principles
        - Promote stool softening
        - Promote comfort

    B. Nursing Interventions
        - Prevent infection.
            ○ Wash hands thoroughly before and after voiding.
            ○ Use a squeeze bottle with warm water or antiseptic solution after each voiding.
            ○ Clean the perineal area from front to back.
            ○ Blot dry, not wipe.
            ○ Use topical application of antiseptic cream or spray sparingly.
            ○ Change perineal pad from front to back after voiding and defecating.
        - Promote comfort.
            ○ Apply ice packs to the perineum for 24 to 48 hr.
            ○ Encourage sitz baths at least twice a day.
            ○ Administer analgesics.
            ○ Administer PCA pump after cesarean birth.
            ○ Apply topical anesthetics to perineal area or witch hazel compresses to the rectal area.

    Ⓝ NCLEX® Connection: Health Promotion and Maintenance, Ante/Intra/Postpartum and Newborn Care

chapter 18

Overview

- Bonding and integration of an infant into the family structure should start during pregnancy, continue into the fourth stage of labor, and throughout hospitalization.
- Assessment of bonding and integration of an infant into the family structure requires that a nurse understand the normal postpartum psychological changes the client undergoes in the attainment of the maternal role and the recognition of deviations. Baby-friendly care can be promoted by delaying nursing procedures during the first hour after birth and through the first attempt of the client to breastfeed to allow for immediate parent-infant contact.
  - A client's emotional and physical condition (unwanted pregnancy, adolescent pregnancy, history of depression, difficult pregnancy and delivery) and the infant's physical condition (prematurity, congenital anomalies) after birth can affect the family's bonding process.
  - Culture, age, and socioeconomic level are factors that can influence the bonding process.
- Miscellaneous Relevant Information
  - Bonding can be delayed secondary to maternal or neonatal factors.

Psychosocial and Maternal Adaptation

- Psychosocial adaptation and maternal adjustment begin during pregnancy as the client goes through commitment, attachment, and preparation for the birth of the newborn. During the first 2 to 6 weeks after birth, the client goes through a period of acquaintance with her newborn, as well as physical restoration. During this time she also focuses on competently caring for her newborn. Finally, the act of achieving maternal identity is accomplished around 4 months following birth. It is important to note that these stages may overlap, and are variable based on maternal, infant, and the environmental factors.
  - Phases of maternal role attainment
    - Dependent: taking-in phase
      - First 24 to 48 hr
      - Focus is on meeting personal needs
      - Rely on others for assistance
      - Excited, talkative; need to review birth experience with others
    - Dependent-independent: taking-hold phase
      - Begins on day 2 or 3; up to 10 days to several weeks
      - Focus on baby care and improving care-giving competency
      - Want to take charge but need acceptance from others
      - Want to learn and practice
    - Interdependent: letting-go phase
      - Focus on family as a unit
      - Resumption of role (intimate partner, individual)

- Nursing assessments include noting the client's condition after birth, observing the maternal adaptation process, assessing maternal emotional readiness to care for the infant, and assessing how comfortable the client appears in providing infant care.
  - Assess for behaviors that facilitate and indicate mother-infant bonding.
    - Considers the infant a family member.
    - Holds the infant face-to-face (en face), maintaining eye contact.
    - Assigns meaning to the infant's behavior and views positively.
    - Identifies the infant's unique characteristics and relates them to those of other family members.
    - Naming the infant indicates that bonding is occurring.
    - Touches the infant and maintains close physical proximity and contact.
    - Provides physical care for the infant such as feeding and diapering.
    - Responds to the infant's cries.
    - Smiles at, talks to, and sings to the infant.
  - Assess for behaviors that impair and indicate a lack of mother-infant bonding.
    - Apathy when the infant cries.
    - Disgust when the infant voids, stools, or spits up.
    - Expresses disappointment in the infant.
    - Turns away from the infant.
    - Does not seek close physical proximity to the infant.
    - Does not talk about the infant's unique features.
    - Handles the infant roughly.
    - Ignores the infant entirely.
  - Assess for signs of mood swings, conflict about maternal role, and/or personal insecurity.
    - Feelings of being "down."
    - Feelings of inadequacy.
    - Feelings of anxiety related to ineffective breastfeeding.
    - Emotional lability with frequent crying.
    - Flat affect and being withdrawn.
    - Feeling unable to care for the infant.
- Nursing interventions to assist with maternal-infant bonding.
  - Facilitate the bonding process by placing the infant skin-to-skin in the en face position with the client immediately after birth.
  - Promote rooming-in as a quiet and private environment that enhances the family bonding process.
  - Promote early initiation of breastfeeding, and encourage the client to recognize infant readiness cues. Offer assistance as needed.
  - Teaching the client about infant care facilitates bonding as the client's confidence improves.
  - Encourage the parents to bond with their infant through cuddling, bathing, feeding, diapering, and inspection.
  - Provide frequent praise, support, and reassurance to the client as she moves toward independence in caring for her infant and adjusting to her maternal role.
  - Encourage the client/parents to express their feelings, fears, and anxieties about caring for their infant.

Paternal Adaptation

- Paternal adaptation takes place as the father develops a parent-infant bond.
  - The father has skin-to-skin contact, holds, and maintains eye-to-eye contact with the infant.
  - The father observes the infant for features similar to his own to validate his claim of the infant.
  - The father talks, sings, and reads to the infant.
- Paternal transition to fatherhood consists of a predictable three-stage process during the first few weeks of transition.
  - Expectations – The father has preconceived ideas about what it will be like to be a father.
  - Reality – The father discovers that his expectations may not be met. Commonly expressed emotions include feeling sad, frustrated, and jealous. He embraces the need to be actively involved in parenting.
  - Transition to mastery – The father decides to become actively involved in the care of the infant.
- The development of the father-infant bond consists of three stages.
  - Making a commitment – The father takes the responsibility of parenting.
  - Becoming connected – The father experiences feelings of attachment to the infant.
  - Making room for the infant – The father modifies his life to include the care of the infant.
- Nursing assessment of paternal adaptation includes observing for the characteristics of father-infant bonding.
- Nursing interventions to assist in the father-infant bonding process.
  - Provide education about infant care when the father is present, and encourage the father to take a hands-on approach.
  - Assist the father in his transition to fatherhood by providing guidance and involving him as a full partner rather than just a helper.
  - Encourage couples to verbalize their concerns and expectations related to infant care.

Sibling Adaptation

- The addition of an infant into the family unit affects everyone in the family, including siblings who may experience a temporary separation from the client. Siblings become aware of changes in the parents' behavior because the infant requires much more of the parents' time.
- Nursing assessment of sibling adaptation to the infant
  - Assess for positive responses from the sibling.
    - Interest and concern for the infant
    - Increased independence
  - Assess for adverse responses from the sibling.
    - Signs of sibling rivalry and jealousy
    - Regression in toileting and sleep habits
    - Aggression toward the infant
    - Increased attention-seeking behaviors and whining

- Nursing interventions to facilitate sibling acceptance of the infant
  - Take the sibling on a tour of the obstetric unit.
  - Encourage the parents to:
    - Let the sibling be one of the first to see the infant.
    - Provide a gift from the infant to give the sibling.
    - Arrange for one parent to spend time with the sibling while the other parent is caring for the infant.
    - Allow older siblings to help in providing care for the infant.
    - Provide the preschooler with a doll to care for.

Complications and Nursing Implications

- Impaired parenting may include the following:
  - Emotional detachment and inability to care for the infant, thus placing the infant at risk for neglect and failure to thrive. Failure to bond with the infant increases the risk of physical and/or emotional abuse.
- Nursing interventions for impaired parenting
  - Emphasize verbal and nonverbal communication skills between the client, caregivers, and the infant.
  - Provide continued assessment of the client's parenting abilities, as well as any other caregivers for the infant.
  - Encourage the continued support of grandparents and other family members.
  - Provide home visits by a nurse and group sessions for discussion regarding infant care and parenting problems.
  - Give the client/caregivers information about social networks that provide a support system where the client and caregivers can seek assistance.
  - Involve outreach programs concerned with self-care, parent-child interactions, child injuries, and failure to thrive.
  - Notify programs that provide prompt and effective community interventions to prevent more serious problems from occurring.

APPLICATION EXERCISES

1. A nurse concludes that the father of an infant is not showing positive signs of parent-infant bonding and appears to be very anxious and nervous when the infant's mother asks him to bring her the infant. Which of the following is an appropriate nursing intervention to promote father-infant bonding?

   A. Hand the father the infant, and suggest that he change the diaper.

   B. Ask the father why he is so anxious and nervous.

   C. Tell the father that he will grow accustomed to the infant.

   D. Provide education about infant care when the father is present.

2. A client in the early postpartum period is very excited and talkative. She is repeatedly telling the nurse every detail of her labor and birth. Because the client will not stop talking, the nurse is having difficulty completing the postpartum assessments. The appropriate action by the nurse is to

   A. come back later when the client is more cooperative.

   B. give the client time to express her feelings.

   C. tell the client she needs to be quiet so the assessment can be completed.

   D. redirect the client's focus so that she will become quiet.

3. A nurse is caring for a client who is 1 day postpartum. The nurse is assessing for maternal adaptation and mother-infant bonding. Which of the following behaviors by the client indicates a need for the nurse to intervene? (Select all that apply.)

   _____ A. Demonstrates apathy when the infant cries

   _____ B. Touches the infant and maintains close physical proximity

   _____ C. Views the infant's behavior as uncooperative during diaper changing

   _____ D. Identifies and relates infant's characteristics to those of family members

   _____ E. Interprets the infant's behavior as meaningful and a way of expressing needs

4. A home-health nurse is conducting a visit to the home of a client who has a 2-month-old infant and a 4-year-old son. The client expresses frustration about the behavior of the 4-year-old who was previously toilet trained and is now frequently wetting himself. The nurse should provide education and explains to the client that

   A. her son was probably not ready for toilet training and should wear training pants.

   B. her son is showing an adverse sibling response.

   C. this indicates the child requires counseling.

   D. this can be resolved by sending the child to preschool.

5. A nurse in the delivery room is planning to promote maternal-infant bonding for a client who just delivered. Which of the following is the priority action by the nurse?

    A. Encourage the parents to touch and explore the neonate's features.

    B. Limit noise and interruption in the delivery room.

    C. Place the neonate at the client's breast.

    D. Place the neonate skin-to-skin on the client's chest.

6. A nurse is leading a parenting class on paternal adaptation for expectant women and their partners. Which concepts on paternal adaptation should the nurse include in the presentation? Use ATI Active Learning Template: Basic Concept to complete this item to include the following:

    A. Related Content:
- Describe three ways the father develops a parent-infant bond.

    B. Underlying Principles:
- Describe three stages of paternal transition to parenthood.
- Describe three stages of the development of the father-infant bond.

    C. Nursing Interventions:
- Describe three actions to assist in the father-infant bonding process.

APPLICATION EXERCISES KEY

1. A. INCORRECT: It is not helpful to push the father into infant care activities without first providing education.

   B. INCORRECT: This is a nontherapeutic statement and presumes the nurse knows what the father is feeling.

   C. INCORRECT: This is a nontherapeutic statement and offers the nurse's opinion.

   D. **CORRECT:** Nursing interventions to promote paternal bonding include providing education about infant care and encouraging the father to take a hands-on approach.

   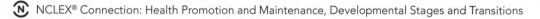 NCLEX® Connection: Health Promotion and Maintenance, Developmental Stages and Transitions

2. A. INCORRECT: The nurse should not delay completing assessments, but continue her activities while encouraging the client to talk.

   B. **CORRECT:** The nurse should recognize that the client in is the taking-in phase, which begins immediately following birth and lasts a few hours to a couple of days.

   C. INCORRECT: It is not necessary for the client to stop talking while the nurse completes the needed assessments.

   D. INCORRECT: The client is in the taking-in phase, which includes talking about the birth experience. The client should be encouraged.

   NCLEX® Connection: Health Promotion and Maintenance, Ante/Intra/Postpartum and Newborn Care

3. A. **CORRECT:** This behavior demonstrates a lack of interest in the infant and impaired maternal-infant bonding.

   B. INCORRECT: Touching the infant and maintaining close proximity are signs of effective maternal-infant bonding.

   C. **CORRECT:** A client's view of her infant as being uncooperative during diaper changing is a sign of impaired maternal-infant bonding.

   D. INCORRECT: Endowing the infant with family characteristics indicates effective maternal-infant bonding.

   E. INCORRECT: Recognizing the infant's behavior as meaningful and a way to express needs is an indication of effective maternal-infant bonding.

   NCLEX® Connection: Psychosocial Integrity, Coping Mechanisms

4. A. INCORRECT: This is not an appropriate intervention by the nurse because it overlooks the child's emotional response to a new family member.

    B. **CORRECT:** Adverse responses by a sibling to a new infant can include regression in toileting habits.

    C. INCORRECT: Recommending that the child receive counseling is not an appropriate nursing intervention for a child who is demonstrating an adverse sibling response.

    D. INCORRECT: Recommending that the child be sent to preschool is not an appropriate nursing intervention for a child who is demonstrating an adverse sibling response.

    Ⓝ NCLEX® Connection: Psychosocial Integrity, Family Dynamics

5. A. INCORRECT: This is an appropriate action, but there is another priority nursing intervention.

    B. INCORRECT: This is an appropriate action, but there is another priority nursing intervention.

    C. INCORRECT: This is an appropriate action, but there is another priority nursing intervention.

    D. **CORRECT:** Placing the neonate in the en face position on the client's chest immediately after birth is the priority nursing intervention to promote maternal-infant bonding.

    Ⓝ NCLEX® Connection: Health Promotion and Maintenance, Developmental Stages and Transitions

6. *Using the ATI Active Learning Template: Basic Concept*

A. Related Content
- Development of parent-infant bond
  - Touching, holding, skin-to-skin contact, and maintaining eye-to-eye contact
  - Recognizing personal features in the infant, and validating his claim to the infant
  - Talking, reading, singing, and verbally interacting with the infant

B. Underlying Principles
- Stages of paternal transition to parenthood
  - Expectations – having preconceived ideas about fatherhood
  - Reality – recognizing expectations may not be met, facing these feelings and then embracing the need to become actively involved in parenting
  - Transition to mastery – taking an active role in parenting
- Development of the father-infant bond
  - Making a commitment and assuming responsibility for parenting
  - Becoming connected and having feelings of attachment to the infant
  - Modifying lifestyle to make room to care for the infant

C. Nursing Interventions
- Provide education about infant care when father is present.
- Encourage the father to take a hands-on role in care when present.
- Provide guidance.
- Involve the father as a full partner, not a helper, in the parenting process.
- Encourage the couple to verbalize their concerns and expectations about infant care.

(N) NCLEX® Connection: Health Promotion and Maintenance, Developmental Stages and Transitions

chapter 19

Overview

- Discharge teaching is an important aspect of postpartum care. It is important for a client to be able to perform self-care and recognize effects that suggest possible complications prior to discharge.

- Discharge planning should be initiated at admission with time spent during the hospitalization on providing client education regarding postpartum self-care.

- A nurse should use a variety of teaching strategies to promote learning. Return demonstrations are important to ensure that adequate learning has taken place.

Assessing a Client's Knowledge of Postpartum Care

- Inquire about the client's current knowledge regarding self-care.

- Assess the client's home support system and who will be there to assist. Include support persons in the educational process.

- Determine the client's readiness for learning and her ability to verbalize or demonstrate the information she has been given.

Nursing Interventions for Postpartum Care

- Provide client teaching on self-care.
  - Perineal care
    - Cleanse the perineal area from front to back with warm water after each voiding and bowel movement.
    - Blot perineal area from front to back.
    - Remove and apply perineal pads from front to back.
  - Breast care
    - Provide breast care for clients who are lactating.
      - Wear a well-fitting, supportive bra continuously for the duration of lactation.
      - Emphasize the importance of hand hygiene prior to breastfeeding to prevent infection.
      - To relieve breast engorgement, have the client completely empty her breasts at each feeding. Allow the infant to nurse on demand, which would be about 8 to 12 times in 24-hr period. Massaging the breasts during feeding can help with emptying. Allow the infant to feed until the breast softens. If the second breast does not soften after the infant's feeding, the breast may be emptied with a breast pump. Alternate breasts with each feeding.

- □ For breast engorgement, apply cool compresses between feedings and apply warm compresses, or take a warm shower prior to breastfeeding. These actions will increase milk flow and promote the letdown reflex.

- □ For flat or inverted nipples, suggest that the client roll the nipples between her fingers just before breastfeeding to help them become more erect and make it easier for the infant to latch on. Use a breast shield between feedings.

- □ For sore nipples, the client should apply a small amount of breast milk to her nipple and allow it to air dry after breastfeeding.

- □ Have the client apply breast creams as prescribed and wear breast shields in her bra to soften her nipples if they are irritated and cracked.

- □ Promote adequate fluid intake to replace fluid lost from breastfeeding as well as to provide an adequate amount of milk for the infant.

- ▪ Breast care for nonlactating clients

  - □ Wear a well-fitting, supportive bra continuously for the first 72 hr.

  - □ Suppression of lactation is necessary for clients who are not breastfeeding. Avoid breast stimulation and running warm water over the breasts for prolonged periods until no longer lactating.

  - □ For breast engorgement, which may occur on the third or fifth postpartum day, apply cold compresses 15 min on and 45 min off. Fresh, cold cabbage leaves can be placed inside the bra. Mild analgesics may be taken for pain and discomfort of breast engorgement.

- ○ Rest/sleep

  - ▪ Plan at least one daily rest period; rest when the infant naps.

- ○ Activity

  - ▪ Do not perform housework requiring heavy lifting for at least 3 weeks. Do not lift anything heavier than the infant.

  - ▪ Avoid sitting for prolonged periods of time with legs crossed (to prevent thrombophlebitis).

  - ▪ Limit stair climbing for the first few weeks postpartum.

  - ▪ Clients who have had a cesarean birth should wait until the 4- to 6-week follow-up visit before performing strenuous exercise, heavy lifting, or excessive stair climbing.

  - ▪ Instruct not to drive for the first 2 weeks postpartum, or while taking opioids for pain control.

- ○ Nutrition

  - ▪ Teach the importance of eating a nutritious diet including all food groups. Encourage a diet high in protein, which will aid in tissue repair. The client should also consume 2,000 to 3,000 mL (2 to 3 L) of fluid each day from food and beverage sources.

  - ▪ Encourage clients who are lactating to add an additional 500 calories/day to their prepregnancy diet. This includes calcium-enriched foods.

- ○ Postpartum exercises

  - ▪ Regain pelvic floor muscle control by performing Kegel exercises. The same muscles are used when starting and stopping the flow of urine. Have the client relax and contract the pelvic floor muscles 10 times 8 times a day.

  - ▪ Teach how to perform pelvic tilt exercises to strengthen back muscles and relieve strain on the lower back. These exercises involve alternately arching and straightening the back.

- ○ Sexual intercourse

  - ▪ Avoid sexual intercourse until the episiotomy/laceration is healed and vaginal discharge has turned white (lochia alba). This usually takes 2 to 4 weeks or until the client is seen by the provider. Over-the-counter lubricants may be needed during the first 6 weeks.

  - ▪ Physiological reactions to sexual activity may be slower and less intense for the first 3 months following birth.

- ○ Contraception

  - ▪ Advise to begin using contraception upon resumption of sexual activity and that pregnancy can occur while breastfeeding even though menses has not returned.

  - ▪ Clients who are lactating should be advised that oral contraceptives should not begin until milk production is well established (usually 4 weeks).

  - ▪ Menses for nonlactating clients may not resume until around 4 to 10 weeks.

  - ▪ Menses for lactating clients may not resume for 3 months or until cessation of breastfeeding.

- • Provide client education on danger signs to report to the provider.

- ○ Chills or fever greater than 38° C (100.4° F) for 2 or more days.

- ○ Change in vaginal discharge with increased amount, large clots, change to a previous lochia color, such as bright red bleeding, and a foul odor.

  - ▪ Normal lochial flow patterns

    - ▫ Bright red vaginal drainage for 2 to 3 days.

    - ▫ Blood-tinged serous vaginal drainage from days 4 to 10.

    - ▫ White vaginal discharge from day 11 to 6 weeks.

- ○ Episiotomy, laceration, or incision pain, that does not resolve with analgesics, foul-smelling drainage, redness, and/or edema.

- ○ Pain or tenderness in the abdominal or pelvic areas that does not resolve with analgesics.

- ○ Breast(s) with localized areas of pain and tenderness with redness and swelling, and/or nipples with cracks or fissures.

- ○ Calves with localized pain and tenderness, redness, and swelling. A lower extremity with either areas of redness and warmth or coolness and paleness.

- ○ Urination with burning, pain, frequency, urgency; urine that is cloudy or has blood.

- • Postpartum depression is when the client feels apathy toward the infant, cannot provide self- or infant-care, or has feelings that she might hurt herself or her infant.

- • The client should be discharged with an appointment set for a postpartum follow-up visit or a number to call and schedule an appointment. Following a vaginal delivery, the follow-up visit should take place in 4 to 6 weeks; following a cesarean birth, the visit should take place in 2 weeks.

- • Date and time of the follow-up appointment should be written and discussed in the discharge instructions.

APPLICATION EXERCISES

1. A nurse is conducting a home visit for a client who is 2 weeks postpartum and breastfeeding. The client reports breast engorgement. Which of the following recommendations should the nurse make?

> A. "Apply cold compresses between feedings."
>
> B. "Take a warm shower right after feedings."
>
> C. "Apply breast milk to the nipples and allow them to air dry."
>
> D. "Use the various infant positions for feedings."

2. A nurse is providing discharge instructions for a client. At 4 weeks postpartum, the client should contact her provider for which of the following client findings?

> A. Scant, nonodorous white vaginal discharge
>
> B. Uterine cramping during breastfeeding
>
> C. Sore nipple with cracks and fissures
>
> D. Decreased response with sexual activity

3. A nurse is conducting a home visit with a client who is 3 months postpartum and breastfeeding. Menses has not yet resumed. The client is discussing contraception with the nurse, stating that she does not want to have another child for a couple of years. The nurse understands that this client needs further instruction if the client makes which of the following statements?

> A. "I have already started using the mini pill for protection."
>
> B. "Because of our beliefs, we are going to use the rhythm method."
>
> C. "I am being refitted for a diaphragm by my doctor next week."
>
> D. "I will begin using birth control when I stop breastfeeding."

4. A nurse is providing care to multiple clients on the postpartum unit. Which of the following clients is at greatest risk for developing a puerperal infection?

> A. A client who has an episiotomy that is erythematous and has extended into a third-degree laceration
>
> B. A client who does not wash her hands between perineal care and breastfeeding
>
> C. A client who is not breastfeeding and is using measures to suppress lactation
>
> D. A client who has a cesarean incision that is well-approximated with no drainage

5. A nurse is providing discharge instructions to a postpartum client following a cesarean birth. The client reports leaking urine every time she sneezes or coughs. Which of the following should the nurse suggest?

    A. Performing sit-ups

    B. Performing pelvic tilt exercises

    C. Doing Kegel exercises

    D. Doing abdominal crunches

6. A nurse is reviewing discharge teaching with a client who is not breastfeeding. What should be included in the teaching? Use the ATI Active Learning Template: Basic Concept to complete this item to include the following sections:

    A. Underlying Principles:
- Breast care: Describe two interventions the client can perform.
- Nutrition: Describe the nutrition and fluid plan the client can use.
- Resumption of sexual intercourse: Describe appropriate actions by the client.
- Danger signs to report to the provider: List two that the client should report.

APPLICATION EXERCISES KEY

1. A. **CORRECT:** Cold compresses applied to the breasts between feedings can help with breast engorgement.

    B. INCORRECT: Taking a warm shower prior to feedings, not immediately after, can assist with the letdown reflex and milk flow.

    C. INCORRECT. Applying breast milk to the nipples and air drying is recommended for the client who has sore nipples; it has no effect on breast engorgement.

    D. INCORRECT: Using the various positions for feedings helps to prevent nipple soreness but has no effect on breast engorgement.

     NCLEX® Connection: Health Promotion and Maintenance, Ante/Intra/Postpartum and Newborn Care

2. A. INCORRECT: Lochia alba, a white vaginal discharge, is normal from the 11th day postpartum to approximately 6 weeks following birth.

    B. INCORRECT: Oxytocin, which is released with breastfeeding, causes the uterus to contract and may cause discomfort.

    C. **CORRECT:** A sore nipple that has cracks and fissures is an indication of mastitis.

    D. INCORRECT: Physiological reactions to sexual activity may be slower and less intense for the first 3 months following birth.

     NCLEX® Connection: Health Promotion and Maintenance, Ante/Intra/Postpartum and Newborn Care

3. A. INCORRECT: Progesterone-only oral contraceptives (mini pills) are a good form of birth control once lactation has been established.

    B. INCORRECT: The rhythm method is a less effective method of birth control, but a client's choice based on personal beliefs should be supported.

    C. INCORRECT: The client is correct in having her diaphragm refitted by the provider, which should be done after a pregnancy and birth or a 7 kg (15 lb) weight change.

    D. **CORRECT:** Lactation does not prevent pregnancy, even if menses has not yet resumed.

     NCLEX® Connection: Health Promotion and Maintenance, Ante/Intra/Postpartum and Newborn Care

4. A. INCORRECT: An episiotomy with a laceration is at risk for an infection, but there is a client who is at greater risk for a puerperal infection.

    B. **CORRECT:** The client who does not wash her hands between perineal care and breastfeeding is at an increased risk for developing mastitis. Therefore, she is most at risk for developing a puerperal infection.

    C. INCORRECT: A client who is suppressing lactation (increases the risk of milk stasis) is at risk for an infection, but there is a client who is at greater risk for a puerperal infection.

    D. INCORRECT: A client who has an abdominal incision is at risk for an infection, but there is a client who is at greater risk for a puerperal infection.

     NCLEX® Connection: Health Promotion and Maintenance, Ante/Intra/Postpartum and Newborn Care

5. A. INCORRECT: Sit-ups should not be performed until after the postpartum follow-up appointment.

    B. INCORRECT: Pelvic tilt exercises consist of the alternate arching and straightening of the back to strengthen the back muscles and relieve back discomfort.

    C. **CORRECT:** Kegel exercises consist of the voluntary contraction and relaxation of the pubococcygeal muscle to strengthen the pelvic muscles, which will assist the client in decreasing urinary stress incontinence that occurs with sneezing and coughing.

    D. INCORRECT: Abdominal crunches should not be performed until after the postpartum follow-up appointment.

     NCLEX® Connection: Health Promotion and Maintenance, Ante/Intra/Postpartum and Newborn Care

6. *Using the ATI Active Learning Template: Basic Concept*

A. Underlying Principles

- Breast Care

  - Wear well-fitting, supportive bra for first 72 hr.

  - Avoid breast stimulation.

  - Avoid running warm water over the breasts for prolonged periods until no longer lactating.

- Nutrition

  - Eat a diet that includes all food groups, and higher protein content.

  - Consume 2,000 to 3,000 (2 to 3 L) of fluid daily from food and beverage sources.

- Sexual Intercourse

  - Avoid sexual intercourse until episiotomy/laceration is healed and vaginal discharge is lochia alba (2 to 4 weeks).

  - Over-the-counter lubricants may be needed.

  - Physiological reactions to sexual activity may be slower and less intense.

- Danger Signs

  - Chills or fever greater than 38° C (100.4° F) for 2 or more days.

  - Change in vaginal discharge with increased amount, large clots, change to previous lochia color, foul odor.

  - Episiotomy, laceration, or incisional pain that does not resolve with analgesics, foul-smelling drainage, redness, and/or edema.

  - Pain or tenderness in the abdominal or pelvic area that does not resolve with analgesics.

  - Breasts with localized areas of pain and tenderness with redness and swelling and/or nipples with cracks or fissures.

  - Calves with localized pain and tenderness, redness, and swelling. Lower extremity with either areas of redness and warmth, or coolness and paleness.

  - Urination with burning, pain, frequency, urgency; urine that is cloudy or bloody.

Ⓝ NCLEX® Connection: Health Promotion and Maintenance, Ante/Intra/Postpartum and Newborn Care

chapter 20

Overview

- Postpartum disorders are unexpected events or occurrences that may happen during the postpartum period. It is imperative for a nurse to have a thorough understanding of each disorder and initiate appropriate nursing interventions to achieve positive outcomes.

- Postpartum disorders reviewed in this chapter include the following:

  ○ Superficial and deep-vein thrombosis, pulmonary embolus, coagulopathies (idiopathic thrombocytopenic purpura and disseminated intravascular coagulation), postpartum hemorrhage, uterine atony, subinvolution of the uterus, inversion of the uterus, retained placenta, and lacerations and/or hematomas.

DEEP-VEIN THROMBOSIS

Overview

- Thrombophlebitis refers to a thrombus that is associated with inflammation.

- Thrombophlebitis of the lower extremities may be of superficial or deep veins, which are most often of the femoral, saphenous, or popliteal veins.

  ○ The postpartum client is at greatest risk for a deep-vein thrombosis (DVT) that may lead to a pulmonary embolism.

Risk Factors

- Pregnancy
- Immobility
- Obesity
- Smoking
- Cesarean birth
- Multiparity
- Greater than 35 years of age
- History of previous thromboembolism
- Diabetes mellitus

Assessment

- Subjective Data
  - Leg pain and tenderness
- Objective Data
  - Physical assessment findings
    - Unilateral area of swelling, warmth, and redness
    - Calf tenderness
  - Diagnostic procedures (noninvasive)
    - Doppler ultrasound scanning
    - Computed tomography
    - Magnetic resonance imaging

Patient-Centered Care

- Nursing Care
  - Prevention of thrombophlebitis
    - Provide the client with education and encouragement pertaining to measures for prevention of DVT.
      - Maintain antiembolism stockings until ambulation established.
      - If bed rest is prolonged longer than 8 hr, perform active and passive range of motion to promote circulation in the legs if warranted.
      - Initiate early and frequent ambulation postpartum.
      - Avoid prolonged periods of standing, sitting, or immobility.
      - Have the client elevate her legs when sitting.
      - Tell the client to avoid crossing her legs, which will reduce the circulation and exacerbate venous stasis.
      - Maintain fluid intake of 2 to 3 L each day from food and beverage sources to prevent dehydration, which causes circulation to be sluggish.
      - Tell the client to discontinue smoking, which is a risk factor.
      - Measure the client's lower extremities for fitted elastic thromboembolic hose to lower extremities.
  - Management of thrombophlebitis
    - Encourage rest.
    - Facilitate bed rest and elevation of the client's extremity above the level of her heart as prescribed (avoid using a knee gatch or pillow under knees).
    - Administer intermittent or continuous warm moist compresses as prescribed.
    - Do NOT massage the affected limb to prevent thrombus from dislodging and becoming an embolus.
    - Measure the client's leg circumferences.
    - Provide thigh-high antiembolism stockings for the client at high risk for venous insufficiency.
    - Administer analgesics (nonsteroidal anti-inflammatory agents).
    - Administer anticoagulants for DVT.

- Medications
  - Heparin
    - Classification
      - Anticoagulant
    - Therapeutic intent
      - Heparin is given IV to prevent formation of other clots and to prevent enlargement of the existing clot.
    - Nursing considerations
      - Initially, IV heparin is administered by continuous infusion for 5 to 7 days with doses adjusted according to coagulation studies. Protamine sulfate, the heparin antidote, should be readily available to counteract the development of heparin-induced antiplatelet antibodies.
      - Monitor aPTT (1.5 to 2.5 times the control level of 30 to 40 seconds).
    - Client education
      - Instruct the client to report bleeding from the gums or nose, increased vaginal bleeding, blood in the urine, and frequent bruising.
  - Warfarin (Coumadin)
    - Classification
      - Anticoagulant
    - Therapeutic intent
      - Warfarin is used for treatment of clots. It is administered orally and is continued by the client for approximately 3 months.
    - Nursing considerations
      - Phytonadione (vitamin K), the warfarin antidote, should be readily available for prolonged clotting times.
      - Monitor PT (1.5 to 2.5 times the control level of 11 to 12.5 seconds) and INR of 2 to 3.
    - Client education
      - Instruct the client to watch for bleeding from the gums or nose, increased vaginal bleeding, blood in the urine, and frequent bruising.
      - Instruct the client to use birth control to avoid pregnancy due to the teratogenic effects of warfarin. Oral contraceptives are contraindicated because of the increased risk for thrombosis.
- Health Promotion and Disease Prevention
  - Client education
    - Provide teaching about precautions to take while receiving anticoagulants.
      - Avoid taking aspirin or ibuprofen (increases bleeding tendencies).
      - Use an electric razor for shaving.
      - Avoid alcohol use (inhibits warfarin).
      - Brush teeth gently using a soft toothbrush.
      - Avoid rubbing or massaging legs.
      - Avoid periods of prolonged sitting or crossing legs.

PULMONARY EMBOLUS

Overview

- An embolus occurs when fragments or an entire clot dislodges and moves into circulation.
- A pulmonary embolism is a complication of DVT that occurs if the embolus moves into the pulmonary artery or one of its branches and lodges in a lung, occluding the vessel and obstructing blood flow to the lungs.

Risk Factors

- Risk factors for pulmonary embolism are the same as those for DVT.

Assessment

- Subjective Data
  - Apprehension
  - Pleuritic chest pain
- Objective Data
  - Dyspnea
  - Tachypnea
  - Hemoptysis
  - Heart murmurs
  - Peripheral edema
  - Distended neck veins
  - Elevated temperature
  - Hypotension
  - Hypoxia
- Diagnostic/Therapeutic Procedures
  - Ventilation/perfusion lung scan
  - Chest radiographic study
  - Radioisotope lung scan
  - Pulmonary angiogram
  - Embolectomy surgically removes the embolus.

Patient-Centered Care

- Nursing Care
  - Place the client in a semi-Fowler's position with the head of the bed elevated to facilitate breathing.
  - Administer oxygen to the client by mask.
  - Medications prescribed include the medications listed under DVT.
    - Thrombolytic therapy to break up blood clots may be prescribed.
      - Alteplase (Activase), streptokinase (Streptase).
      - Similar side effects and contraindications as anticoagulants.

COAGULOPATHIES (IDIOPATHIC THROMBOCYTOPENIC PURPURA AND DISSEMINATED INTRAVASCULAR COAGULATION)

Overview

- Idiopathic thrombocytopenic purpura (ITP) is a coagulopathy that is an autoimmune disorder in which the life span of platelets is decreased by antiplatelet antibodies. This can result in severe hemorrhage following a cesarean birth or lacerations.
- Disseminated intravascular coagulation (DIC) is a coagulopathy in which clotting and anticlotting mechanisms occur at the same time.
- The client is at risk for both internal and external bleeding, as well as damage to organs resulting from ischemia caused by microclots.
- Coagulopathies are suspected when the usual measures to stimulate uterine contractions fail to stop vaginal bleeding.

Risk Factors

- Risk factors for ITP are genetic in origin.
- Risk factors for DIC can occur secondary to other complications to include the following:
  - Abruptio placenta
  - Amniotic fluid embolism
  - Missed abortion
  - Fetal death in utero (fetus has died but is retained in the uterus for at least 6 weeks)
  - Severe preeclampsia or eclampsia (gestational hypertension)
  - Septicemia
  - Cardiopulmonary arrest
  - Hemorrhage
  - Hydatidiform mole

Assessment

- Objective Data
  - Physical assessment findings
    - Unusual spontaneous bleeding from the client's gums and nose (epistaxis)
    - Oozing, trickling, or flow of blood from incision, lacerations, or episiotomy
    - Petechiae and ecchymoses
    - Excessive bleeding from venipuncture, injection sites, or slight traumas
    - Tachycardia, hypotension, and diaphoresis
    - Oliguria
- Laboratory Tests
  - CBC with differential
  - Blood typing and crossmatch
  - Clotting factors
    - Platelet levels (thrombocytopenia)
    - Fibrinogen levels (decreased)
    - PT (increased)
    - Fibrin split product levels (increased)
- Therapeutic Procedures
  - A splenectomy may be performed by the provider if ITP does not respond to medical management.
  - Surgical intervention (hysterectomy) for DIC is performed by the provider as indicated.

Patient-Centered Care

- Nursing Care
  - Nursing assessments for ITP and DIC
    - Skin, venipuncture, injection sites, lacerations, and episiotomy for bleeding.
    - Vital signs and hemodynamic status.
    - Urinary output usually by insertion of an indwelling urinary catheter.
    - Transfuse platelets.
    - Assist in preparing the client for a splenectomy if ITP does not respond to medical management and provide postsurgical care.
    - Nursing interventions for DIC focus on assessing for and correcting the underlying cause (removal of dead fetus or placental abruption, treatment of infection, preeclampsia, or eclampsia).
      - Administer fluid volume replacement, which may include blood and blood products.
      - Administer pharmacologic interventions including antibiotics, vasoactive medications, and uterotonic agents as prescribed.
      - Administer supplemental oxygen.
      - Provide protection from injury.

POSTPARTUM HEMORRHAGE

Overview

- Postpartum hemorrhage is considered to occur if the client loses more than 500 mL of blood after a vaginal birth or more than 1,000 mL of blood after a cesarean birth. Two complications that can occur following postpartum hemorrhage include hypovolemic shock and anemia.

Risk Factors

- Uterine atony
- Complications during pregnancy (e.g., placenta previa, abruptio placenta)
- Precipitous delivery
- Administration of magnesium sulfate therapy during labor
- Lacerations and hematomas
- Inversion of uterus
- Subinvolution of the uterus
- Retained placental fragments
- Coagulopathies (DIC)

Assessment

- Subjective Data
  - Increase or change in lochial pattern (return to previous stage, large clots)
- Objective Data
  - Physical assessment findings
    - Uterine atony
    - Blood clots larger than a quarter
    - Perineal pad saturation in 15 min or less
    - Constant oozing, trickling, or frank flow of bright red blood from the vagina
    - Tachycardia and hypotension
    - Skin pale, cool, and clammy with loss of turgor and pale mucous membranes
    - Oliguria
  - Laboratory tests
    - Hgb and Hct
    - Coagulation profile (PT)
    - Blood type and crossmatch

Patient-Centered Care

- Nursing Care
  - Monitor vital signs.
  - Assess for source of bleeding.
    - Assess fundus for height, firmness, and position. If uterus is boggy, massage fundus to increase muscle contraction.
    - Assess lochia for color, quantity, and clots.
    - Assess for signs of bleeding from lacerations, episiotomy site, or hematomas.
  - Assess bladder for distention.
    - Insert an indwelling urinary catheter to assess the client's kidney function and obtain an accurate measurement of urinary output.
  - Maintain or initiate IV fluids to replace fluid volume loss with IV isotonic solutions, such as lactated Ringer's or 0.9% sodium chloride; colloid volume expanders, such as albumin; and blood products (packed RBCs and fresh frozen plasma).
  - Provide oxygen to the client at 2 to 3 L/min per nasal cannula as prescribed, and monitor oxygen saturation.
  - Elevate the client's legs to a 20° to 30° angle to increase venous return.
- Medications
  - Oxytocin (Pitocin)
    - Classification
      - Uterine stimulant
    - Therapeutic intent
      - Promotes uterine contractions
    - Nursing considerations
      - Assess uterine tone and vaginal bleeding.
        - Monitor the client for adverse reactions of water intoxication, such as lightheadedness, nausea, vomiting, headache, and malaise. These reactions can progress to cerebral edema with seizures, coma, and death.
  - Methylergonovine (Methergine)
    - Classification
      - Uterine stimulant
    - Therapeutic intent
      - Controls postpartum hemorrhage
    - Nursing considerations
      - Assess uterine tone and vaginal bleeding. Do not administer to clients who have hypertension.
      - Monitor the client for adverse reactions including hypertension, nausea, vomiting, and headache.

- ○ Misoprostol (Cytotec)
  - ▪ Classification
    - ▫ Uterine stimulant
  - ▪ Therapeutic intent
    - ▫ Controls postpartum hemorrhage.
  - ▪ Nursing considerations
    - ▫ Assess uterine tone and vaginal bleeding.
- ○ Carboprost tromethamine (Hemabate)
  - ▪ Classification
    - ▫ Uterine stimulant
  - ▪ Therapeutic intent
    - ▫ Controls postpartum hemorrhage.
  - ▪ Nursing considerations
    - ▫ Assess uterine tone and vaginal bleeding.
      - ‣ Monitor for adverse reactions including fever, chills, headache, nausea, vomiting, and diarrhea.
- Health Promotion and Disease Prevention
  - ○ Client education
    - ▪ Instruct the client to limit physical activity to conserve strength, and to increase iron and protein intake to promote the rebuilding of RBC volume.

UTERINE ATONY

Overview

- Uterine atony results from the inability of the uterine muscle to contract adequately after birth. This can lead to postpartum hemorrhage.

Risk Factors

- Retained placental fragments
- Prolonged labor
- Oxytocin (Pitocin) induction or augmentation of labor
- Overdistention of the uterine muscle (multiparity, multiple gestations, polyhydramnios [hydramnios], macrosomic fetus)
- Precipitous labor
- Magnesium sulfate administration as a tocolytic
- Anesthesia and analgesia administration
- Trauma during labor and birth from operative delivery (forceps-assisted or vacuum-assisted birth, cesarean birth)

Assessment

- Subjective Data
  - Increased vaginal bleeding
- Objective Data
  - Physical assessment findings
    - A uterus that is larger than normal and boggy with possible lateral displacement on palpation
    - Prolonged lochial discharge
    - Irregular or excessive bleeding
    - Tachycardia and hypotension
    - Skin that is pale, cool, and clammy with loss of turgor and pale mucous membranes
  - Diagnostic procedures
    - Bimanual compression or manual exploration of the uterine cavity for retained placental fragments by the provider
    - Surgical management such as a hysterectomy

Patient-Centered Care

- Nursing Care
  - Ensure that the client's urinary bladder is empty.
  - Monitor
    - Fundal height, consistency, and location.
    - Lochia for quantity, color, and consistency.
    - Perform fundal massage if indicated.
    - If the uterus becomes firm, continue assessing hemodynamic status.
    - If uterine atony persists, anticipate surgical intervention, such as a hysterectomy.
  - Express clots that may have accumulated in the uterus, but only after the uterus is firmly contracted.

    - It is critical not to express clots prior to the uterus becoming firmly contracted because pushing on an uncontracted uterus can invert the uterus and result in extensive hemorrhage.
  - Monitor vital signs.
  - Maintain or initiate IV fluids.
  - Provide oxygen to the client at 2 to 3 L/min per nasal cannula.
- Medications (as noted above for postpartum hemorrhage)
- Health Promotion and Disease Prevention
  - Client education
    - Instruct the client to limit physical activity to conserve strength and to increase iron and protein intake to promote the rebuilding of RBC volume.

SUBINVOLUTION OF THE UTERUS

Overview

- Subinvolution is when the uterus remains enlarged with continued lochial discharge and may result in postpartum hemorrhage.

Risk Factors

- Pelvic infection and endometritis
- Retained placental fragments not completely expelled from the uterus

Assessment

- Subjective Data
  - Increased vaginal bleeding
- Objective Data
  - Physical assessment findings
    - A uterus that is enlarged and higher than normal in the abdomen relative to the umbilicus.
    - A boggy uterus.
    - Prolonged lochia discharge with irregular or excessive bleeding.
  - Laboratory tests
    - Blood, intracervical, and intrauterine bacterial cultures to check for evidence of infection and/or endometritis.
  - Diagnostic procedures
    - Dilation and curettage (D&C) is performed by the provider to remove retained placental fragments if indicated.

Patient-Centered Care

- Nursing Care
  - Monitor fundal position and consistency.
  - Monitor lochia for color, amount, consistency, and odor.
  - Monitor vital signs.
  - Encourage the client to use activities that can enhance uterine involution.
    - Breastfeeding
    - Early and frequent ambulation
    - Frequent voiding
- Medications
  - Oxytocin (Pitocin)
- Classification
  - Uterine stimulant
- Therapeutic Intent
  - To promote uterine contractions and expel the retained fragments of placenta.

- Nursing Considerations
  - Assess uterine tone and vaginal bleeding.
  - Monitor for adverse reactions of water intoxication, such as lightheadedness, nausea, vomiting, headache, and malaise, which can progress to cerebral edema with seizures, coma, and death.
  - Antibiotic therapy
    - May be prescribed to prevent or treat infection.

INVERSION OF THE UTERUS

Overview

- Inversion of the uterus is the turning inside out of the uterus and may be partial or complete. Uterine inversion is an emergency situation that can result in postpartum hemorrhage and requires immediate intervention.

Risk Factors

- Retained placenta
- Uterine atony
- Excessive fundal pressure
- Abnormally adherent placental tissue
- Multiparity
- Fundal implantation of the placenta
- Extreme traction applied to the umbilical cord
- Leiomyomas (a benign uterine fibroid tumor)

Assessment

- Subjective Data
  - Pain in lower abdomen
- Objective Data
  - Physical assessment findings
    - Vaginal bleeding
      - Complete inversion as evidenced by a large, red, rounded mass that protrudes 20 to 30 cm outside the introitus
      - Partial inversion as evidenced by the palpation of a smooth mass through the dilated cervix
    - Dizziness
    - Low blood pressure
    - Pallor
  - Diagnostic procedures
    - Manual replacement of the uterus into the uterine cavity and repositioning of the uterus by the provider

Patient-Centered Care

- Nursing Care
  - Assess for an inverted uterus by:
    - Visualizing the introitus.
    - Performing a pelvic exam.
    - Maintaining IV fluids.
    - Administering oxygen.
  - Stop oxytocin (Pitocin) if it is being administered at the time uterine inversion occurred.
  - Avoid excessive traction on the umbilical cord.
  - Anticipate surgery if nonsurgical interventions and management are unsuccessful.
  - Medications
    - Terbutaline (Brethine)
      - Classification
        - Tocolytic
      - Therapeutic intent
        - To relax the uterus prior to the provider's attempt at replacement of the uterus into the uterine cavity and uterus repositioning
  - Nursing considerations
    - Following replacement of the uterus into the uterine cavity
      - Closely observe the client's response to treatment and assess for stabilization of hemodynamic status.
      - Avoid aggressive fundal massage.
      - Administer oxytocics as prescribed.
      - Administer broad-spectrum antibiotics for infection prophylaxis.
  - Client education
    - Inform the client that a cesarean birth will be needed for subsequent pregnancies.

RETAINED PLACENTA

Overview

- The placenta or fragments of the placenta remain in the uterus and prevents the uterus from contracting, which can lead to uterine atony or subinvolution.

Risk Factors

- Partial separation of a normal placenta.
- Entrapment of a partially or completely separated placenta by a constricting ring of the uterus.
- Excessive traction on the umbilical cord prior to complete separation of the placenta.
- Placental tissue that is abnormally adherent to the uterine wall.
- Common in preterm births between 20 and 24 weeks of gestation.

Assessment

- Objective Data
  - Physical assessment findings
    - Uterine atony, subinvolution, or inversion.
    - Excessive bleeding or blood clots larger than a quarter.
    - The return of lochia rubra once lochia has progressed to serosa alba.
    - Malodorous lochia or vaginal discharge.
    - Elevated temperature.
  - Laboratory tests
    - Hgb and Hct
  - Diagnostic procedures
    - Manual separation and removal of the placenta is done by the provider.
    - D&C if oxytocics are ineffective in expelling the placental fragments.

Patient-Centered Care

- Nursing Care
  - Monitor the uterus for fundal height, consistency, and position.
  - Monitor lochia for color, amount, consistency, and odor.
  - Monitor vital signs.
  - Maintain or initiate IV fluids.
  - Provide oxygen to the client at 2 to 3 L/min per nasal cannula.
  - Anticipate surgical interventions, such as a hysterectomy, if postpartum bleeding is present and continues.
- Medications
  - Oxytocin (Pitocin)
    - To expel retained fragments of the placenta
      - Classification
        - Uterine stimulant
      - Therapeutic intent
        - Promotes uterine contractions and expel the retained fragments of placenta.
  - Nursing considerations
    - Assess uterine tone and vaginal bleeding.
    - Monitor for adverse reactions of water intoxication, such as lightheadedness, nausea, vomiting, headache, and malaise, which can progress to cerebral edema with seizures, coma, and death.

- ○ Terbutaline (Brethine)
  - ▪ Classification
    - ▫ Tocolytic
  - ▪ Therapeutic intent
    - ▫ Relaxes the uterus prior to D&C if placental expulsion with oxytocics is unsuccessful.
- • Health Promotion and Disease Prevention
  - ○ Client education
    - ▪ Instruct the client to limit physical activity to conserve strength, and to increase iron and protein intake to promote the rebuilding of RBC volume.

LACERATIONS AND/OR HEMATOMAS

Overview

- • Lacerations that occur during labor and birth consist of the tearing of soft tissues in the birth canal and adjacent structures including the cervical, vaginal, vulvar, perineal, and/or rectal areas.
- • An episiotomy may extend and become a third- or fourth-degree laceration.
- • A hematoma is a collection of 250 to 500 mL of clotted blood within tissues that may appear as a bulging bluish mass. Hematomas may occur in the pelvic region or higher up in the vagina or broad ligament.
- • Pain, rather than noticeable bleeding, is the distinguishable symptom of hematomas.
- • The client is at risk for hemorrhage or infection due to a laceration or hematoma.

Risk Factors

- • Operative vaginal birth (forceps-assisted, vacuum assisted birth).
- • Precipitous birth.
- • Cephalopelvic disproportion.
- • Size (macrosomic infant) and abnormal presentation or position of the fetus.
- • Prolonged pressure of the fetal head on the vaginal mucosa.
- • Previous scarring of the birth canal from infection, injury, or operation.
- • Clients who are nulliparous are at a greater risk for injury due to firmer and less resistant tissue.
- • Women who have light skin, especially those with reddish hair, have less distensible tissue than women who are dark skin.

Assessment

- Subjective Data
  - Laceration
    - Sensation of oozing or trickling of blood
    - Excessive rubra lochia (with or without clots)
  - Hematoma
    - Pain
    - Pressure sensation in rectum (urge to defecate) or vagina
    - Difficulty voiding
- Objective Data
  - Physical assessment findings
    - Laceration
      - Vaginal bleeding even though the uterus is firm and contracted
      - Continuous slow trickle of bright red blood from vagina, laceration, episiotomy
    - Hematoma
      - Bulging, bluish mass or area of red-purple discoloration on vulva, perineum, or rectum
  - Therapeutic procedures
    - Repair and suturing of the episiotomy or lacerations is done by the provider.
    - Ligation of the bleeding vessel or surgical incision for evacuation of the clotted blood from the hematoma is done by the provider.

Patient-Centered Care

- Nursing Care
  - Assess pain.
  - Visually or manually inspect the vulva, perineum, and rectum for lacerations and/or hematomas.
  - Assess an episiotomy for extension into a third- or fourth-degree laceration.
  - Evaluate lochia.
  - Continue to assess vital signs and hemodynamic status.
  - Attempt to identify the source of the bleeding.
  - Assist the provider with repair procedures.
  - Use ice packs to treat small hematomas.
  - Administer prescribed pain medication.
  - Encourage sitz baths and frequent perineal hygiene.

APPLICATION EXERCISES

1. A nurse is caring for a postpartum client. The nurse should understand that which of the following findings are the earliest indication of hypovolemia caused by hemorrhage?

    A. Increasing pulse and decreasing blood pressure

    B. Dizziness and increasing respiratory rate

    C. Cool, clammy skin, and pale mucous membranes

    D. Altered mental status and level of consciousness

2. A nurse educator on the postpartum unit is reviewing risk factors for postpartum hemorrhage with a group of nurses. Which of the following should be included in the discussion? (Select all that apply.)

    _X_ A. Precipitous delivery

    _X_ B. Lacerations

    _X_ C. Inversion of the uterus

    ___ D. Oligohydramnios

    _X_ E. Retained placental fragments

3. A nurse on the postpartum unit is performing a physical assessment of a client who is being admitted with a suspected deep-vein thrombosis (DVT). Which of the following clinical findings should the nurse anticipate the client will exhibit? (Select all that apply.)

    _X_ A. Calf tenderness to palpation

    _X_ B. Swelling of the extremity

    _X_ C. Elevated temperature

    _X_ D. Area of warmth

    ___ E. Report of nausea

4. A nurse on the postpartum unit is planning care for a client who has thrombophlebitis. Which of the following nursing interventions should the nurse include in the plan of care?

    A. Apply cold compresses to the affected extremity.

    B. Massage the affected extremity.

    C. Allow the client to ambulate.

    D. Measure leg circumferences.

5. A nurse is caring for a client who has disseminated intravascular coagulation (DIC). Which of the following antepartum complications should the nurse understand is a risk factor for this client?

A. Preeclampsia

B. Thrombophlebitis

C. Placenta previa

D. Hyperemesis gravidarum

6. A nurse is planning care for a client who has a deep-vein thrombosis (DVT). What nursing interventions should be incorporated into the plan of care? Use the ATI Active Learning Template: Systems Disorder to complete this item to include the following sections:

A. Description of the Disorder: Describe the disease process and location.

B. Risk Factors: Describe four risk factors for the disorder.

C. Client Education: Describe four teaching points for prevention of a DVT.

D. Medications: Describe two medications and their related laboratory tests.

APPLICATION EXERCISES KEY

1. A. **CORRECT:** A rising pulse rate and decreasing blood pressure are often the first indications of inadequate blood volume.

    B. INCORRECT: Dizziness and increased respiratory rate are findings that occur in hypovolemia, but they are not the earliest indicators.

    C. INCORRECT: Skin that is cool, clammy, and pale along with pale mucous membranes are changes that occur in the physical status of a client who has decreased blood volume, but they are not the first indicators of inadequate blood volume.

    D. INCORRECT: Altered mental status and changes in level of consciousness are late manifestations of decreased blood volume, which leads to hypoxia and low oxygen saturation.

    Ⓝ NCLEX® Connection: Physiological Adaptations, Alterations in Body Systems

2. A. **CORRECT:** A rapid, precipitous delivery is a risk factor for postpartum hemorrhage.

    B. **CORRECT:** The presence of lacerations is a risk factor for postpartum hemorrhage.

    C. **CORRECT:** Inversion of the uterus in a risk factor for postpartum hemorrhage.

    D. INCORRECT: Oligohydramnios does not place a client at risk for postpartum hemorrhage.

    E. **CORRECT:** Retained placental fragments is a risk factor for postpartum hemorrhage.

    Ⓝ NCLEX® Connection: Health Promotion and Maintenance, Ante/Intra/Postpartum and Newborn Care

3. A. **CORRECT:** A client report of calf tenderness to palpation is an expected finding in a client who has a DVT.

    B. **CORRECT:** Swelling of the affected extremity is an expected finding in a client who has a DVT.

    C. **CORRECT:** Elevated temperature is an expected finding in a client who has a DVT.

    D. **CORRECT:** An area of warmth over the thrombus is an expected finding in a client who has a DVT.

    E. INCORRECT: A report of nausea is not an expected finding in a client who has a DVT.

    Ⓝ NCLEX® Connection: Physiological Adaptations, Illness Management

4.   A. INCORRECT: The nurse should plan to apply warm compresses to the affected extremity.

     B. INCORRECT: The nurse should not massage the affected extremity. This action may result in dislodgement of the clot.

     C. INCORRECT: The client should be encouraged to rest with the affected extremity elevated.

     D. **CORRECT:** The nurse should plan to measure the circumference of the leg to assess for changes in the client's condition.

     (N) NCLEX® Connection: Physiological Adaptations, Hemodynamics

5.   A. **CORRECT:** DIC may occur secondary in a client who has preeclampsia.

     B. INCORRECT: Thrombophlebitis is not a risk factor for DIC.

     C. INCORRECT: Placenta previa is not a risk factor for DIC.

     D. INCORRECT: Hyperemesis gravidarum is not a risk factor for DIC.

     (N) NCLEX® Connection: Physiological Adaptations, Alterations in Body Systems

6.   *Using the ATI Active Learning Template: Systems Disorder*

     A. Description of the Disorder: DVT refers to a thrombus that is associated with inflammation. It may occur in a superficial or deep vein (femoral, saphenous, or popliteal).

     B. Risk Factors

- Pregnancy
- Immobility
- Obesity
- Smoking
- Cesarean birth
- Multiparity
- Older than 35 years of age
- History of previous thromboembolism
- Diabetes mellitus

     C. Client Education

- Wear antiembolic stockings until ambulation established.
- Perform active range of motion when on bed rest for longer than 8 hr.
- Initiate early and frequent postpartum ambulation.
- Avoid prolonged periods of standing, sitting, or immobility.
- Elevate the legs when sitting.
- Avoid crossing legs.
- Maintain 2 to 3 L of daily fluid intake from food and beverage sources.
- Discontinue smoking

     D. Medications

- Heparin – aPTT
- Warfarin (Coumadin) – PT and INR

     (N) NCLEX® Connection: Physiological Adaptations, Hemodynamics

chapter 21

Overview

- Postpartum infections are complications that may occur up to 28 days following childbirth, or a spontaneous or induced abortion. Fever of 38° C (100.4° F) or higher for 2 consecutive days during the first 10 days of the postpartum period is indicative of a postpartum infection and requires further investigation. The infection may be present in the bladder, uterus, wound, or breast of a postpartum client. The major complication of puerperal infection is septicemia.

- Uterine infection, wound infection, mastitis, and a urinary tract infection are examples of postpartum infections. Early identification and prompt treatment are necessary to promote positive outcomes.

INFECTIONS (ENDOMETRITIS, MASTITIS, AND WOUND INFECTIONS)

Overview

- Uterine infection is also referred to as endometritis. Endometritis is an infection of the uterine lining or endometrium. It is the most frequently occurring puerperal infection.

- Endometritis usually begins on the second to fifth postpartum day, generally starting as a localized infection at the placental attachment site and spreading to include the entire uterine endometrium.

- Sites of wound infections include cesarean incisions, episiotomies, lacerations, and/or any trauma wounds present in the birth canal following labor and birth.

- Mastitis is an infection of the breast involving the interlobular connective tissue and is usually unilateral. Mastitis may progress to an abscess if untreated.

  ○ It occurs most commonly in mothers breastfeeding for the first time and well after the establishment of milk flow, which is usually 2 to 4 weeks after delivery.

  ○ *Staphylococcus aureus* is usually the infecting organism.

    View Image: Mastitis

Risk Factors

- The immediate postpartum period following birth is a time of increased risk for all women for micro-organisms entering the reproductive tract and migrating into the blood and other parts of the body, which can result in life-threatening septicemia.
  - Risk factors
    - Cervical dilation that provides the uterus with exposure to the external environment through the vagina
    - Well-supplied exposed blood vessels
    - Wounds from lacerations, incisions, and/or hematomas
    - Alkalinity of amniotic fluid, blood, and lochia during pregnancy and the early postpartum period, decreasing the acidity of the vaginal secretions
- Risk factors for endometritis
  - Cesarean birth
  - Retained placental fragments and manual extraction of the placenta
  - Prolonged rupture of membranes
  - Chorioamnionitis
  - Internal fetal/uterine pressure monitoring
  - Multiple vaginal examinations after rupture of membranes
  - Prolonged labor
  - Postpartum hemorrhage
- Risk factors for mastitis
  - Milk stasis from a blocked duct
  - Nipple trauma and cracked or fissured nipples
  - Poor breastfeeding technique with improper latching of the infant onto the breast, which can lead to sore and cracked nipples
  - Decrease in breastfeeding frequency due to supplementation with bottle feeding
  - Poor hygiene and inadequate handwashing when handling perineal pads and touching the breasts

Assessment

- Subjective Data
  - Puerperal infections
    - Flulike symptoms such as body aches, chills, fever, and malaise
    - Anorexia and nausea
  - Endometritis
    - Pelvic pain
    - Chills
    - Fatigue
    - Loss of appetite

- ○ Mastitis
  - ▪ Painful or tender, localized hard mass, and reddened area usually on one breast
  - ▪ Chills
  - ▪ Fatigue
- Objective Data
  - ○ Physical assessment findings
    - ▪ Puerperal infections
      - □ Elevated temperature of at least 38° C (100.4° F) for 2 or more consecutive days
      - □ Tachycardia
    - ▪ Endometritis
      - □ Uterine tenderness and enlargement
      - □ Dark, profuse lochia
      - □ Lochia that is either malodorous or purulent
      - □ Temperature greater than 38° C (100.4° F) typically on the third to fourth postpartum day
      - □ Tachycardia
    - ▪ Wound infection
      - □ Wound warmth, erythema, tenderness, pain, edema, seropurulent drainage, and wound dehiscence (separation of wound or incision edges) or evisceration (protrusion of internal contents through the separated wound edges)
      - □ Temperature greater than 38° C (100.4° F) for 2 or more consecutive days
    - ▪ Mastitis
      - □ Axillary adenopathy in the affected side (enlarged tender axillary lymph nodes) with an area of inflammation that may be red, swollen, warm, and tender
  - ○ Laboratory tests
    - ▪ Blood, intracervical, or intrauterine bacterial cultures to reveal the offending organism
    - ▪ WBC count (leukocytosis)
    - ▪ RBC sedimentation rate (distinctly increased)
    - ▪ RBC count (anemia)
  - ○ Therapeutic procedures
    - ▪ The provider may need to open and drain the wound or perform wound debridement if indicated.

Patient-Centered Care

- Nursing Care
  - ○ Obtain frequent vital signs.
  - ○ Assess pain.
  - ○ Assess fundal height, position, and consistency.
  - ○ Observe lochia for color, quantity, and consistency.

○ Inspect incisions, episiotomy, and lacerations.

○ Inspect breasts.

○ Nursing interventions for puerperal infections

▪ Use aseptic technique for appropriate procedures, proper hand hygiene, and don gloves for labor, birth, and postpartum cares.

▪ Provide client education about preventative measures to include thorough handwashing and good perineal hygiene.

▪ Maintain or initiate IV access.

▪ Administer IV broad-spectrum antibiotic therapy (penicillins or cephalosporins) as prescribed.

▪ Provide comfort measures, such as warm blankets or cool compresses, depending on the findings.

▪ Educate the client about signs of worsening conditions to report and the importance of adherence to the treatment plan with the completion of a full course of antibiotics.

▪ Encourage a diet high in protein to promote tissue healing.

○ Nursing interventions for endometritis

▪ Collect vaginal and blood cultures.

▪ Administer IV antibiotics as prescribed.

▪ Administer analgesics as prescribed.

▪ Teach the client hand hygiene techniques.

▪ Encourage client to maintain interaction with her infant to facilitate bonding.

○ Nursing interventions for wound infection

▪ Perform wound care.

▪ Administer IV antibiotics as prescribed.

▪ Provide or encourage comfort measures such as sitz baths, perineal care, and warm or cold compresses.

▪ Teach the client good hand hygiene techniques (changing perineal pads from front to back, performing thorough hand hygiene prior to and after perineal care).

○ Nursing interventions for mastitis

▪ Provide the client with education regarding breast hygiene to prevent and manage mastitis.

□ Instruct to thoroughly wash hands prior to breastfeeding.

□ Instruct to maintain cleanliness of breasts with frequent changes of breast pads.

□ Encourage allowing nipples to air-dry.

□ Teach proper infant positioning and latching-on techniques, including both the nipple and the areola. The client should release the infant's grasp on the nipple prior to removing the infant from the breast.

□ Instruct the client about completely emptying her breasts with each feeding to prevent milk stasis, which provides a medium for bacterial growth.

□ Encourage using ice packs or warm packs on affected breasts for discomfort.

        □ Instruct the client to continue breastfeeding frequently (at least every 2 to 4 hr), especially on the affected side. Instruct the client to manually express breast milk or use a breast pump if breastfeeding is too painful.

        □ Instruct the client to begin breastfeeding from the unaffected breast first to initiate the letdown reflex in the affected breast that is distended or tender.

        □ Encourage rest, analgesics, and fluid intake of at least 3,000 mL per day.

        □ Encourage the client to wear a well-fitting bra for support.

        □ Tell the client to report redness and fever.

        □ Administer antibiotics, and teach the client the importance of completing the entire course of antibiotics as prescribed.

- Medications for endometritis
  - Clindamycin (Cleocin)
    - Classification and therapeutic intent
      - □ Antibiotic used in the treatment of bacterial infections
    - Client education
      - □ Educate the client to take all the medication as prescribed.
      - □ Tell the client to notify the provider of the development of watery, bloody diarrhea.
      - □ Tell the client to notify the provider if the client is breastfeeding.

URINARY TRACT INFECTION

Overview

- Urinary tract infections (UTIs) are a common postpartum infection secondary to bladder trauma incurred during the delivery or a break in aseptic technique during bladder catheterization.
- A potential complication of a UTI is the progression to pyelonephritis with permanent kidney damage leading to kidney failure.

Risk Factors

- Postpartal hypotonic bladder and/or urethra (urinary stasis and retention)
- Epidural anesthesia
- Urinary bladder catheterization
- Frequent pelvic examinations
- Genital tract injuries
- History of UTIs
- Cesarean birth

Assessment

- Subjective Data
  - ○ Reports of urgency, frequency, dysuria, and discomfort in the pelvic area
  - ○ Fever
  - ○ Chills
  - ○ Malaise
- Objective Data
  - ○ Physical assessment findings
    - Change in vital signs, elevated temperature
    - Urine (cloudy, blood-tinged, malodorous, sediment visible)
    - Urinary retention
    - Pain in the suprapubic area
    - Pain at the costovertebral angle (pyelonephritis)
  - ○ Diagnostic procedures
    - Urinalysis for WBCs, RBCs, protein, bacteria

Patient-Centered Care

- Nursing Care
  - ○ Obtain either a random or clean-catch urine sample.
  - ○ Administer antibiotics and teach the client the importance of completing the entire course of antibiotics as prescribed.
  - ○ Teach the client proper perineal hygiene, such as wiping from front to back.
  - ○ Encourage the client to increase her fluid intake to 3,000 mL/day to dilute the bacteria and flush her bladder.

  - ○ Recommend that the client drink cranberry and prune juice to promote urine acidification, which inhibits bacterial multiplication.

APPLICATION EXERCISES

1. A nurse on the postpartum unit is caring for several clients. The nurse should recognize that the greatest risk for development of a postpartum infection is the client who

    A. experienced a precipitous labor less than 3 hr in duration.

    B. had premature rupture of membranes and prolonged labor.

    C. delivered a large for gestational age infant.

    D. had a boggy uterus that was not well-contracted.

2. A nurse is teaching a client who is breastfeeding and has mastitis. Which of the following is an appropriate statement by the nurse?

    A. "Limit the amount of time the infant nurses on each breast."

    B. "Nurse the infant only on the unaffected breast until resolved."

    C. "Completely empty each breast at each feeding or use a pump."

    D. "Wear a tight-fitting bra until lactation has ceased."

3. A nurse is reviewing discharge teaching with a client who has a urinary tract infection. Which of the following statements by the client indicates understanding of the teaching? (Select all that apply.)

    _____ A. "I will perform peri care and apply a perineal pad in a back-to-front direction."

    ___X___ B. "I will drink cranberry and prune juices to make my urine more acidic."

    ___X___ C. "I will drink large amounts of fluids to flush the bacteria from my urinary tract."

    _____ D. "I will go back to breastfeeding after I have finished taking the antibiotic."

    ___X___ E. "I will take Tylenol for any discomfort."

4. A nurse is caring for a client who has mastitis. Which of the following is the typical causative agent of mastitis?

    A. *Staphylococcus aureus*

    B. *Chlamydia trachomatis*

    C. *Klebsiella pneumonia*

    D. *Clostridium perfringens*

5. A nurse is preparing to administer clindamycin hydrochloride (Cleocin) 600 mg IV intermittent bolus in 50 mL of 0.9% sodium chloride over 30 min. The nurse should set the IV infusion pump to deliver how many mL/hr? (Round the answer to the nearest whole number.)

100 mL

6. A nurse educator is reviewing care of a client who has endometritis with a group of newly hired nurses. What should be included in the review? Use the ATI Active Learning Template: Systems Disorder to complete this item to include the following:

    A. Description of the Disorder

    B. Objective and Subjective Data: Describe at least three of each.

    C. Nursing Care: Describe at least three nursing interventions.

APPLICATION EXERCISES KEY

1. A. INCORRECT: A precipitous labor places the client at risk for trauma and lacerations during delivery, but there is another client who is at greater risk for postpartum infection.

    B. **CORRECT:** Premature rupture of membranes with prolonged labor poses the greatest risk for developing a postpartum infection because the birth canal was open, allowing pathogens to enter.

    C. INCORRECT: Delivery of a large infant places the client at risk for a postpartum infection, but there is another client who is at greater risk.

    D. INCORRECT: A boggy uterus that did not remain well-contracted places the client at risk for a postpartum infection, but there is another client who is at greater risk.

     NCLEX® Connection: Health Promotion and Maintenance, Ante/Intra/Postpartum and Newborn Care

2. A. INCORRECT: Frequent, on-demand breastfeeding should be encouraged to promote milk flow.

    B. INCORRECT: The client should be instructed to continue breastfeeding, especially on the affected side.

    C. **CORRECT:** Instruct the client to completely empty each breast at each feeding to prevent milk stasis, which provides a medium for bacterial growth.

    D. INCORRECT: The client should wear a well-fitting bra, not one that is too tight or a binder.

     NCLEX® Connection: Health Promotion and Maintenance, Ante/Intra/Postpartum and Newborn Care

3. A. INCORRECT: Perineal cleansing and pad application should be done front to back, not back to front.

    B. **CORRECT:** Acidification of urine inhibits bacterial multiplication.

    C. **CORRECT:** Increased fluid intake can help to flush the bacteria from the urinary tract.

    D. INCORRECT: Breastfeeding does not have to be delayed until the course of antibiotics is completed.

    E. **CORRECT:** Acetaminophen (Tylenol) is taken to reduce discomfort and pain associated with a urinary tract infection.

     NCLEX® Connection: Basic Care and Comfort, Elimination

4. A. **CORRECT:** *Staphylococcus aureus*, *Escherichia coli*, and streptococcus are usually the infecting agents that enter the breast due to sore or cracked nipples, which results in mastitis.

    B. INCORRECT: *Chlamydia trachomatis* is a STI but not the causative agent of mastitis.

    C. INCORRECT: *Klebsiella pneumonia* is a causative agent of pneumonia.

    D. INCORRECT: *Clostridium perfringens* can cause wound infections but is not a causative agent of mastitis.

     NCLEX® Connection: Reduction of Risk Potential, System Specific Assessments

5. The nurse should set the IV pump to deliver **100 mL/hr**.

Using Ratio Proportion, Desired Over Have, and Dimensional Analysis

STEP 1: *What is the unit of measurement to calculate?*
mL/hr

STEP 2: *What is the volume needed? Volume needed = Volume.*
50 mL

STEP 3: *What is the total infusion time? Time available = Time.*
30 min

STEP 4: *Should the nurse convert the units of measurement?*
No (mL = mL)
Yes (min ≠ hr)
$$\frac{1 \text{ hr}}{60 \text{ min}} = \frac{X \text{ hr}}{30 \text{ min}}$$
X = 0.5

STEP 5: *Set up an equation and solve for X.*
$$\frac{\text{Volume (mL)}}{\text{Time (hr)}} = X$$
$$\frac{50 \text{ mL}}{0.5 \text{ hr}} = X \text{ mL/hr}$$
100 = X

STEP 6: *Round if necessary.*

STEP 7: *Reassess to determine whether the IV flow rate makes sense.*
If the amount prescribed is 50 mL to infuse over 30 min (0.5 hr), it makes sense to administer 100 mL/hr. The nurse should set the IV pump to deliver clindamycin hydrochloride 600 mg in 50 mL of 0.9% sodium chloride at 100 mL/hr.

Ⓝ NCLEX® Connection: Pharmacological and Parenteral Therapies, Dosage Calculation

6. *Using the ATI Active Learning Template: Systems Disorder*

   A. Description of the Disorder

   - Endometritis is an infection of the uterine lining or endometrium. It usually begins on the second to fifth postpartum day as a localized infection at the placental attachment site and spreads to include the entire endometrium. It is the most frequently occurring puerperal infection.

   B. Objective Data and Subjective Data

   - Objective Data
     - Uterine tenderness and enlargement
     - Dark, profuse lochia
     - Malodorous or purulent lochia
     - Temperature greater than 38° C (100.4° F) on the third or fourth postpartum day
     - Tachycardia
   - Subjective Data
     - Pelvic pain
     - Chills
     - Fatigue, loss of appetite

   C. Nursing Care

   - Collect vaginal and blood cultures.
   - Administer IV antibiotics as prescribed.
   - Administer analgesics as prescribed.
   - Teach client hand hygiene techniques.
   - Encourage client interaction with her infant to facilitate bonding.

Ⓝ NCLEX® Connection: Physiological Adaptations, Alterations in Body Systems

chapter **22**

Overview

- Postpartum blues can occur in approximately 50% to 70% of women during the first few days after birth and generally continues for up to 10 days. It is characterized by tearfulness, insomnia, lack of appetite, and feeling of letdown. A mother may experience an intense fear and/or anxiety, anger, and inability to cope with the slightest problems and become despondent. Postpartum blues typically resolves in 10 days without intervention.

- Postpartum depression occurs within 6 months of delivery and is characterized by persistent feelings of sadness and intense mood swings. It occurs in 10% to 15% of new mothers and usually does not resolve without intervention. It is similar to nonpostpartum mood disorders.

- Postpartum psychosis develops within the first 2 to 3 weeks of the postpartum period. Clients who have a history of bipolar disorder are at a higher risk. The symptoms are severe and may include confusion, disorientation, hallucinations, delusions, obsessive behaviors, and paranoia. The client may attempt to harm herself or her infant.

  ○ A nurse should monitor the client for suicidal or delusional thoughts. The infant should be monitored for failure to thrive secondary to an inability of the mother to provide care for her newborn.

Risk Factors

- Hormonal changes with a rapid decline in estrogen and progesterone levels
- Postpartum physical discomfort and/or pain
- Individual socioeconomic factors
- Decreased social support system
- Anxiety about assuming new role as a mother
- Unplanned or unwanted pregnancy
- History of previous depressive episode
- Low self-esteem
- History of domestic violence

Assessment

- Subjective Data
  - Postpartum blues
    - Feelings of sadness
    - Lack of appetite
    - Sleep pattern disturbances
    - Feeling of inadequacies
    - Intense mood swings
  - Postpartum depression
    - Feelings of guilt and inadequacies
    - Irritability
    - Anxiety
    - Fatigue persisting beyond a reasonable amount of time
    - Feeling of loss
    - Lack of appetite
    - Persistent feelings of sadness
    - Intense mood swings
    - Sleep pattern disturbances
  - Postpartum psychosis
    - Pronounced sadness
    - Disorientation
    - Confusion
    - Paranoia
- Objective Data
  - Physical assessment findings
    - Postpartum blues
      - Crying
    - Postpartum depression
      - Crying
      - Weight loss
      - Flat affect
      - Irritability
      - Rejection of the infant
      - Severe anxiety and panic attack
    - Postpartum psychosis
      - Behaviors indicating hallucinations or delusional thoughts of self harm or harming the infant

Patient-Centered Care

- Nursing Care

  ○ Monitor interactions between the client and her infant. Encourage bonding activities.

  ○ Monitor the client's mood and affect.

  ○ Reinforce that feeling down in the postpartum period is normal and self-limiting. Encourage the client to notify her provider if the condition persists.

  ○ Encourage the client to communicate feelings, validate and address personal conflicts, and reinforce personal power and autonomy.

  ○ Reinforce the importance of compliance with any prescribed medication regimen.

  ○ Contact a community resource to schedule a follow-up visit after discharge for clients who are at high risk for postpartum depression.

- Medications

  ○ Antidepressants may be prescribed by the provider if indicated.

  ○ Antipsychotics and mood stabilizers may be prescribed for clients who have postpartum psychosis.

- Care After Discharge

  ○ Advise the client to get plenty of rest and to nap when the infant sleeps.

  ○ Reinforce the importance of the client taking time out for herself.

  ○ Schedule a follow-up visit prior to the traditional postpartum visit for clients who are at risk for developing postpartum depression.

  ○ Provide information about community resources such as La Leche League or community mental health centers.

  ○ Encourage the client to seek counseling, and make referrals to social agencies as indicated.

APPLICATION EXERCISES

1. A nurse is assessing a postpartum client who is exhibiting tearfulness, insomnia, lack of appetite, and a feeling of letdown. The nurse knows these findings are characteristics of

    A. postpartum fatigue.

    B. postpartum psychosis.

    C. the letting-go phase.

    D. postpartum depression.

2. A nurse is caring for a client who has postpartum depression. Which of the following are expected findings? (Select all that apply.)

    A. Disappointment in the characteristics of the infant

    B. Concerns about lack of income to pay bills

    C. Anxiety about assuming a new role as a mother

    D. Rapid decline in estrogen and progesterone

    E. Postpartum physical discomfort and/or pain

3. A nurse is caring for a postpartum client who delivered her third infant 2 days ago. The nurse recognizes that which of the following findings are suggestive of postpartum depression? (Select all that apply.)

    A. Fatigue

    B. Insomnia

    C. Euphoria

    D. Flat affect

    E. Crying

4. A nurse manager is reviewing a protocol for the care of a client who has postpartum depression. What should be included in this protocol? Use the ATI Active Learning Template: Systems Disorder to complete this item to include the following sections:

    A. Description of Disorder

    B. Medications

    C. Nursing Care: Describe four nursing interventions.

    D. Care After Discharge: Describe two teaching points for the client.

APPLICATION EXERCISES KEY

1. A. INCORRECT: Postpartum fatigue results from the work of labor. It is normally self-limiting.

   B. INCORRECT: The client who has postpartum psychosis will exhibit pronounced feelings of sadness, confusion, disorientation, hallucinations, delusions, and paranoia, and may attempt to harm herself or her infant.

   C. INCORRECT: The letting-go phase is the phase in which the client assumes her position at home and her new maternal role, focusing on the forward movement of the family unit.

   D. **CORRECT:** Postpartum depression in the client is characterized by tearfulness, insomnia, lack of appetite, and feeling let down.

    NCLEX® Connection: Psychosocial Integrity, Coping Mechanisms

2. A. INCORRECT: Disappointment in the characteristics of the infant would be an indication of impaired mother-infant bonding.

   B. **CORRECT:** Feelings of financial inadequacy to provide for family is a finding associated with postpartum depression.

   C. **CORRECT:** A client's anxiety about assuming a new role as a mother is a finding associated with postpartum depression.

   D. **CORRECT:** The rapid decline in estrogen and progesterone is a finding associated with postpartum depression.

   E. **CORRECT:** Physical discomfort and/or pain is a finding associated with postpartum depression.

    NCLEX® Connection: Health Promotion and Maintenance, Ante/Intra/Postpartum and Newborn Care

3. A. **CORRECT:** Fatigue is a finding suggestive of postpartum depression.

   B. **CORRECT:** Insomnia is a finding suggestive of postpartum depression.

   C. INCORRECT: Euphoria is not associated with postpartum depression.

   D. **CORRECT:** A flat affect is a finding suggestive of postpartum depression.

   E. **CORRECT:** Crying is a finding suggestive of postpartum depression.

    NCLEX® Connection: Health Promotion and Maintenance, Ante/Intra/Postpartum and Newborn Care

4. *Using the ATI Active Learning Template: Systems Disorder*

    A. Description of Disorder
       • Postpartum depression occurs within 6 months of delivery. It is characterized by persistent feelings of sadness and intense mood swings. It occurs in 10% to 15% of new mothers and usually does not resolve without intervention. It is similar to nonpostpartum mood disorders.

    B. Medications
       • Antidepressants

    C. Nursing Care
       • Monitor client-infant interactions; encourage bonding activities.
       • Monitor client's mood and affect.
       • Encourage verbalization of feelings; validate and address person conflicts; reinforce personal power and autonomy.
       • Reinforce compliance with medication regimen.
       • Provide referral, and schedule appointment with an appropriate community resource.

    D. Care After Discharge
       • Get plenty of rest; nap when the infant sleeps.
       • Take time for herself.
       • Seek counseling, and use resources provided by referred community agencies.

    Ⓝ NCLEX® Connection: Psychosocial Integrity, Coping Mechanisms

UNIT 4   Newborn Nursing Care

SECTIONS
> Low-Risk Newborn
> Complications of the Newborn

NCLEX® CONNECTIONS

When reviewing the chapters in this unit, keep in mind the relevant sections of the NCLEX® outline, in particular:

Client Needs: Health Promotion and Maintenance	Client Needs: Basic Care and Comfort	Client Needs: Reduction of Risk Potential

> Relevant topics/tasks include:
» Ante/Intra/Postpartum and Newborn Care
  > Provide newborn care and education.
» Techniques of Physical Assessment
  > Apply knowledge of nursing procedures and psychomotor skills to techniques of physical assessment.
	> Relevant topics/tasks include:
	» Nonpharmacological Comfort Interventions
	  > Apply knowledge of pathophysiology to nonpharmacological comfort/palliative care interventions.
	» Nutrition and Oral Hydration
	  > Manage the client's nutritional intake (e.g., adjust diet, monitor height and weight).
		> Relevant topics/tasks include:
		» Changes/Abnormalities in Vital Signs
		  > Apply knowledge of client pathophysiology when measuring vital signs.
		» Laboratory Values
		  > Identify laboratory values for ABGs, BUN, cholesterol, glucose, hematocrit, hemoglobin, glycosylated hemoglobin, platelets, potassium, sodium, WBC, creatinine, PT, PTT and APTT, INR.
		» System Specific Assessment
		  > Assess the client for signs of hypoglycemia or hyperglycemia.

chapter 23

Overview

- Understanding physiologic responses of a newborn to birth and physical assessment findings are imperative for providing nursing care following the birth of a newborn. Apgar scoring, physical examination of the newborn, New Ballard Scale (gestational age assessment), normal newborn vital signs and measurements, classifications of a newborn by gestational age and weight, diagnostic and therapeutic procedures, and complications of a newborn will be addressed in this chapter.

Physiologic Response of Newborn to Birth

- Adjustments to extrauterine life occur as a newborn's respiratory and circulatory systems are required to rapidly adjust to life outside of the uterus.
- The establishment of respiratory function with the cutting of the umbilical cord is the most critical extrauterine adjustment as air inflates the lungs with the first breath.
- Circulatory changes after birth occur with the expulsion of the placenta and the cutting of the umbilical cord as a newborn begins breathing independently. The three shunts (ductus arteriosus, ductus venosus, and foramen ovale) functionally close during a newborn's transition to extrauterine life with the flow of oxygenated blood in the lungs and readjustment of atrial blood pressure in the heart.

Physical Assessment of Newborn Following Birth

- Apgar scoring and a brief physical exam is done immediately following birth to rule out abnormalities. An Apgar score is assigned based on a quick review of systems that is completed at 1 and 5 min of life. This allows the nurse to rapidly assess extrauterine adaptation and intervene with appropriate nursing actions.
  - 0 to 3 indicates severe distress
  - 4 to 6 indicates moderate distress
  - 7 to 10 indicates no distress

SCORE	0	1	2
Heart rate	› Absent	› Less than 100	› Greater than 100
Respiratory rate	› Absent	› Slow, weak cry	› Good cry
Muscle tone	› Flaccid	› Some flexion	› Well-flexed
Reflex irritability	› None	› Grimace	› Cry
Color	› Blue, pale	› Pink body, cyanotic hands and feet (acrocyanosis)	› Completely pink

 View Video: Apgar Scoring

○ Equipment for newborn assessment

- Bulb syringe – Used for suctioning excess mucus from the mouth and nose.

- Stethoscope with a pediatric head – Used to evaluate heart rate, breath sounds, and bowel sounds.

- Axillary thermometer – Used to monitor temperature and prevent hypothermia. Rectal temperatures are avoided because they can injure the delicate rectal mucosa; an initial rectal temperature may be obtained to evaluate for anal abnormalities.

- Blood pressure cuff 2.5 cm wide – Palpation or electronic method. Blood pressure may be done in all four extremities if evaluating the newborn for cardiac problems.

- Scale with protective cover in place – Scale should be at 0; weight should include pounds, ounces, and grams.

- Tape measure in centimeters – Measure from crown to heel of foot for length. Measure head circumference at greatest diameter (occipital to frontal). Measure chest circumference beginning at the nipple line, and abdominal circumference above the umbilicus.

- Clean gloves – Worn for all physical assessments until discharge.

• The nurse performs a quick initial assessment to review the newborn's systems and to observe for any abnormalities.

○ External assessment – Skin color, peeling, birthmarks, foot creases, breast tissue, nasal patency, and meconium staining (may indicate fetal hypoxia)

○ Chest – Point of maximal impulse location, ease of breathing, auscultation for heart rate and quality of tones and respirations for crackles, wheezes, and equality of bilateral breath sounds

○ Abdomen – Rounded abdomen and umbilical cord for one vein and two arteries

○ Neurologic – Muscle tone and reflex reaction (Moro reflex); palpation for the presence and size of fontanels and sutures; assessment of fontanels for fullness or bulge

○ Other observations – Inspection for gross structural malformations

• A gestational age assessment is performed within 2 to 12 hr of birth. Neonatal morbidity and mortality are related to gestational age and birth weight. This assessment involves taking measurements of the newborn and the use of the New Ballard Scale. This scale provides an estimation of gestational age and a baseline to assess growth and development.

○ Expected reference ranges of physical measurements

- Weight – 2,500 to 4,000 g

- Length – 45 to 55 cm (18 to 22 in)

- Head circumference – 32 to 36.8 cm (12.6 to 14.5 in)

- Chest circumference – 30 to 33 cm (12 to 13 in)

○ New Ballard Scale – A newborn maturity rating scale that assesses neuromuscular and physical maturity. Each individual assessment parameter displays at least six ranges of development along a continuum. Each range of development within an assessment is assigned a number value from -1 to 5. The totals are added to give a maturity rating in weeks gestation (a score of 35 indicates 38 weeks of gestation).

 View Video: Gestational Age Assessment

- Neuromuscular maturity assesses:
  - Posture ranging from fully extended to fully flexed (0 to 4).
  - Square window formation with the neonate's wrist (-1 to 4).
  - Arm recoil, where the neonate's arm is passively extended and spontaneously returns to flexion (0 to 4).
  - Popliteal angle, which is the degree of the angle to which the newborn's knees can extend (-1 to 5).
  - Scarf sign, which is crossing the neonate's arm over the chest (-1 to 4).
  - Heel to ear, which is how far the neonate's heels reach to her ears (-1 to 4).
- Physical maturity assesses:
  - Skin texture, ranging from sticky and transparent, to leathery, cracked, and wrinkled (-1 to 5).
  - Lanugo presence and amount, ranging from none, sparse, abundant, thinning, bald, or mostly bald (-1 to 4).
  - Plantar surface creases, ranging from less than 40 to 50 mm to creases over the entire sole (-1 to 4).
  - Breast tissue amount, ranging from imperceptible, to full areola with a 5 to 10 mm bud (-1 to 4).
  - Eyes and ears for amount of eye opening and ear cartilage present (-1 to 4).
  - Genitalia development, ranging from flat smooth scrotum to pendulous testes with deep rugae for males (-1 to 4), and prominent clitoris with flat labia to the labia majora covering the labia minora and clitoris for females (-1 to 4).

- Following physical assessment, classification of the newborn by gestational age and birth weight is then determined.
  - Appropriate for gestational age (AGA) – Weight is between the 10th and 90th percentile.
  - Small for gestational age (SGA) – Weight is below the 10th percentile.
  - Large for gestational age (LGA) – Weight is above the 90th percentile.
  - Low birth weight (LBW) – Weight of 2,500 g or less at birth.
  - Intrauterine growth restriction (IUGR) – Growth rate does not meet expected norms.
  - Term – Birth between the beginning of week 38 and prior to the end of 42 weeks of gestation.
  - Preterm or premature – Born prior to the completion of 37 weeks of gestation.
  - Postterm (postdate) – Born after the completion of 42 weeks of gestation.
  - Postmature – Born after the completion of 42 weeks of gestation with evidence of placental insufficiency.

- Vital signs are checked in the following sequence: respirations, heart rate, blood pressure, and temperature. The nurse observes the respiratory rate first before the newborn becomes active or agitated by use of the stethoscope, thermometer, and/or the blood pressure cuff.
  - Respiratory rate increases from 30 to 60/min with short periods of apnea (less than 15 seconds) occurring most frequently during the rapid eye movement sleep cycle. Periods of apnea lasting longer than 15 seconds should be evaluated. Crackles and wheezing are symptoms of fluid or infection in the lungs. Grunting and nasal flaring are signs of respiratory distress.
  - Heart rate should be 100 to 160/min with brief fluctuations above and below this range depending on activity level (crying, sleeping). Apical pulse rate is assessed for a full minute, preferably when the newborn is sleeping. The pediatric stethoscope head is placed on the fourth or fifth intercostal space at the left midclavicular line over the apex of the newborn's heart. Heart murmurs are documented and reported.

- ○ Blood pressure should be 60 to 80 mm Hg systolic and 40 to 50 mm Hg diastolic.
- ○ Temperature should be 36.5° to 37.2° C (97.7° to 98.9° F) axillary. The newborn is at risk for hypothermia and hyperthermia until thermoregulation (ability to produce heat and maintain normal body temperature) stabilizes. If the newborn becomes chilled (cold stress), oxygen demands can increase and acidosis can occur.
- A more extensive physical exam is performed on the neonate within 24 hr of birth. Vital signs are obtained. A head-to-toe assessment is performed. Neurological and behavioral assessments are completed by eliciting reflexes and observing responses. Laboratory data is monitored.
- Physical exam from head to toe
  - ○ Posture
    - Lying in a curled-up position with arms and legs in moderate flexion
    - Resistant to extension of extremities
  - ○ Skin
    - Skin color should be pink or acrocyanotic with no jaundice present on the first day. Secondary to increased bilirubin, jaundice may appear on the third day of life, but then decrease spontaneously.
    - Skin turgor should be present, showing that the newborn is well hydrated. The skin should spring back immediately when pinched.
    - Texture should be dry, soft, and smooth, showing good hydration. Cracks in hands and feet may be present. In full-term newborns, desquamation (peeling) occurs a few days after birth.
    - Vernix caseosa (protective, thick, cheesy covering) amounts vary, with more present in creases and skin folds.
    - Lanugo (fine downy hair) varies regarding the amount present. It is usually found on the pinnas, forehead, and shoulders.
    - Normal deviations
      - □ Milia (small raised white spots on the nose, chin, and forehead) may be present. These spots disappear spontaneously without treatment (parents should not squeeze the spots).
      - □ Mongolian spots (bluish purple spots of pigmentation) are commonly noted on the shoulders, back, and buttocks. These spots are frequently present on newborns who have dark skin. Be sure the parents are aware of Mongolian spots, and document location and presence.
      - □ Telangiectatic nevi (stork bites) are flat pink or red marks that easily blanch and are found on the back of the neck, nose, upper eyelids, and middle of the forehead. They usually fade by the second year of life.
      - □ Nevus flammeus (port wine stain) is a capillary angioma below the surface of the skin that is purple or red, varies in size and shape, is commonly seen on the face, and does not blanch or disappear.
      - □ Erythema toxicum (erythema neonatorum) is a pink rash that appears suddenly anywhere on the body of a term newborn during the first 3 weeks. This is frequently referred to as newborn rash. No treatment is required.

○ Head

- Should be 2 to 3 cm larger than chest circumference. If the head circumference is greater than or equal to 4 cm larger than the chest circumference, this can be an indication of hydrocephalus (excessive cerebral fluid within the brain cavity surrounding the brain). If the head circumference is less than or equal to 32 cm, this can be an indication of microcephaly (abnormally small head).

- Anterior fontanel should be palpated and approximately 5 cm on average and diamond shaped. Posterior fontanel is smaller and triangle shaped. Fontanels should be soft and flat. Fontanels may bulge when the newborn cries, coughs, or vomits, and are flat when the newborn is quiet. Bulging fontanels may indicate increased intracranial pressure, infection, or hemorrhage. Depressed fontanels may indicate dehydration.

- Sutures should be palpable, separated, and may be overlapping (molding), a normal occurrence resulting from head compression during labor.

- Caput succedaneum (localized swelling of the soft tissues of the scalp caused by pressure on the head during labor) is an expected finding that may be palpated as a soft edematous mass and may cross over the suture line. Caput succedaneum usually resolves in 3 to 4 days and does not require treatment.

- Cephalohematoma is a collection of blood between the periosteum and the skull bone that it covers. It does not cross the suture line. It results from trauma during birth such as pressure of the fetal head against the maternal pelvis in a prolonged difficult labor or forceps delivery. It appears in the first 1 to 2 days after birth and resolves in 2 to 3 weeks.

View Images
› Caput Succedaneum   › Cephalohematoma

○ Eyes

- Assess eyes for symmetry in size and shape.

- Each eye and the space between the eyes should equal one-third of the total distance between the outer canthus of both eyes to rule out chromosomal abnormalities such as Down syndrome.

- Eyes are usually blue or gray. Permanent eye color is established within 3 to 12 months.

- Lacrimal glands are immature, resulting in tearless crying.

- Subconjunctival hemorrhages may result from pressure during birth.

- Pupillary and red reflex are present.

- Eyeball movement will demonstrate random, jerky movements.

○ Ears

- When examining the placement of ears, draw an imaginary line through the inner to the outer canthus of the newborn's eye. The eye should be even with the upper tip of the pinna of the newborn's ear. Ears that are low-set can indicate a chromosome abnormality such as Down syndrome or a kidney disorder.

- Cartilage should be firm and well formed. Lack of cartilage indicates prematurity.

- The newborn should respond to voices and other sounds.

- Inspect ears for skin tags.

○ Nose

- Should be midline, flat, and broad with lack of a bridge.

- Some mucus should be present, but with no drainage.

- Newborns are obligate nose breathers and do not develop the response of opening the mouth with a nasal obstruction until 3 weeks after birth. Therefore, a nasal blockage may result in flaring of the nares, cyanosis, or asphyxia.

- Newborns sneeze to clear nasal passages.

○ Mouth

- Assess for palate closure and strength of sucking.

- Lip movements should be symmetrical.

- Saliva should be scant. Excessive saliva may indicate a tracheoesophageal fistula.

- Epstein's pearls (small white cysts found on the gums and at the junction of the soft and hard palates) are expected findings. They result from the accumulation of epithelial cells and disappear a few weeks after birth.

- Tongue should move freely, be symmetrical in shape, and not protrude. (A protruding tongue may be a sign of Down syndrome.)

- Soft and hard palate should be intact.

- Gums and tongue should be pink. Gray-white patches on the tongue and gums can indicate thrush, a fungal infection caused by Candida albicans, sometimes acquired from the mother's vaginal secretions.

○ Neck

- Neck should be short, thick, surrounded by skin folds, and exhibit no webbing.

- Neck should move freely from side to side and up and down.

- Absence of head control may indicate prematurity or Down syndrome.

○ Chest

- Chest should be barrel-shaped.

- Respirations are primarily diaphragmatic.

- Clavicles should be intact.

- Absence of retractions.

- Nipples should be prominent, well formed, and symmetrical.

- Breast nodule should be approximately 6 mm.

○ Abdomen

- Umbilical cord should be odorless and exhibit no intestinal structures.

- Abdomen should be round, dome-shaped, and nondistended.

- Bowel sounds should be present 1 to 2 hr following birth.

○ Anogenital

- Anus should be present, patent, and not covered by a membrane.

- Meconium should be passed within 24 hr after birth.

- Genitalia of a male newborn should include rugae on the scrotum.

- Testes should be present in scrotum.

- Male urinary meatus is located at penile tip.
- Genitalia of a female should include labia majora covering the labia minora and clitoris, and are usually edematous.
- Vaginal blood-tinged discharge may occur in female newborns, which is caused by maternal pregnancy hormones. This is an expected finding.
- A hymenal tag should be present.
- Urine should be passed within 24 hr after birth. Uric acid crystals will produce a rust color in the urine the first couple of days of life.

○ Extremities

- Assess for full range, symmetry of motion, and spontaneous movements.
- Extremities should be flexed.
- Assess for bowed legs and flat feet, which should be present because lateral muscles are more developed than the medial muscles.
- No click should be heard when abducting the hips.
- Gluteal folds should be symmetrical.
- Soles should be well-lined over two-thirds of the feet.
- Nail beds should be pink, and no extra digits are present.

○ Spine

- Spine should be straight, flat, midline and easily flexed.

○ Reflexes

REFLEX	EXPECTED FINDING	EXPECTED AGE
Sucking and rooting reflex	› Elicited by stroking the cheek or edge of mouth. Newborn turns the head toward the side that is touched and starts to suck.	Birth to 4 months
Palmar grasp	› Elicited by placing an object in the newborn's palm. The newborn grasps the object.	Birth to 6 months
Plantar grasp	› Elicited by touching the sole of the foot. The newborn responds by curling toes downward.	Birth to 8 months
Moro reflex	› Moro reflex by striking a flat surface that the newborn is lying on, or allowing the head and trunk of the newborn in a semisitting position to fall backward to an angle of at least 30°. Arms and legs symmetrically extend and then abduct while fingers spread to form a "C."	Birth to 4 months
Startle reflex	› This reflex is elicited by clamping hands or by a loud noise. The newborn will abduct arms at the elbows, and the hands will remain unclenched.	Birth to 4 months
Tonic neck reflex (fencer position)	› The newborn extends arm and leg on the side when head is turned to that side with flexion of arm and leg of opposite side. › The newborn turns head to one side. The newborn responds by extending arm and leg on that side, and flexing arm and leg on opposite side.	Birth to 3 to 4 months

REFLEX	EXPECTED FINDING	EXPECTED AGE
Babinski's reflex	› Elicited by stroking outer edge of sole of the foot, moving up toward toes. Toes will fan upward and out.	Birth to 1 year
Stepping	› Elicited by holding the newborn upright with feet touching a flat surface. The newborn responds with stepping movements.	Birth to 4 weeks

- ○ Senses
  - ▪ Vision – Should be able to focus on objects 9 to 12 inches away from face. This is approximately the distance from the mother's face when the newborn is breastfeeding. The eyes are sensitive to light; therefore, newborns prefer dim lighting. Pupils are reactive to light, and the blink reflex is easily stimulated. The newborn can track high-contrast objects and prefers bright colors and patterns.
  - ▪ Hearing – Similar to that of an adult once the amniotic fluid drains from the ears. Newborns exhibit selective listening to familiar voices and rhythms of intrauterine life. The newborn turns toward the general direction of a sound.
  - ▪ Touch – Should respond to tactile messages of pain and touch. The mouth is the area most sensitive to touch in the newborn.
  - ▪ Taste – Can taste and prefers sweets over salty, sour, or bitter.
  - ▪ Smell – Highly developed sense of smell, prefer sweet smells, and can recognize the smell of the mother.
  - ▪ Habitation – Protective mechanism whereby newborn becomes accustomed to environmental stimuli. Response to a constant or repetitive stimulus is decreased. Allows newborn to select stimuli that promotes continued learning, avoiding overload.
- • Provide education to the mother and family about the neonate's appearance, and give reassurance about expected findings that the family may be concerned about (e.g., milia, Epstein's pearls, caput succedaneum).

Diagnostic and Therapeutic Procedures Following Birth

- • Cord blood is collected at birth. Laboratory tests are conducted to determine ABO blood type and Rh status if the mother's blood type is "O" or she is Rh-negative. A CBC may be done by a capillary stick to evaluate for anemia, polycythemia, infection, or clotting problems. Blood glucose is done to evaluate for hypoglycemia.

EXPECTED LABORATORY VALUES			
Hgb	14 to 24 g/dL	Platelets	150,000 to 300,000/mm^3
Hct	44% to 64%	Glucose	40 to 60 mg/dL
RBC count	4,800 to 7,100,000/mm^3	Bilirubin	0 to 6 mg/dL on day 1
Leukocytes	9,000 to 30,000/mm^3		8 mg/dL or less on day 2
			12 mg/dL or less on day 3

Complications

- Airway obstruction related to mucus
  - Mouth and nose are suctioned with a bulb syringe. Gentle percussion over the chest can help loosen secretions.
- Hypothermia
  - Monitor for an axillary temperature of less than 36.5° C (97.7° F).
  - If temperature is unstable, place the newborn in a radiant warmer, and maintain skin temperature at approximately 36.5° C (97.7° F).
  - Assess axillary temperature every hour until stable.
  - All exams and assessments should be performed under a radiant warmer.
- Inadequate oxygen supply related to obstructed airway, poorly functioning cardiopulmonary system, or hypothermia
  - Monitor respirations and skin color for cyanosis.
  - Stabilize the body temperature or clear airway as indicated, administer oxygen, and if needed, prepare for resuscitation.

APPLICATION EXERCISES

1. A nurse is caring for a newborn who was born at 38 weeks of gestation, weighs 3,200 g, and is in the 60th percentile for weight. Based on the weight and gestational age, the nurse should classify this neonate as

    A. low birth weight.

    B. appropriate for gestational age.

    C. small for gestational age.

    D. large for gestational age.

2. A nurse is completing a newborn assessment and observes small white nodules on the roof of the newborn's mouth. This finding is a characteristic of which of the following conditions?

    A. Mongolian spots

    B. Milia spots

    C. Erythema toxicum

    D. Epstein's pearls

3. A nurse is assessing the reflexes of a newborn. In checking for the Moro reflex, the nurse should perform which of the following?

    A. Make a loud noise such as clapping hands together over the newborn's crib.

    B. Stimulate the pads of the newborn's hands with stroking or massage.

    C. Stimulate the soles of the newborn's feet on the outer lateral surface of each foot.

    D. Hold the newborn in a semisitting position, then allow the newborn's head and trunk to fall backward.

4. A nurse is completing an assessment. Which of the following data indicate the newborn is adapting to extrauterine life? (Select all that apply.)

    _____ A. Expiratory grunting

    _____ B. Inspiratory nasal flaring

    _____ C. Apnea for 10-second periods

    _____ D. Obligatory nose breathing

    _____ E. Crackles and wheezing

5. A nurse is preparing to bathe a newborn and observes a bluish marking across the newborn's lower back. The nurse should understand that this mark is

    A. frequently seen in newborns who have dark skin.

    B. a finding indicating hyperbilirubinemia.

    C. a forceps mark from an operative delivery.

    D. related to prolonged birth or trauma during delivery.

6. A nurse in the nursery is admitting a newborn 2 hr following birth. What nursing actions should the nurse use to evaluate newborn physical development? Use the ATI Active Learning Template: Growth and Development to complete this item to include the following sections:

    A. Physical Development:
- Describe at least three tools for assessment.
- Describe four reflex responses present at birth and how they are elicited.
- Describe newborn heart rate and how it is assessed.

APPLICATION EXERCISES KEY

1. A. INCORRECT: A newborn who has a low birth weight would weigh less than 2,500 g.

    B. **CORRECT:** This newborn is classified as appropriate for gestational age because the weight is between the 10th and 90th percentile.

    C. INCORRECT: A newborn who is small for gestational age would weigh below the 10th percentile.

    D. INCORRECT: A newborn who is large for gestational age would weigh above the 90th percentile.

    Ⓝ NCLEX® Connection: Health Promotion and Maintenance, Developmental Stages and Transitions

2. A. INCORRECT: Mongolian spots are dark areas observed in dark-skinned newborns.

    B. INCORRECT: Milia are small white bumps that occur on the nose due to clogged sebaceous glands.

    C. INCORRECT: Erythema toxicum is a transient maculopapular rash seen in newborns.

    D. **CORRECT:** Epstein's pearls are small white nodules that appear on the roof of a newborn's mouth.

    Ⓝ NCLEX® Connection: Health Promotion and Maintenance, Aging Process

3. A. INCORRECT: Clapping hands elicits the startle reflex.

    B. INCORRECT: Stimulating the pads of the newborn's hands elicits the grasp reflex.

    C. INCORRECT: Stimulating the outer lateral portion of the newborn's soles elicits Babinski's reflex.

    D. **CORRECT:** The Moro reflex is elicited by holding the newborn in a semi-sitting position and then allowing the head and trunk to fall backward.

    Ⓝ NCLEX® Connection: Health Promotion and Maintenance, Developmental Stages and Transitions

4. A. INCORRECT: Expiratory grunting is a manifestation of respiratory distress.

    B. INCORRECT: Nasal flaring is a manifestation of respiratory distress.

    C. **CORRECT:** Periods of apnea lasting less than 15 seconds are an expected finding.

    D. **CORRECT:** Newborns are obligatory nose breathers.

    E. INCORRECT: Crackles and wheezing are symptoms of fluid or infection in the lungs.

    Ⓝ NCLEX® Connection: Health Promotion and Maintenance, Aging Process

5.   A. **CORRECT:** Mongolian spots are commonly found over the lumbosacral area of newborns who have dark skin and are of African American, Asian, or Native American origin.

   B. INCORRECT: Hyperbilirubinemia would present as jaundice.

   C. INCORRECT: Forceps marks would most likely present as a cephalohematoma.

   D. INCORRECT: Birth trauma would present as ecchymosis.

   (N) NCLEX® Connection: Health Promotion and Maintenance, Aging Process

6.   *Using the ATI Active Learning Template: Growth and Development*

   A. Physical Development
   - Assessment tools
     - Brief initial systems assessment
     - Gestational age assessment – Physical measurements and New Ballard Scale
     - Vital signs
     - Head-to-toe physical assessment
   - Reflexes
     - Sucking and rooting – Turns head to side that is touched and begins to suck when cheek or edge of mouth is stroked.
     - Palmar grasp – Grasps object when placed in palm.
     - Plantar grasp – Toes curl downward when sole of the foot is touched.
     - Moro – Arms and legs symmetrically extend and then abduct while fingers spread to form a "C" when infant's head and trunk are allowed to fall backward to an angle of at least 30°.
     - Tonic neck (fencer position) – Extends arm and leg on same side when head is turned to that side, and flexes arm and leg of opposite side.
     - Babinski's – Toes fan upward and out when outer edge of sole of foot is stroked, moving up toward toes.
     - Stepping – Makes stepping movements when held upright with feet touching flat surface.
   - Heart rate
     - 100 to 160/min with brief fluctuations above and below, depending on activity level.
     - When newborn is sleeping, place pediatric stethoscope head on fourth or fifth intercostal space at the left midclavicular line over apex of the heart. Listen for a full minute.
     - Note any murmurs.

   (N) NCLEX® Connection: Health Promotion and Maintenance, Developmental Stages and Transitions

chapter 24

Overview

- Newborn care consists of stabilization and/or resuscitation. This may include establishing a patent airway, maintaining adequate oxygenation, and thermoregulation for the maintenance of body temperature. A physical assessment will be done every 8 hr or as needed (physical examination, measurements, and monitoring laboratory studies). Nursing interventions and family teaching (umbilical cord care, prophylactic measures, newborn screening, newborn feedings and bathing, and fostering baby-friendly activities) are integrated into a newborn's plan of care.

Assessment

- Physical Assessment

  - Vital signs should be checked on admission/birth and every 30 min x 2, every 1 hr x 2, and then every 8 hr.

  - Weight should be checked daily at the same time, using the same scale.

  - Inspect the newborn's umbilical cord. Observe for any bleeding from the cord, and ensure that the cord is clamped securely to prevent hemorrhage.

  - In the first 6 to 8 hr of life as body systems stabilize and pass through periods of adjustment, observe for periods of reactivity.

    - First period of reactivity – The newborn is alert, exhibits exploring activity, makes sucking sounds, and has a rapid heart rate and respiratory rate. Heart rate may be as high as 160 to 180/min, but will stabilize at a baseline of 100 to 120/min during a period that lasts 15 to 30 min after birth.

    - Period of relative inactivity – The newborn will become quiet and begin to rest and sleep. The heart rate and respirations will decrease, and this period will last from 30 min to 2 hr after birth.

    - Second period of reactivity – The newborn reawakens, becomes responsive again, and often gags and chokes on mucus that has accumulated in his mouth. This period usually occurs 2 to 8 hr after birth and may last 10 min to several hours.

  - Using the facility's preferred pain assessment tool, conduct a pain assessment on the newborn every 8 to 12 hr and following painful procedures.

- Laboratory Tests
  - ○ Hgb and Hct, if prescribed
  - ○ Blood glucose for hypoglycemia, per facility policy or as prescribed
  - ○ Metabolic screening
    - Newborn genetic screening is mandated in all states. A capillary heel stick should be done 24 hr following birth. For results to be accurate, the newborn must have received formula or breast milk for at least 24 hr. If the newborn is discharged before 24 hr of age, the test should be repeated in 1 to 2 weeks.
    - All states require testing for phenylketonuria (PKU). PKU is a defect in protein metabolism in which the accumulation of the amino acid phenylalanine can result in mental retardation. (Treatment in the first 2 months of life can prevent retardation.)
  - ○ Other genetic testing that may be done includes: galactosemia, cystic fibrosis, maple syrup urine disease, hypothyroidism, and sickle cell disease.
  - ○ Collecting blood samples
    - Heel stick blood samples are obtained by the nurse, who dons clean gloves.
    - Warm the newborn's heel first to increase circulation.
    - Cleanse the area with an appropriate antiseptic, and allow for drying.
    - A spring-activated lancet is used so that the skin incision is made quickly and painlessly.
    - The outer aspect of the heel should be used, and the lancet should go no deeper than 2.4 mm to prevent necrotizing osteochondritis resulting from penetration of bone with the lancet.
    - Follow facility protocol for specimen collection, equipment to be used, and labeling of specimens.
    - Apply pressure with dry gauze (do not use alcohol because it will cause bleeding to continue) until bleeding stops, and cover with an adhesive bandage.
    - Cuddle and comfort the newborn when the procedure is completed to reassure the newborn and promote feelings of safety.
- Diagnostic Procedures
  - ○ Newborn hearing screening is required in most states. Newborns are screened so that deafness can be detected and treated early.

Patient-Centered Care

- Nursing Care
  - ○ Stabilize and/or give resuscitation to the newborn.
  - ○ Monitor for signs and symptoms of respiratory complications.
    - Bradypnea – respirations less than 25/min
    - Tachypnea – respirations greater than 60/min
    - Abnormal breath sounds – expiratory grunting, crackles, and wheezes
    - Respiratory distress – nasal flaring, retractions, grunting, and labored breathing

○ Interventions for stabilization and resuscitation of airway

- The newborn is able to clear most secretions in air passages by the cough reflex. Routine suctioning of the mouth first, then the nasal passages with a bulb syringe, is done to remove excess mucus in the respiratory tract.

- Newborns delivered by cesarean birth are more susceptible to fluid remaining in the lungs than newborns who were delivered vaginally.

- If bulb suctioning is unsuccessful, mechanical suction and/or back blows and chest thrusts may be used, as well as the institution of emergency procedures.

- The bulb syringe should be kept with the newborn, and the newborn's family should be instructed on its use. Family members should be asked to perform a demonstration to show that they understand bulb syringe techniques.

  □ Compress bulb before insertion into one side of the mouth.

  □ Avoid center of the mouth to prevent stimulating gag reflex.

  □ Aspirate mouth first, one nostril, then second nostril.

○ Identification (using two identifiers) is applied to the newborn immediately after birth by the nurse. It is an important safety measure to prevent the newborn from being given to the wrong parents, switched, or abducted.

- The newborn, mother, and mother's partner are identified by plastic identification wristbands with permanent locks that must be cut to be removed. Identification bands should include the newborn's name, sex, date, time of birth, and mother's health record number. The newborn should have one band placed on the ankle and one on the wrist. In addition, the newborn's footprints and mother's thumbprints are taken. The above information is also included with the footprint sheet.

- Each time the newborn is taken to the parents, the identification band should be verified against the mother's identification band.

- All facility staff who assist in caring for the newborn are required to wear photo identification badges.

- The newborn is not to be given to anyone who does not have a photo identification badge that distinguishes that person as a staff member of the facility maternal-newborn unit.

- Many facilities have locked maternal-newborn units that require staff to permit entrance or exit. Some facilities have a sensor device on the ID band or umbilical cord clamp that sounds an alarm if the newborn is removed from the facility.

○ Thermoregulation provides a neutral thermal environment that helps a newborn maintain a normal core temperature with minimal oxygen consumption and caloric expenditure. A newborn has a relatively large surface-to-weight ratio, reduced metabolism per unit area, blood vessels closer to the surface, and small amounts of insulation. The newborn keeps warm by metabolizing brown fat, which is unique to newborns, but only within a very narrow temperature range. Becoming chilled (cold stress) can increase the newborn's oxygen demands and rapidly use up brown fat reserves. Therefore, monitoring temperature regulation is important.

- Monitor for hypothermia in the newborn.

  □ Axillary temperature of less than 36.5° C (97.7° F)

  □ Cyanosis

  □ Increased respiratory rate

- Interventions to maintain thermoregulation
  - Core temperature varies within newborns, but it should be kept around 36.5° C (97.7° F). Heat loss occurs by four mechanisms.
    - Conduction – Loss of body heat resulting from direct contact with a cooler surface. Preheat a radiant warmer, warm a stethoscope and other instruments, and pad a scale before weighing the newborn. The newborn should be placed directly on the mother's abdomen and covered with a warm blanket.
    - Convection – Flow of heat from the body surface to cooler environmental air. Place the bassinet out of the direct line of a fan or air conditioning vent, swaddle the newborn in a blanket, and keep the head covered. Any procedure done with the newborn uncovered should be performed under a radiant heat source.
    - Evaporation – Loss of heat as surface liquid is converted to vapor. Gently rub the newborn dry with a warm sterile blanket (adhering to standard precautions) immediately after delivery. If thermoregulation is unstable, postpone the initial bath until the newborn's skin temperature is 36.5° C (97.7° F). When bathing, expose only one body part at a time, washing and drying thoroughly.
    - Radiation – Loss of heat from the body surface to a cooler solid surface that is close to, but not in direct contact. Keep the newborn and examining tables away from windows and air conditioners.
  - Temperature stabilizes at 37° C (98.6° F) within 4 hr after birth if chilling is prevented.
- Bathing can begin once the newborn's temperature has stabilized to at least 36.5° C (97.7° F). A complete sponge bath should be given within the first 1 to 2 hr after birth under a radiant heat source to prevent heat loss. If necessary, the first bath will be postponed until thermoregulation stabilizes.
  - Gloves should be worn until the newborn's first bath to avoid exposure to body secretions.
- Feedings may be started immediately following birth.
  - Breastfeeding is initiated as soon as possible after birth as part of baby-friendly initiatives.
  - Formula feeding usually is started at about 2 to 4 hr of age. A few sips of sterile water may be given to assess sucking and swallowing reflexes and ensure that there are no anomalies, such as a tracheoesophageal fistula, prior to initiating formula.
    - The newborn is fed on demand, which is normally every 3 to 4 hr for bottle-fed newborns and more frequently for breastfed newborns.
    - Monitor and document feedings per facility protocol.
- Sleep-wake states are variations of consciousness in the newborn consisting of six states along a continuum comprised of: deep sleep, light sleep, drowsy, quiet alert, active alert, and extreme irritability (crying).

  - Newborns sleep approximately 17 hr a day, an average of 4 hr at a time. Newborns are positioned supine, "safe sleep," to decrease the incidence of sudden infant death syndrome (SIDS).
    - No bumper pads, loose linens, or toys should be placed in the bassinet.
    - Mothers should sleep in close proximity but not in a shared space. Higher incidence rates are noted for SIDS and suffocation with bed sharing.
    - Educate parents about the need for immunizations as a measure to prevent SIDS.

- ○ Monitor elimination habits.

  - Newborns should void once within 24 hr of birth. They should void 6 to 10 times a day after 4 days of life.

  - Meconium should be passed within the first 24 hr after birth. The newborn will then continue to stool 3 to 4 times a day depending on whether he is being breast- or bottle-fed.

  - The stools of newborns who are breastfed may appear yellow and seedy. These stools are lighter in color and looser than the stools of newborns who are formula-fed.

- ○ Monitor and document output.

  - Keep the perineal area clean and dry. The ammonia in urine is irritating to the skin and can cause diaper rash.

  - After each diaper change, cleanse the perineal area with clear water or water with a mild soap. Diaper wipes with alcohol should be avoided. Pat dry, and apply triple antibiotic ointment, petroleum jelly, or zinc oxide, depending on facility protocol.

- ○ Infection control is essential in preventing cross-contamination from newborn to newborn and between newborns and staff. Newborns are at risk for infection during the first few months of life because of immature immune systems.

  - Provide individual bassinets equipped with a thermometer, diapers, T-shirts, and bathing supplies.

  - All personnel caring for a newborn should scrub with antimicrobial soap from elbows to finger tips before entering the nursery. In between care of the newborn, the nurse should follow facility hygiene protocols. Cover gowns or special uniforms are used to avoid direct contact with clothes.

- ○ Provide family education and promote family-newborn attachment.

  - Provide family education while performing all nursing care. Encourage family involvement, allowing the mother and family to perform newborn care with direct supervision and support by the nurse.

  - Encourage mothers and family to hold the newborn so that they can experience eye-to-eye contact and interaction.

  - Foster sibling interaction in newborn care.

- • Medications

  - ○ Erythromycin (Romycin)

    - Prophylactic eye care is the mandatory instillation of antibiotic ointment into the eyes to prevent ophthalmia neonatorum. Infections can be transmitted during descent through the birth canal. Ophthalmia neonatorum is caused by Neisseria gonorrhoeae or Chlamydia trachomatis and can cause blindness.

    - Nursing Considerations and Client Education

      - □ Forms of erythromycin and tetracycline are the medications of choice.

      - □ Use a single-dose unit to avoid cross-contamination.

      - □ Apply a 1 to 2 cm ribbon of ointment to the lower conjunctival sac of each eye, starting from the inner canthus and moving outward.

- A possible side effect is chemical conjunctivitis, causing redness, swelling, drainage, and temporarily blurred vision for 24 to 48 hr. Reassure the parents that this will resolve on its own.
- Application may be delayed for 1 hr after birth to facilitate baby-friendly activities during the first period of newborn reactivity.
○ Vitamin K (Aquamephyton)
- Administered to prevent hemorrhagic disorders. Vitamin K is not produced in the gastrointestinal tract of the newborn until around day 8. Vitamin K is produced in the colon by bacteria that forms once formula or breast milk is introduced into the gut of the newborn.
- Nursing Considerations and Client Education
- Administer 0.5 to 1 mg intramuscularly into the vastus lateralis (where muscle development is adequate) within 1 hr after birth.
○ Hepatitis B Immunization
- Provides protection against hepatitis B.
- Nursing Considerations and Client Education
- Recommended to be given to all newborns; informed consent must be obtained.
- For newborns born to healthy women, recommended dosage schedule is at birth, 1 month, and 6 months.
- For women infected with hepatitis B, hepatitis B immunoglobulin (HBIG) and the hepatitis B vaccine is given within 12 hr of birth. The hepatitis B vaccine is given alone at 1 month, 2 months, and 12 months.
- It is important NOT to give the vitamin K and the hepatitis B injections in the same thigh. Sites should be alternated.
○ Topical Antimicrobial Therapy
- May be used for prevention of infection and to promote drying of the umbilical cord stump.
- Nursing Considerations
- Assess stump and base of cord for edema, erythema, and drainage with each diaper change.
- Care for the cord as prescribed by the provider. This may include applying triple dye or cleansing with neutral pH cleanser and sterile water. The cord should be kept clean and dry to prevent infection.
- Bathing infant by submerging in water should not occur until the cord has fallen off.

Complications

- Cold stress (ineffective thermoregulation) can lead to hypoxia, acidosis, and hypoglycemia. Newborns with respiratory distress are at a higher risk for hypothermia.

  - Nursing Actions

    - Monitor for manifestations of cold stress (cyanotic trunk, depressed respirations).

    - The newborn should be warmed slowly over a period of 2 to 4 hr. Correct hypoxia by administering oxygen. Correct acidosis and hypoglycemia.

- Hypoglycemia frequently occurs in the first few hours of life secondary to the use of energy to establish respirations and maintain body heat. Newborns of mothers who have diabetes mellitus, are small or large for gestational age, are less than 37 weeks of gestation, or are greater than 42 weeks of gestation, are at risk for hypoglycemia and should have blood glucose monitored within the first 2 hr of life. Follow facility protocols regarding frequency of assessing blood glucose levels.

  - Nursing Actions

    - Monitor for jitteriness; twitching; a weak, high-pitched cry; irregular respiratory effort; cyanosis; lethargy; eye rolling; seizures; and a blood glucose level less than 40 mg/dL by heel stick.

    - Give formula immediately or have the mother breastfeed to elevate blood glucose. Brain damage can result if brain cells are depleted of glucose.

- Hemorrhage due to improper cord care or placement of clamp

  - Nursing Actions

    - Ensure that the clamp is tight; if seepage of blood is noted, a second clamp should be applied.

    - Notify the provider if bleeding continues.

APPLICATION EXERCISES

1. A nurse is preparing to administer prophylactic eye ointment to a newborn to treat ophthalmia neonatorum. Which of the following medications should the nurse anticipate administering?

    A. Ofloxacin (Floxin)

    B. Nystatin (Mycostatin)

    C. Erythromycin (Romycin)

    D. Ceftriaxone (Rocephin)

2. A newborn was not dried completely after delivery. The nurse should understand that which of the following mechanisms causes the newborn to lose heat?

    A. Conduction

    B. Convection

    C. Evaporation

    D. Radiation

3. When performing nursing care for a newborn after birth, which of the following nursing interventions is the highest priority?

    A. Initiating breastfeeding

    B. Performing the initial bath

    C. Giving a vitamin K injection

    D. Covering the newborn's head with a cap

4. A nurse is preparing to administer a vitamin K (Aquamephyton) injection to a newborn. Which of the following is an appropriate response by the nurse to the newborn's mother regarding why this medication is given?

    A. "It assists with blood clotting."

    B. "It promotes maturation of the bowel."

    C. "It is a preventative vaccine."

    D. "It provides immunity."

5. A nurse is taking a newborn to a mother for breastfeeding. Which of the following is an appropriate action for the nurse to take for security purposes?

    A. Ask the mother to state her full name.

    B. Look at the name on the newborn's bassinet.

    (C) Match the mother's identification band with the newborn's band.

    D. Compare name on the bassinet and room number.

6. A nurse is conducting a class for parents on care of the newborn. What should be included in this class? Use the ATI Active Learning Template: Basic Concept to complete this item to include the following sections:

    A. Stabilization of Airway:
- Underlying principles: Describe three mechanisms that promote airway clearance.
- Nursing Interventions: Describe appropriate bulb syringe technique.

APPLICATION EXERCISES KEY

1. A. **INCORRECT:** Ofloxacin is an antibiotic, but it is not used for ophthalmia neonatorum.

    B. **INCORRECT:** Nystatin is used to treat *Candida albicans*, an oral yeast infection.

    C. **CORRECT:** One medication of choice for ophthalmia neonatorum is erythromycin ophthalmic ointment 0.5%. This antibiotic provides prophylaxis against *Neisseria gonorrhoeae* and *Chlamydia trachomatis*.

    D. **INCORRECT:** Ceftriaxone is an antibiotic, but it is not used for ophthalmia neonatorum.

    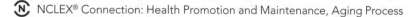 NCLEX® Connection: Health Promotion and Maintenance, Aging Process

2. A. **INCORRECT:** Conduction is the loss of heat from the body surface area to cooler surfaces that the newborn may be in contact with.

    B. **INCORRECT:** Convection is the flow of heat from the body surface area to cooler air.

    C. **CORRECT:** Evaporation is the loss of heat that occurs when a liquid is converted to a vapor. In a newborn, heat loss by evaporation occurs as a result of vaporization of the moisture from the skin.

    D. **INCORRECT:** Radiation is the loss of heat to a cooler surface that is not in direct contact with the newborn.

    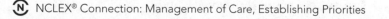 NCLEX® Connection: Health Promotion and Maintenance, Aging Process

3. A. **INCORRECT:** Initiating breastfeeding is important following birth, but it is not the priority action.

    B. **INCORRECT:** Initial baths aren't given until the newborn's temperature is stable. It is not the priority action.

    C. **INCORRECT:** Vitamin K can be given immediately after birth, but it is not the priority action.

    D. **CORRECT:** The greatest risk to the newborn is cold stress. Therefore the highest priority intervention is to prevent heat loss. Covering the newborn's head with a cap prevents cold stress due to excessive evaporative heat loss.

    NCLEX® Connection: Management of Care, Establishing Priorities

4. A. **CORRECT:** Vitamin K is deficient in a newborn because the colon is sterile. Until bacteria are present to stimulate vitamin K production, the newborn is at risk for hemorrhagic disease.

    B. INCORRECT: Vitamin K does not assist the bowel to mature.

    C. INCORRECT: Vitamin K is not part of the vaccines that are administered.

    D. INCORRECT: Vitamin K does not provide immunity.

    (N) NCLEX® Connection: Pharmacological and Parenteral Therapies, Medication Administration

5. A. INCORRECT: Asking the mother to state her full name is not appropriate verification because two identifiers should be used.

    B. INCORRECT: Looking at the name on the bassinet is not appropriate verification because two identifiers should be used.

    C. **CORRECT:** Each time the newborn is taken to the mother, the identification band should be verified against the mother's identification band.

    D. INCORRECT: Comparing the name on the bassinet with the room number is not appropriate verification because it does not include two identifiers involving the mother and newborn.

    (N) NCLEX® Connection: Safety and Infection Control, Accident/Error/Injury Prevention

6. *Using the ATI Active Learning Template: Basic Concept*

    A. Stabilization of Airway

    - Underlying Principles: Mechanisms that promote airway clearance
      - Infant's cough reflex
      - Mechanical suctioning, back blows/chest thrusts
      - Use of the bulb syringe for suctioning
    - Nursing Interventions: Bulb syringe technique
      - Depress the bulb
      - Insert syringe into side of mouth, avoiding center of the mouth
      - Suction mouth first, then one nostril, then second nostril

    (N) NCLEX® Connection: Health Promotion and Maintenance, Ante/Intra/Postpartum and Newborn Care

Overview

- Acquiring an understanding of the nutritional needs of newborns (breastfeeding, bottle feeding) is essential. Nutrition considerations, complications, and interventions will be discussed in this chapter.

Nutritional Needs for the Newborn

- Desirable growth and development of the newborn is enhanced by good nutrition. Feeding the newborn provides an opportunity for parents to meet the newborn's nutritional needs as well as an opportunity for them to bond with the newborn. Whether the mother chooses to breast or bottle feed, nurses should provide education and support.

- Normal newborn weight loss immediately after birth and subsequent weight gain should be as follows:

NEWBORN WEIGHT LOSS/GAIN
› Loss of 5% to 10% immediately after birth (regain 10 to 14 days after birth)
› Gain of 110 to 200 g/week for first 3 months

- Healthy newborns need a fluid intake of 100 to 140 mL/kg/24 hr. Newborns do not need to be given water because they receive sufficient water from either breast milk or formula.

- Adequate caloric intake is essential to provide energy for growth, digestion, metabolic needs, and activity. For the first 3 months, the newborn requires 110 kcal/kg/day. From 3 to 6 months, the requirement decreases to 100 kcal/kg/day. Both breast milk and formula provide 20 kcal/oz.

- Carbohydrates should make up 40% to 50% of the newborn's total caloric intake. The most abundant carbohydrate in breast milk or formula is lactose.

- At least 15% of calories must come from fat (triglycerides). The fat in breast milk is easier to digest than the fat in cow's milk.

- For adequate growth and development, a newborn must receive 2.25 to 4 g/kg of protein per day.

- Breast milk contains the vitamins necessary to provide adequate newborn nutrition. Recommendations are to provide 400 IU of vitamin D daily, starting in the first week of life. Infant formula has vitamins added to the formulation, but vitamin D supplements also are recommended. Mothers who are breastfeeding and are vegetarians who exclude meat, fish, and dairy products should provide vitamin B_{12} supplementation to their newborns.

- The mineral content of commercial newborn formula and breast milk is adequate with the exception of iron and fluoride.

  ○ Iron is low in all forms of milk, but it is absorbed better from breast milk. Newborns who only breastfeed for the first 6 months maintain adequate Hgb levels and do not need any additional iron supplementation. After 6 months of age, all newborns need to be fed iron-fortified cereal and other foods rich in iron. Newborns who are formula fed should receive iron-fortified newborn formula until 12 months of age. Mothers who breastfeed their newborns are encouraged to do so for the newborn's first 12 months of life.

  ○ Fluoride levels in breast milk and formulas are low. A fluoride supplement should be given to newborns not receiving fluoridated water after 6 months of age.

- Solids are not introduced until 6 months of age. If introduced too early, food allergies may develop.

Breastfeeding

- Breastfeeding is the optimal source of nutrition for newborns. Breastfeeding is recommended exclusively for the first 6 months of age by the American Academy of Pediatrics. Newborns should be breastfed every 2 to 3 hr. Parents should awaken the newborn to feed at least every 3 hr during the day and at least every 4 hr during the night until the newborn is feeding well and gaining weight adequately. Breastfeeding should occur 8 to 12 times within a 24-hr window. Then, a feed-on-demand schedule may be followed.

- Colostrum is secreted from the mother's breasts during postpartum days 1 to 3. It contains the IgA immunoglobulin that provides passive immunity to the newborn.

- Nursing interventions can help a new mother be successful in breastfeeding. This includes the provision of adequate calories and fluids to support breastfeeding. The practice of rooming-in, allowing mothers and newborns to remain together, should be encouraged as part of baby-friendly initiatives. Lactation consultants can improve the mother's efforts and success in breastfeeding.

- Advantages of breastfeeding – Parents should be presented with factual information about the nutritional and immunological needs of their newborn. The nurse should present information about both breastfeeding and bottle feeding in a nonjudgmental manner. The optimal time to provide newborn nutritional information is during pregnancy, so that the parents make a decision prior to hospital admission.

  ○ Benefits of breastfeeding

    ▪ Reduces the risk of infection by providing IgA antibodies, lysozymes, leukocytes, macrophages, and lactoferrin that prevents infections.

    ▪ Promotes rapid brain growth due to large amounts of lactose.

    ▪ Provides protein and nitrogen for neurological cell building and improves the newborn's ability to regulate calcium and phosphorus levels.

    ▪ Contains electrolytes and minerals.

    ▪ Breast milk is easy for the newborn to digest.

    ▪ Breastfeeding is convenient and inexpensive.

    ▪ Reduces incidence of sudden infant death syndrome (SIDS), allergies, and childhood obesity.

    ▪ Promotes maternal-infant bonding.

- Nursing Interventions to Promote Successful Breastfeeding
  - Place the newborn skin-to-skin on the mother's abdomen immediately after birth. Initiate breastfeeding as soon as possible or within the first 30 min following delivery.
  - Explain breastfeeding techniques to the mother. Have the mother wash her hands, get comfortable, and have caffeine-free, nonalcoholic fluids to drink during breastfeeding.
  - Explain the let-down reflex (stimulation of maternal nipple releases oxytocin that causes the let-down of milk).
  - Reassure the mother that uterine cramps are normal during breastfeeding, resulting from oxytocin, which also promote uterine involution.
  - Express a few drops of colostrum or milk and spread it over the nipple to lubricate the nipple and entice the newborn.
  - Show the mother the proper latch-on position. Have her support the breast in one hand with the thumb on top and four fingers underneath. With the newborn's mouth in front of the nipple, the newborn can be stimulated to open his mouth by tickling his lower lip with the tip of the nipple. The mother pulls the newborn to the nipple with his mouth covering part of the areola as well as the nipple.

 View Images: Breastfeeding Techniques

  - Explain to the mother that when her newborn is latched on correctly, his nose, cheeks, and chin will be touching her breast.
  - Demonstrate the four basic breastfeeding positions: football, cradle or modified cradle, across the lap, and side-lying.
  - Encourage the mother to breastfeed at least 15 to 20 min/breast to ensure that her newborn receives adequate fat and protein, which is richest in the breast milk as it empties the breast.
  - Avoid educating mothers regarding the duration of newborn feedings. Mothers should be instructed to evaluate when the newborn has completed the feeding, including slowing of newborn suckling, a softened breast, or sleeping.
  - Explain to the mother that newborns will nurse on demand after a pattern is established.
  - Show the mother how to insert a finger in the side of the newborn's mouth to break the suction from the nipple prior to removing the newborn from the breast to prevent nipple trauma.
  - Show the mother how to burp the newborn when she alternates breasts. The newborn should be burped either over the shoulder or in an upright position with his chin supported. The mother should gently pat the newborn on his back to elicit a burp.
  - Tell the mother to begin the newborn's next feeding with the breast she stopped feeding him with in the previous feeding.
  - Tell the mother how to tell if her newborn is receiving adequate feeding (gaining weight, voiding 6 to 8 diapers a day, and contentedness between feedings).
  - Explain to the mother that the newborn may have loose, pale, and/or yellow stools during breastfeeding, and that this is normal.
  - Tell the mother to avoid nipple confusion in the newborn by not offering supplemental formula, pacifier, or soothers. Supplementation can be provided using a small feeding or syringe feeding, if needed.
  - Tell the mother to always place her newborn on his back after feedings.

- Promote rooming-in efforts.

- Offer referral to breastfeeding support groups.

- Contact a lactation consultant to offer additional recommendations and support, especially to mothers who have concerns about adequate breast milk or mothers who have been unsuccessful with breastfeeding in the past.

Q
EBP

- Herbal products, such as fenugreek, and prescription medications, such as metoclopramide (Reglan), have been reported to increase breast milk production. There is insufficient data to confirm or deny their effect on lactation. Mothers should check with the provider before taking over-the-counter or prescription medications.

- Nursing Interventions to Promote Successful Storage of Breast Milk Obtained by a Breast Pump

  - Inform the mother that breast milk can still be provided to the newborn during periods of separation by using a breast pump.

    - Breast pumps can be manual, electric, or battery-operated and pumped directly into a bottle or freezer bag.

    - One or both breasts can be pumped, and suction is adjustable for comfort.

  - Teach the parents that breast milk must be stored according to guidelines for proper containers, labeling, refrigerating, and freezing.

    - Breast milk may be stored at room temperature under very clean conditions for up to 8 hr. It may be refrigerated in sterile bottles for use within 8 days, or may be frozen in sterile containers in the freezer compartment of a two-door refrigerator for up to 6 months. Breast milk may be stored in a deep freezer for 12 months.

    - Thawing the milk in the refrigerator for 24 hr is the best way to preserve the immunoglobulins present in it. It also can be thawed by holding the container under running lukewarm water or placing it in a container of lukewarm water. The bottle should be rotated often, but not shaken when thawing in this manner.

    - Thawing by microwave is contraindicated because it destroys some of the immune factors and lysozymes contained in the milk. Microwave thawing also leads to the development of hot spots in the milk because of uneven heating, which can burn the newborn.

    - Do not refreeze thawed milk.

    - Used portions of breast milk must be discarded.

Bottle feeding

- Formula feeding can be a successful and adequate source of nutrition if the mother chooses not to breastfeed. The newborn should be fed every 3 to 4 hr. Parents should awaken the newborn to feed at least every 3 hr during the day and at least every 4 hr during the night until the newborn is feeding well and gaining weight adequately. Then, a feed-on-demand schedule may be followed.

- Nursing Interventions to Promote Successful Bottle Feeding

  - Teach the parents how to prepare formula, bottles, and nipples. Review the importance of handwashing prior to formula preparation.

  - Teach the parents about the different forms of formula (ready-to-feed, concentrated, and powder) and how to prepare each correctly.

  - Bottles can be put in the dishwasher or washed by hand in hot soapy water using a good bottle and nipple brush.

- ○ Teach parents to wash the lid of a can of concentrated formula with hot soapy water before opening it.

- ○ Instruct parents to use tap water to mix concentrated or powder formula. If the water source is questionable, tap water should be boiled first.

- ○ Instruct parents that prepared formula can be refrigerated for up to 48 hr.

- ○ Teach the parents to check the flow of formula from the bottle to ensure it is not coming out too slow or too fast.

- ○ Show the parents how to cradle the newborn in their arms in a semi-upright position. The newborn should not be placed in the supine position during bottle feeding because of the danger of aspiration. Newborns who bottle feed do best when held close and at a 45° angle.

- ○ Instruct the mother how to place the nipple on top of the newborn's tongue.

- ○ Keep the nipple filled with formula to prevent the newborn from swallowing air.

- ○ Always hold the bottle and never prop the bottle for feeding.

- ○ Newborns should be burped several times during a feeding, usually after each ½ to 1 oz of formula or breast milk.

- ○ Place the newborn on his back after feedings.

- ○ Tell the parents to discard any unused formula remaining in the bottle when the newborn is finished feeding due to the possibility of bacterial contamination.

- ○ Teach the parents how to tell if their newborn is being adequately fed (gaining weight; bowel movements are yellow, soft and formed; infant will stool after every feeding, and after a couple of weeks, movements decrease to 1 to 2 per day; voiding 6 to 8 times per day; and satisfaction between feedings).

Risk Factors for Impaired Newborn Nutrition

- Risk factors for failure to thrive (newborn) can be related to ineffective feeding patterns of the newborn or inadequate breastfeeding by the mother.
  - ○ Newborn factor
    - Inadequate breastfeeding
    - Illness
    - Infection
    - Malabsorption
    - Other conditions that increase the newborn's energy needs
  - ○ Maternal factor
    - Inadequate or slow milk production
    - Inadequate emptying of the breast
    - Inappropriate timing of feeding
    - Inadequate breast tissue
    - Pain with feeding
    - Maternal hemorrhage
    - Illness
    - Infections

Monitoring Newborn for Adequate Growth

- Monitor the newborn for adequate growth and weight gain.
  - Weights are done daily in the newborn nursery and then usually at 2 days of age after discharge for newborns who are breastfed and 6 weeks of age for newborns who are formula fed. Growth is assessed by placing the newborn's weight on a growth chart. Adequate growth should be within the 10th to 90th percentile. Poor weight gain would be below 10% and too much weight gain would be above 90%.
  - The newborn's length and head circumference are also routinely monitored.
- Assessment of newborn nutrition begins during pregnancy and continues after birth by reviewing the parents' attitudes and choices about their newborn's feeding. Breastfeeding is the preferred method. However, if the mother chooses not to breastfeed, she must not be made to feel guilty.
  - Newborn
    - Maturity level
    - History of labor and delivery
    - Birth trauma
    - Maternal risk factors
    - Congenital defects
    - Physical stability
    - State of alertness
    - Presence of bowel sounds
  - Mother
    - Previous experience with breastfeeding
    - Knowledge about breastfeeding
    - Cultural factors
    - Feelings about breastfeeding
    - Physical features of breasts
    - Physical/psychological readiness
    - Support of family and significant others
- Assess the mother's ability to feed her newborn, whether by breast or bottle.
- Calculate the newborn's 24-hr I&O, if indicated, to ensure adequate nutrition.

Intervening for Newborn Nutrition

- Provide the mother with education about feeding-readiness cues exhibited by newborns and encourage the mother to begin feeding her newborn upon cues rather than waiting until the newborn is crying. Cues include the following:
  - Hand-to-mouth or hand-to-hand movements
  - Sucking motions
  - Rooting
  - Mouthing

Complications for Newborn Nutrition

- There may be special considerations when a newborn has difficulty receiving adequate nutrition. Nursing interventions can often help these newborns receive adequate nutrition.
  - ○ Newborns who are sleepy
    - ▪ Unwrap the newborn.
    - ▪ Change the newborn's diaper.
    - ▪ Hold the newborn upright and turn him from side to side.
    - ▪ Talk to the newborn.
    - ▪ Massage the newborn's back, and rub his hands and feet.
    - ▪ Apply a cool cloth to the newborn's face.
  - ○ Newborns who are fussy
    - ▪ Swaddle the newborn.
    - ▪ Hold the newborn close, move, and rock him gently.
    - ▪ Reduce the newborn's environmental stimuli.
    - ▪ Place the newborn skin to skin.
- Failure to thrive is slow weight gain. A newborn usually falls below the 5th percentile on the growth chart.

  - ○ Newborns who are breastfeeding
    - ▪ Evaluate positioning and latch-on during breastfeeding.
    - ▪ Massage the breast during feeding.
    - ▪ Determine feeding patterns and length of feedings.
    - ▪ If the newborn is spitting up, the newborn may have an allergy to dairy products. Determine the maternal intake of dairy products. The mother may need to eliminate dairy from her diet. Instruct her to consume other food sources high in calcium or calcium supplements.
  - ○ Newborns who are formula feeding
    - ▪ Evaluate how much and how often the newborn is feeding.
    - ▪ If the newborn is spitting up or vomiting, he may have an allergy or intolerance to cow milk-based formula and may require a soy-based formula.

APPLICATION EXERCISES

1. A nurse is giving instructions to a mother about how to breastfeed her newborn. Which of the following actions by the mother indicates understanding of the teaching?

    A. The mother places a few drops of water on her nipple before feeding.

    B. The mother gently removes her nipple from the infant's mouth to break the suction.

    C. When she is ready to breastfeed, the mother gently strokes the newborn's cheek with her finger.

    D. When latched on, the infant's nose, cheek, and chin are touching the breast.

2. A nurse is teaching a group of new parents about proper techniques for bottle feeding. Which of the following instructions should the nurse provide?

    A. Burp the newborn at the end of the feeding.

    B. Hold the newborn close in a supine position.

    C. Keep the nipple full of formula throughout the feeding.

    D. Refrigerate any unused formula.

3. A nurse is caring for a newborn. Which of the following actions by the newborn indicates readiness to feed?

    A. Spits up clear mucus

    B. Attempts to place his hand in his mouth

    C. Turns his head toward sounds

    D. Lies quietly with his eyes open

4. A nurse is reviewing formula preparation with parents who plan to bottle feed their newborn. Which of the following should be included in the teaching? (Select all that apply.)

    _____ A. Use a disinfectant wipe to clean the lid of the formula can.

    _____ B. Store prepared formula in the refrigerator for up to 72 hr.

    __X__ C. Place used bottles in the dishwasher.

    __X__ D. Check the nipple for appropriate flow of formula.

    __X__ E. Use tap water to dilute concentrated formula.

5. A nurse is reviewing breastfeeding positions with the mother of a newborn. Which of the following is an appropriate position for the nurse to discuss?

    A. Over-the-shoulder position

    B. Supine position

    C. Chin-supported position

    D. Cradle position

6. A nurse is teaching about the use of a breast pump and storing breast milk with a group of new mothers. What should be included in the teaching? Use the ATI Active Learning Template: Basic Concept to complete this item to include the following:

    A. Related Content:
- List the types of breast pumps.
- Describe use of the pump.

    B. Nursing Interventions:
- Describe storage and freezing of milk.
- Describe procedures for thawing milk.

APPLICATION EXERCISES KEY

1. A. INCORRECT: The infant is enticed to suck when the mother spreads colostrum on the nipple.

    B. INCORRECT: The mother should insert a finger in the side of the newborn's mouth to break the suction before removing her nipple.

    C. INCORRECT: The mother should stroke the newborn's lips with her nipple to promote sucking.

    D. **CORRECT:** Effective latching-on includes the infant's nose, cheek and chin touching the mother's breast.

    Ⓝ NCLEX® Connection: Health Promotion and Maintenance, Ante/Intra/Postpartum and Newborn Care

2. A. INCORRECT: The newborn should be burped after each ½ oz of formula.

    B. INCORRECT: The newborn should be cradled in a semi-upright position.

    C. **CORRECT:** The nipple should always be kept full of formula to prevent the newborn from sucking in air during the feeding.

    D. INCORRECT: Any unused formula should be discarded due to the possibility of bacterial contamination.

    Ⓝ NCLEX® Connection: Health Promotion and Maintenance, Ante/Intra/Postpartum and Newborn Care

3. A. INCORRECT: Spitting up, coughing, or gagging on mucus is an attempt by the newborn to clear his airway.

    B. **CORRECT:** Readiness-to-feed cues include the newborn making hand-to-mouth and hand-to-hand movements, sucking motions, rooting, and mouthing.

    C. INCORRECT: The infant turns his head toward sounds in the environment as a sensory response indicating normal central nervous system functioning.

    D. INCORRECT: Lying quietly with eyes open is an alerting behavior, indicating normal newborn reactivity.

    Ⓝ NCLEX® Connection: Health Promotion and Maintenance, Aging Process

4. A. INCORRECT: Chemicals from the disinfectant wipe can remain on the lid during opening and mix with the formula.

    B. INCORRECT: Once formula is prepared, it can be refrigerated for up to 48 hr.

    C. **CORRECT:** Bottles can be placed in a dishwasher or washed by hand in hot soapy water using a good bottle brush.

    D. **CORRECT:** The flow of formula from the nipple should be checked to determine that it is not too fast or too slow.

    E. **CORRECT:** Tap water is used to mix concentrated or powder formula. If the water is from a questionable source, it should be boiled first.

    Ⓝ NCLEX® Connection: Health Promotion and Maintenance, Ante/Intra/Postpartum and Newborn Care

5.   A. INCORRECT: An over-the-shoulder position can be used when burping the newborn.

    B. INCORRECT: The supine position is appropriate for the sleeping newborn.

    C. INCORRECT: Holding the newborn upright with the chin supported is a position that can be used when burping the newborn.

    D. **CORRECT:** The cradle position for breastfeeding includes the mother laying the newborn across her forearm with her hand supporting the lower back and buttocks.

    (N) NCLEX® Connection: Health Promotion and Maintenance, Ante/Intra/Postpartum and Newborn Care

6.   *Using the ATI Active Learning Template: Basic Concept*

    A. Related Content

- Types of breast pumps
  - Manual
  - Electric
  - Battery-operated
- Use of the pump – Pumping of one or both breasts using adjustable suction for comfort to obtain breast milk for storage in a bottle or freezer bag

    B. Nursing Interventions

- Storage
  - Store at room temperature under very clean conditions for up to 8 hr.
  - Refrigerate in sterile bottles for use within 8 days.
  - Freeze in sterile containers in the freezer of a two-door refrigerator for up to 6 months.
  - Store in a deep freezer for up to 12 months.
- Thawing
  - Thaw milk in the refrigerator for 24 hr to preserve immunoglobulins.
  - Hold container under running lukewarm water or place in a pan of lukewarm water; bottle should be rotated, but not shaken.
  - Do not thaw in a microwave.

    (N) NCLEX® Connection: Health Promotion and Maintenance, Ante/Intra/Postpartum and Newborn Care

chapter 26

UNIT 4	NEWBORN NURSING CARE
	SECTION: LOW-RISK NEWBORN
CHAPTER 26	Nursing Care and Discharge Teaching

Overview

- Discharge teaching and newborn care including bathing, umbilical cord care, circumcision, car seat safety, environmental safety, newborn behaviors, feeding, elimination and signs of illness to report to the provider will be discussed in this chapter.

- Prior to discharge, a nurse should provide anticipatory guidance to prepare new parents to care for their newborn at home. Mothers and newborns are normally discharged once the newborn is 6 to 48 hr old. Serious complications can result if improper discharge instructions are given to the parents prior to taking the newborn home.

- A nurse should inquire about the family's current experience and knowledge regarding newborn care, anticipate the learning needs of the parents, and assess their readiness for learning to provide education about newborn care.

- Parents should be made aware of general guidelines about newborn behavior and care. These guidelines include causes of crying in the newborn, quieting techniques, sleeping patterns, hunger cues, and feeding, bathing, and clothing the newborn.

- Parents need to be aware of the importance of well-newborn checkups, immunization schedules, and when to call the provider for signs of illness.

- Providing a safe protective environment at home should be stressed to new parents and should include instruction about proper car seat usage, which is a very important part of the discharge instruction process.

- Assessment of the family's readiness to care for the newborn at home

  - Previous newborn experience and knowledge

  - Parent-newborn attachment

  - Adjustment to the parental role

  - Social support

  - Educational needs

  - Sibling rivalry issues

  - Readiness of the parents to have their home and lifestyle altered to accommodate their newborn

  - Parents' ability to verbalize and demonstrate newborn care following teaching

Interventions for Home Care of the Newborn

- Through verbal discussion, pamphlets, and demonstration, the nurse provides education to the client and family regarding newborn behavior, quieting techniques, newborn care, signs of newborn well-being and illness, and issues of newborn safety.

- Crying
  - Inform the parents that newborns cry when they are hungry, need to be burped, are overstimulated, wet, cold, hot, tired, or bored. Assure the mother that, in time, she will learn what her newborn's cry means. The mother should be instructed not to feed her newborn every time he cries. Overfeeding can lead to stomach aches and diarrhea. After checking the newborn, it is okay to let a newborn cry for short periods of time.

- Quieting Techniques
  - Swaddling
  - Close skin contact
  - Nonnutritive sucking with pacifier
  - Rhythmic noises to simulate utero sounds
  - Movement (a car ride, vibrating chair, infant swing, rocking newborn)
  - Placing the newborn on his stomach across a holder's lap while gently bouncing legs
  - En face position for eye contact
  - Stimulation

- Sleep-Wake Cycle
  - Reinforce to the parents that placing the newborn in the supine position for sleeping greatly decreases the risk of sudden infant death syndrome.
  - Most newborns sleep 17 out of every 24 hr with periods of wakefulness increasing. By 4 weeks of age, the newborn may remain awake from one feeding to the next.
  - Many parents believe that adding solid food to the newborn's diet will help with sleep patterns. During the first 6 months of life, the American Academy of Pediatrics recommends only breastfeeding. Most newborns will sleep through the night without a feeding by 4 to 5 months of age. The provider will instruct the parents when to add solid food to the newborn's diet.
  - Keep the newborn's environment quiet and dark at night.
  - Place the newborn in a crib or bassinet to sleep. The newborn should never sleep in the parents' bed due to the risk of suffocation.
  - Most newborns get their days and nights mixed up. Provide basic suggestions for helping the parents develop a predictable routine. Bring the newborn out into the center of the action in the afternoon, and keep him there for the rest of the evening. Bathe him right before bedtime so that he feels soothed. Give him his last feeding around 2300, and then place him into a crib or bassinet.
  - When awake, the newborn can be placed on his abdomen to promote muscle development for crawling. The infant should be supervised.
  - For nighttime feedings and diaper changes, keep a small night-light on to avoid having to turn on bright lights. Speak softly, and handle the newborn gently so that he goes back to sleep easily.

- Oral and nasal suctioning: Review correct technique with the parents.

- Positioning and Holding of Newborn (Head Support)
  - Teach the parents that the newborn has minimal head control. The head should be supported when the newborn is lifted because it is larger and heavier then the rest of the body.
  - Four basic ways to hold the newborn
    - Cradle hold – Cradle the newborn's head in the bend of the elbow. This permits eye-to-eye contact and is a good position for feeding.
    - Upright position – Hold the newborn upright, and face him toward the holder while supporting his head, upper back, and buttocks.
    - Football hold – Support half of the newborn's body in the holder's forearm with the newborn's head and neck resting in the palm of the hand. This is a good position for breastfeeding and when shampooing the newborn's hair.
    - Colic hold – Place the newborn facedown along the holder's forearm with the hand firmly between the newborn's legs. The newborn's cheek should be by the holder's elbow on the outside. The newborn should be able to see the ground, and the holder's arm should be close to the body, using it to brace and steady the newborn. This is a good position for quieting a fussy newborn.

Q
EBP
- Swaddling
  - Parents should be shown how to swaddle their newborn. Swaddling the newborn snugly in a receiving blanket helps the newborn to feel more secure. Swaddling brings the newborn's extremities in closer to his trunk, which is similar to the intrauterine position.
- Bathing
  - After the initial bath, the newborn's face, diaper area, and skin folds are cleansed daily. Complete bathing is performed 2 to 3 times a week using a mild soap that does not contain hexachlorophene.
  - Bathing by immersion is not done until the newborn's umbilical cord has fallen off and the circumcision has healed on males. Wash the area around the cord, taking care not to get the cord wet. Move from the cleanest to dirtiest part of the newborn's body, beginning with his eyes, face, and head; proceed to the chest, arms, and legs; and wash the groin area last.
  - Teach the parents proper newborn bathing techniques by a demonstration. Have the parents return the demonstration.
  - Bathing should take place at the convenience of the parents, but not immediately after feeding to prevent spitting up and vomiting.
  - Organize all equipment so that the newborn is not left unattended. Never leave the newborn alone in the tub or sink.
  - Make sure the hot water heater is set at 49° C (120.2° F) or less. The room should be warm, and the bath water should be 36.6° to 37.2° C (98° to 99° F). Test the water for comfort on inner wrist prior to bathing the newborn.
  - Avoid drafts or chilling of the newborn. Expose only the body part being bathed, and dry the newborn thoroughly to prevent chilling and heat loss.
  - The newborn's eyes should be cleaned using a clean portion of the wash cloth. Clear water should be used to clean each eye, moving from the inner to the outer canthus.
  - Each area of the newborn's body should be washed, rinsed, and dried, with no soap left on the skin.

○ Wrap the newborn in a towel, and swaddle him in a football hold to shampoo his head. Rinse shampoo from the newborn's head, and dry to avoid chilling.

○ In male newborns, to cleanse an uncircumcised penis, wash with soap and water and rinse the penis. The foreskin should not be forced back or constriction may result.

○ In female newborns, wash the vulva by wiping from front to back to prevent contamination of the vagina or urethra from rectal bacteria.

○ Do not use lotions, oils, or powders, because they can alter a newborn's skin and provide a medium for bacterial growth or cause an allergic reaction. Powder should be avoided because it can cause respiratory problems if inhaled by the newborn.

• Feeding/Elimination

○ Mothers who are breastfeeding should be seen by the lactation consultant.

○ The newborn is offered the breast immediately after birth and frequently thereafter. Newborns who are breastfed will average 15 to 20 min per breast and 30 to 40 min for the total feeding. Feedings should be 8 to 12 times in a 24-hr period. Feeding for a newborn who is breastfeeding should be on demand or every 2 to 3 hr. Newborns who are formula fed also should be fed on demand or every 3 to 4 hr.

○ Inform parents that adhering to specific timing of feedings is to be avoided. Parents should be instructed to recognize when the newborn has completed the feeding. No other fluids are offered to the newborn unless indicated by the provider.

○ The mother's milk supply is equal to the demand of the newborn. Eventually, the newborn will empty a breast within 5 to 10 min, but may need to continue to suck to meet comfort needs.

○ Frequent feedings (every 2 hr may be indicated), and manual expression of milk to initiate flow may be needed.

○ Most newborns spit up a small amount after feedings. Keep the newborn upright and quiet for a few minutes after feedings.

○ Newborns should have 6 to 8 wet diapers a day with adequate feedings and may have 3 to 4 stools per day.

• Diapering

○ To avoid diaper rash, the newborn's diaper area should be kept clean and dry. Diapers should be changed frequently, and the perineal area cleaned with warm water or wipes and dried thoroughly to prevent skin breakdown.

• Cord Care

○ Before discharge, the cord clamp is removed.

○ Prevent cord infection by keeping the cord dry, and keep the top of the diaper folded underneath it.

○ Sponge baths are given until the cord falls off, which occurs around 10 to 14 days after birth. Tub bathing and submersion can follow.

○ Cord infection (complication of improper cord care) can result if the cord is not kept clean and dry.

▪ Monitor for symptoms of a cord that is moist and red, has a foul odor, or has purulent drainage.

▪ Notify the provider immediately if findings of cord infection are present.

- Circumcision Care
    - Circumcision is the surgical removal of the foreskin of the penis.
        - Circumcision is a personal choice made by the newborn's family for reasons of hygiene, religious conviction (Jewish male on eighth day after birth), tradition, culture, or social norms. Parents should make a well-informed decision in consultation with the provider.
        - Contraindications for circumcision include newborns born with hypospadias (abnormal positioning of urethra on ventral undersurface of the penis) and epispadias (urethral canal terminates on dorsum of penis) because the prepuce skin may be needed for surgical repair of the defect. Familial history of bleeding disorders is also a contraindication.
        - Circumcision should not be done immediately following birth because the newborn's level of vitamin K is at a low point, and the newborn would be at risk for hemorrhage.
        - Advocates of circumcision state that circumcision promotes a penis with clean glans, minimizes the risk of phimosis later in life, and reduces the risk of penile cancer and cervical cancer in sexual partners.
    - Diagnostic and therapeutic procedures and management
        - Anesthesia is required for circumcision. Types of anesthesia include a ring block, dorsal-penile nerve block, and topical anesthetic (eutectic mixture of local anesthetics). Oral sucrose, oral acetaminophen, and nonpharmacologic methods, such as swaddling and nonnutritive sucking, may be employed prior to the procedure.
        - Surgical methods for removing the foreskin include the Yellen, Mogen, and Gomco clamps, and Plastibell.
            - The provider applies the Yellen, Mogen, or Gomco clamp to the penis, loosens the foreskin, and inserts the cone under the foreskin to provide a cutting surface for removal of the foreskin and to protect the penis. The wound is covered with sterile petroleum gauze to prevent infection and control bleeding.
            - The provider slides the Plastibell device between the foreskin and the glans of the penis. The provider ties a suture tightly around the foreskin at the coronal edge of the glans. This applies pressure as the excess foreskin is removed from the penis. After 5 to 7 days, the Plastibell drops off, leaving a clean, healed excision. No petroleum is used for circumcision with the Plastibell.
    - Nursing assessments
        - Preprocedure – The newborn should be assessed for:
            - A history of bleeding tendencies in the family (hemophilia and clotting disorders).
            - Hypospadias or epispadias.
            - Ambiguous genitalia (when the newborn has genitalia that may include both male and female characteristics).
            - Illness or infection.
        - Postprocedure – The newborn should be assessed for:
            - Bleeding every 15 min for the first hour and then every hour for at least 12 hr.
            - The first voiding.

- ○ Nursing interventions
  - ■ Preprocedure – Parent teaching
    - □ Signed informed consent form from parents is needed.
    - □ Explain to the parents that the newborn will not be able to be bottle feed for up to 4 hr prior to the procedure to prevent vomiting and aspiration based on the preferences of the provider. Newborns who are breastfed may nurse up until the procedure.
    - □ Explain that the newborn is restrained on a special board during the procedure.
  - ■ Gather and prepare supplies.
  - ■ Administer medication to newborn as prescribed.
  - ■ Assist with procedure
    - □ Place the newborn on the restraining board, and provide a radiant heat source to prevent cold stress. Do not leave the newborn unattended. Have bulb syringe readily available.
    - □ Comfort the newborn as needed.
    - □ Document time and type of circumcision, excessive bleeding, and newborn voiding following procedure.
- ○ Postprocedure care
  - ■ Remove the newborn from the restraining board and swaddle to provide comfort.
  - ■ Monitor for bleeding and voiding per facility protocol. Apply gauze lightly to penis if bleeding or oozing is observed.
  - ■ Fan fold diapers to prevent pressure on the circumcised area.
- ○ Postprocedure parent teaching
  - ■ Teach the parents to keep the area clean. Change the newborn's diaper at least every 4 hr, and clean the penis with warm water with each diaper change. With clamp procedures, apply petroleum jelly with each diaper change for at least 24 hr after the circumcision to keep the diaper from adhering to the penis.
  - ■ Avoid wrapping the penis in tight gauze, which can impair circulation to the glans.
  - ■ A tub bath should not be given until the circumcision is healed. Until then, warm water should be trickled gently over the penis.
  - ■ Notify the provider if there is any redness, discharge, swelling, strong odor, tenderness, decrease in urination, or excessive crying from the newborn.
  - ■ Tell the parents that a film of yellowish mucus may form over the glans by day 2 and it is important not to wash it off.
  - ■ Teach the parents to avoid using premoistened towelettes to clean the penis because they contain alcohol.
  - ■ Inform the parents that the newborn may be fussy or may sleep for several hours after the circumcision. Provide comfort measures for 24 to 48 hr, to include acetaminophen (Tylenol) as prescribed.
  - ■ Inform the parents that the circumcision will heal completely within a couple of weeks.

- ○ Complications and nursing management
  - ▪ Hemorrhage
    - □ Monitor the newborn for bleeding.
    - □ Provide gentle pressure on the penis using a small gauze square. Gelfoam powder or a sponge may be applied to stop bleeding. If bleeding persists, notify the provider that a blood vessel may need to be ligated. Have a nurse continue to hold pressure until the provider arrives while another nurse prepares the circumcision tray and suture material.
  - ▪ Cold stress/hypoglycemia
    - □ Monitor the newborn for excessive loss of heat resulting in increased respirations and lowered body temperature.
    - □ Swaddle and feed the newborn as soon as the procedure is over.
  - ▪ Other complications
    - □ Report any frank bleeding, foul-smelling drainage, or lack of voiding to the provider.
    - □ Provide discharge instructions to the parents about manifestations of infection, comfort measures, medications, and when to notify the provider.
- Clothing
  - ○ Instruct the parents about how to properly clothe their newborn. The best clothing is soft and made of cotton. Clothes should be washed separately with mild detergent and hot water. Dress lightly for indoors and on hot days. Too many layers of clothing or blankets can make the newborn too hot. On cold days, cover the newborn's head when outdoors. A general rule is to dress the newborn as the parents would dress themselves.
- Home Safety
  - ○ Never leave the newborn unattended with pets or other small children.
  - ○ Keep small objects (coins) out of the reach of newborns due to choking hazard.
  - ○ Never leave the newborn alone on a bed, couch, or table. Newborns move enough to reach the edge and fall off.
  - ○ Never place the newborn on his stomach to sleep during the first few months of life. The back-lying position is the position of choice. The newborn can be placed on his abdomen when awake and being supervised.
  - ○ Never provide a newborn with a soft surface to sleep on (pillows and waterbed). The newborn's mattress should be firm. Never put pillows, toys, bumper pads, or loose blankets in a crib. Crib linens should be tight-fitting.
  - ○ Do not tie anything around the newborn's neck.
  - ○ Monitor the safety of the newborn's crib. The space between the mattress and sides of the crib should be less than 2 fingerbreadths. The slats on the crib should be no more than 5.1 cm (2.25 in) apart.
  - ○ The newborn's crib or playpen should be away from window blinds and drapery cords. Newborns can become strangled in them.
  - ○ The bassinet or crib should be placed on an inner wall, not next to a window, to prevent cold stress by radiation.
  - ○ If an infant carrier is placed on a high place, such as a table, always be within arm's reach.
  - ○ Smoke detectors should be on every floor of a home and should be checked monthly to ensure that they are working. Batteries should be changed yearly. (Change batteries when daylight savings time occurs or on a child's birthday.)

○ Eliminate potential fire hazards. Keep a crib and playpen away from heaters, radiators, and heat vents. Linens could catch fire if they come into contact with heat sources.

○ Control the temperature and humidity of the newborn's environment by providing adequate ventilation.

○ Avoid exposing the newborn to cigarette smoke in a home or elsewhere. Secondhand exposure increases the newborn's risk of developing respiratory illnesses.

○ All visitors should wash their hands before touching the newborn. Any individual who has an infection should be kept away from the newborn.

○ Carefully handle the newborn. Do not toss the newborn up in the air or swing him by his extremities.

○ Provide community resources to clients who may need additional and ongoing assessment and instruction on newborn care (adolescent parents).

- Car Seat Safety

  ○ Use an approved rear-facing car seat in the back seat, preferably in the middle, (away from air bags and side impact) to transport the newborn. Keep infants in rear-facing car seats until age 2 or until the child reaches the maximum height and weight for the seat. Do not use a used or secondhand car seat.

- Newborn Wellness Checkups

  ○ Parents should be advised that their newborn will require well-newborn checkups at 2 weeks to 6 weeks of age, and then every 2 months until 6 months of age. Newborns who are breastfed usually have a weight check around 2 days after discharge.

  ○ The schedule for immunizations should be reviewed with the parents. The nurse should stress the importance of receiving these immunizations on a schedule for the newborn to be protected against diphtheria, tetanus, pertussis, hepatitis B, *Haemophilus influenzae*, polio, measles, mumps, rubella, influenza, rotavirus, pneumococcal, and varicella.

- Signs of Illness to Report

  ○ Parents should be instructed regarding the signs of illness and to report them immediately.

    ■ A fever above 38° C (100.4° F) or a temperature below 36.6° C (97.9° F)

    ■ Poor feeding or little interest in food

    ■ Forceful vomiting or frequent vomiting

    ■ Decreased urination

    ■ Diarrhea or decreased bowel movements

    ■ Labored breathing with flared nostrils or an absence of breathing for greater than 15 seconds

    ■ Jaundice

    ■ Cyanosis

    ■ Lethargy

    ■ Inconsolable crying

    ■ Difficulty waking

    ■ Bleeding or purulent drainage around umbilical cord or circumcision

    ■ Drainage developing in eyes.

- Parents should be encouraged to seek CPR training.

Complications Related to Newborn Home Care

- Complications stemming from improper understanding of discharge instructions may include:
  - An infected cord or circumcision from improper care or tub bathing too soon.
  - Falls; suffocation; strangulation; burns resulting in injuries, fractures, aspiration; or even death due to improper safety precautions.
  - Respiratory infections due to passive smoke or inhaled powders.
  - Improper or no use of a car seat resulting in injuries or death.
  - Serious infections due to lack of noncompliance with immunization schedule.

APPLICATION EXERCISES

1. A nurse is reviewing care of the umbilical cord with the parent of a newborn. Which of the following should be included in the teaching?

  A. Cover the cord with a small gauze square.

  B. Trickle clean water over the cord with each diaper change.

  C. Apply hydrogen peroxide to the cord twice a day.

  D. Keep the diaper folded below the cord.

2. A nurse is providing discharge teaching to the parents of a newborn regarding circumcision care. Which of the following statements made by a parent indicates a need for further clarification?

  A. "His circumcision will heal within a couple of weeks."

  B. "I do not need to remove the yellow mucus that will form."

  C. "I will clean his penis with each diaper change."

  D. "I will give him a tub bath within a couple of days."

3. A nurse is reviewing contraindications for circumcision with a newly hired nurse. Which of the following are contraindications? (Select all that apply.)

  ___X___ A. Hypospadias

  _____ B. Hydrocele

  ___X___ C. Familiar history of hemophilia

  _____ D. Hyperbilirubinemia

  ___X___ E. Epispadias

4. A nurse is caring for a newborn immediately following a circumcision using a Gomco procedure. Which of the following is an appropriate nursing intervention?

  A. Apply Gelfoam powder to the site.

  B. Place the newborn in the prone position.

  C. Apply petroleum gauze to the site.

  D. Avoid changing the diaper until the first voiding.

5. A nurse is reviewing car seat safety with the parents of a newborn. The nurse instructs the parents to restrain the newborn in a car seat in the

    A. front seat, rear-facing position.

    B. front seat, forward-facing position.

    C. back seat, rear-facing position.

    D. back seat, forward-facing position.

6. A nurse is leading a discussion with a group of parents on bathing a newborn. What should be included in this discussion? Use the ATI Active Learning Template: Basic Concept to complete this item to include the following sections:

    A. Nursing Interventions:
   - Describe two interventions that relate to general skin care.
   - Describe two interventions that relate to promoting infant safety.
   - Describe two interventions that relate to the correct order of giving a bath.
   - Describe two interventions that prevent complications in the newborn.

APPLICATION EXERCISES KEY

1. A. INCORRECT: Covering the cord with a gauze square prevents the cord from drying and encourages infection.

    B. INCORRECT: The cord should be kept clean and dry, and water should not be applied to the cord.

    C. INCORRECT: The cord should be kept clean and dry. Hydrogen peroxide is not applied to the cord site.

    D. **CORRECT:** Folding the diaper below the cord prevents urine from the diaper penetrating the cord site.

    Ⓝ NCLEX® Connection: Health Promotion and Maintenance, Aging Process

2. A. INCORRECT: The circumcision will heal within a couple of weeks. This statement reflects understanding of the teaching.

    B. INCORRECT: The yellow mucus should remain in place as part of the healing process.

    C. INCORRECT: The penis should be cleaned with warm water with each diaper change.

    D. **CORRECT:** A tub bath should not be given until the circumcision is healed, which occurs within a couple of weeks.

    Ⓝ NCLEX® Connection: Health Promotion and Maintenance, Ante/Intra/Postpartum and Newborn Care

3. A. **CORRECT:** Hypospadias involves a defect in the location of the urethral opening and is a contraindication to circumcision.

    B. INCORRECT: Hydrocele, a collection of fluid in the scrotal sac, is not a contraindication to circumcision.

    C. **CORRECT:** A family history of hemophilia is a contraindication for circumcision.

    D. INCORRECT: Hyperbilirubinemia is not a contraindication for circumcision.

    E. **CORRECT:** Epispadias involves a defect in the location of the urethral opening and is a contraindication to circumcision.

    Ⓝ NCLEX® Connection: Health Promotion and Maintenance, Aging Process

4. A. INCORRECT: Gelfoam powder is used to control bleeding when there is a risk for hemorrhage.

    B. INCORRECT: Newborns should not be placed in the prone position.

    C. **CORRECT:** Petroleum gauze is applied to the site for 24 hr to prevent the skin edges from sticking to the diaper.

    D. INCORRECT: Diapers are changed more frequently to inspect the site.

    Ⓝ NCLEX® Connection: Health Promotion and Maintenance, Aging Process

5.   A. INCORRECT: This is not an appropriate position for the car seat.

B. INCORRECT: This is not an appropriate position for the car seat.

C. **CORRECT:** The newborn should be restrained in a car seat in a rear-facing position in the back seat until 2 years of age.

D. INCORRECT: This is not an appropriate position for the car seat.

 NCLEX® Connection: Safety and Infection Control, Accident/Error/Injury Prevention

6.   *Using ATI Active Learning Template: Basic Concept*

A. Nursing Interventions

- Skin Care

  ○ The eyes are cleaned using a clean portion of the wash cloth.

  ○ The newborn should be washed, rinsed, and dried with no soap left on the skin.

  ○ Use a mild soap that does not contain hexachlorophene.

- Infant Safety

  ○ Do not leave the newborn unattended during the bath.

  ○ Hot water heater should be set at 49° C (120.2° F) or less.

  ○ The room should be warm, and the bath water should be at 36.6° to 37.2° C (98° to 99° F).

  ○ Bath water should be tested on the inner wrist prior to use.

- Order of Giving the Bath

  ○ Move from the cleanest to the dirtiest areas of the newborn's body, which includes starting with the eyes, face, and head; proceeding to the chest, arms, and legs; and washing the groin area last.

  ○ The eyes are cleaned by moving from the inner to the outer canthus.

- Preventing Complications

  ○ Bathing by immersion is not done until the umbilical cord falls off and the circumcision is healed.

  ○ Do not bathe the newborn immediately after feeding to prevent spitting up and vomiting.

  ○ After cleansing the uncircumcised newborn male, the foreskin should not be forced back.

  ○ In female newborns, wash the vulva by wiping from front to back.

  ○ Do not use lotions, oils, or powders.

 NCLEX® Connection: Health Promotion and Maintenance, Ante/Intra/Postpartum and Newborn Care

chapter 27

Overview

- This chapter highlights the assessment and management of newborn complications. Assessment, risk factors, and collaborative care will be discussed. It is essential for a nurse to immediately identify complications and implement appropriate interventions. Ongoing emotional support to a client and significant other is also imperative to the plan of care.

- The complications neonatal substance withdrawal, hypoglycemia, respiratory distress syndrome (RDS)/asphyxia/meconium aspiration, preterm newborn, small for gestational age (SGA) newborn, large for gestational age (LGA)/macrosomic newborn, postterm newborn, neonatal infection/sepsis (sepsis neonatorum), birth trauma or injury, hyperbilirubinemia, and congenital anomalies will be detailed in this chapter.

NEONATAL SUBSTANCE WITHDRAWAL

Overview

- Maternal substance use during pregnancy consists of any use of alcohol or drugs. Intrauterine drug exposure can cause anomalies, neurobehavioral changes, and evidence of withdrawal in the neonate. These changes depend on the specific drug or combination of drugs used, dosage, route of administration, metabolism and excretion by the mother and her fetus, timing of drug exposure, and the length of drug exposure.

- Substance withdrawal in the newborn occurs when the mother uses drugs that have addictive properties during pregnancy. This includes illegal drugs, alcohol, tobacco, and prescription drugs.

- Fetal alcohol syndrome (FAS) results from the chronic or periodic intake of alcohol during pregnancy. Alcohol is considered teratogenic, so the daily intake of alcohol increases the risk of FAS.

- Newborns who have FAS are at risk for specific congenital physical defects, along with long-term complications that include the following:

  ○ Feeding problems

  ○ Central nervous system dysfunction (mental retardation, cerebral palsy)

  ○ Behavioral difficulties such as hyperactivity

  ○ Language abnormalities

  ○ Future substance use

  ○ Delayed growth and development

  ○ Poor maternal-newborn bonding

Risk Factors

- Mother using substances prior to knowing she is pregnant
- Maternal substance use and addiction

Assessment

- Objective Data
  - Physical assessment findings
    - Monitor the neonate for abstinence syndrome (withdrawal) and increased wakefulness using the neonatal abstinence scoring system that assesses for and scores the following:
      - CNS – increased wakefulness, a high-pitched, shrill cry, incessant crying, irritability, tremors, hyperactive with an increased Moro reflex, increased deep-tendon reflexes, increased muscle tone, abrasions and/or excoriations on the face and knees, and convulsions.
      - Metabolic, vasomotor, and respiratory findings – nasal congestion with flaring, frequent yawning, skin mottling, tachypnea greater than 60/min, sweating, and a temperature greater than 37.2° C (99° F).
      - Gastrointestinal – poor feeding, regurgitation (projectile vomiting), diarrhea, and excessive, uncoordinated, and constant sucking.
    - Opiate withdrawal
      - Can last for 2 to 3 weeks
      - Manifestations of neonatal abstinence syndrome – rapid changes in mood, hypersensitivity to noise and external stimuli, dehydration, and poor weight gain
    - Heroin withdrawal
      - Manifestations of neonatal abstinence syndrome – low birth weight and SGA, decreased Moro reflexes (rather than increased), and hypothermia or hyperthermia.
    - Methadone withdrawal
      - Manifestations of neonatal abstinence syndrome – an increased incidence of seizures, sleep pattern disturbances, higher birth weights, and higher risk of sudden infant death syndrome (SIDS)
    - Marijuana withdrawal
      - Preterm birth and meconium staining.
    - Amphetamine withdrawal
      - Clinical findings – Preterm or SGA, drowsiness, jitteriness, sleep pattern disturbances, respiratory distress, frequent infections, poor weight gain, emotional disturbances, and delayed growth and development
    - Fetal alcohol syndrome
      - Clinical findings
        - Facial anomalies include eyes with epicanthal folds, strabismus, and ptosis; mouth with a poor suck, small teeth, and cleft lip or palate
        - Deafness
        - Abnormal palmar creases and irregular hair

- ▸ Many vital organ anomalies, such as heart defects, including atrial and ventricular septal defects, tetralogy of Fallot, and patent-ductus arteriosus
- ▸ Developmental delays and neurologic abnormalities
- ▸ Prenatal and postnatal growth retardation
- ▸ Sleep disturbances
  - ▪ Tobacco
    - ▫ Clinical findings – prematurity, low birth weight, increased risk for SIDS, increased risk for bronchitis, pneumonia, and developmental delays

Patient-Centered Care

- Nursing Care
  - ○ Nursing care for maternal substance use and neonatal effects or withdrawal include the following in addition to normal newborn care.
    - ▪ Perform a neonatal abstinence scoring system assessment, as prescribed by the provider.
    - ▪ Elicit and assess the newborn's reflexes.
    - ▪ Monitor the newborn's ability to feed and digest intake.
    - ▪ Monitor the newborn's fluids and electrolytes with skin turgor, mucous membranes, fontanels, and I&O.
    - ▪ Observe the newborn's behavior.
- Laboratory Tests
  - ○ Blood tests should be done to differentiate between neonatal drug withdrawal and central nervous system irritability.
    - ▪ CBC
    - ▪ Blood glucose
    - ▪ Calcium
    - ▪ Magnesium
    - ▪ Thyroid-stimulating hormone, thyroxine, triiodothyronine
    - ▪ Drug screen of urine or meconium to reveal the agent used by the mother
    - ▪ Hair analysis
- Diagnostic Procedures
  - ○ Chest x-ray for FAS to rule out congenital heart defects
- Medications
  - ○ Phenobarbital (Solfoton)
    - ▪ Classification
      - ▫ Anticonvulsant
    - ▪ Intended effect
      - ▫ It is prescribed to decrease CNS irritability and control seizures for newborns who have alcohol or opioid addiction.

- Nursing considerations
  - Assess IV site frequently.
  - Check for any medication incompatibilities.
  - Decrease environmental stimuli.
  - Cluster cares for newborn to minimize stimulation.
  - Swaddle the newborn to reduce self-stimulation and protect the skin from abrasions.
  - Monitor and maintain fluids and electrolytes.
  - Administer frequent, small feedings of high-calorie formula – may require gavage feedings.
  - Elevate the newborn's head during and following feedings, and burp the newborn to reduce vomiting and aspiration.
  - Try various nipples to compensate for a poor suck reflex.
  - Have suction available to reduce the risk for aspiration.
  - For newborns who are addicted to cocaine, avoid eye contact and use vertical rocking and a pacifier.
  - Prevent infection.
  - Initiate a consult with child protective services.
  - Consult lactation services to evaluate whether breastfeeding is desired or contraindicated to avoid passing narcotics in breast milk. Methadone is not contraindicated during breastfeeding.
- Health Promotion and Disease Prevention
  - Client education
    - Refer the mother to a drug and/or alcohol treatment center.
    - Discuss the importance of SIDS prevention activities due to the increased rate in newborns of mothers who used methadone.

HYPOGLYCEMIA

Overview

- Hypoglycemia is a serum glucose level of less than 40 mg/dL. Routine assessment of all newborns, especially newborns who are LGA and SGA, should include monitoring for hypoglycemia.
- Hypoglycemia – differs for a newborn who is preterm or term. Hypoglycemia occurring in the first 3 days of life in the term newborn is defined as a blood glucose level of less than 40 mg/dL. In the preterm newborn, hypoglycemia is defined as a blood glucose level of less than 25 mg/dL.
- Untreated hypoglycemia can result in seizures, brain damage, and/or death.

Risk Factors

- Maternal diabetes mellitus
- Preterm infant
- LGA or SGA
- Stress at birth, such as cold stress and asphyxia
- Maternal epidural anesthesia

Assessment

- Objective Data
  - Physical assessment findings
    - Poor feeding
    - Jitteriness/tremors
    - Hypothermia
    - Diaphoresis
    - Weak shrill cry
    - Lethargy
    - Flaccid muscle tone
    - Seizures/coma
    - Irregular respirations
    - Cyanosis
    - Apnea
  - Laboratory tests and diagnostic procedures
    - Two consecutive plasma glucose levels less than 40 mg/dL in a newborn who is term, and less than 25 mg/dL in a newborn who is preterm

Patient-Centered Care

- Nursing Care
  - Obtain blood by heel stick for glucose monitoring.
  - Provide frequent oral and/or gavage feedings, or continuous parenteral nutrition early after birth to treat hypoglycemia.
  - Monitor the neonate's blood glucose level closely per facility protocol.
  - Monitor IV if the neonate is unable to feed orally.

RESPIRATORY DISTRESS SYNDROME (RDS)/ASPHYXIA/MECONIUM ASPIRATION

Overview

- Respiratory distress syndrome (RDS) occurs as a result of surfactant deficiency in the lungs and is characterized by poor gas exchange and ventilatory failure.
- Surfactant is a phospholipid that assists in alveoli expansion. Surfactant keeps alveoli from collapsing and allows gas exchange to occur.
- Atelectasis (collapsing of a portion of lung) increases the work of breathing. As a result, respiratory acidosis and hypoxemia can develop.

- Birth weight alone is not an indicator of fetal lung maturity.
- Complications from RDS are related to oxygen therapy and mechanical ventilation.
  - Pneumothorax
  - Pneumomediastinum
  - Retinopathy of prematurity
  - Bronchopulmonary dysplasia
  - Infection
  - Intraventricular hemorrhage

Risk Factors

- Preterm gestation
- Perinatal asphyxia (meconium staining, cord prolapse, nuchal cord)
- Maternal diabetes mellitus
- Premature rupture of membranes
- Maternal use of barbiturates or narcotics close to birth
- Maternal hypotension
- Cesarean birth without labor
- Hydrops fetalis (massive edema of the fetus caused by hyperbilirubinemia)
- Maternal bleeding during the third trimester

Assessment

- Objective Data
  - Physical assessment findings
    - Tachypnea (respiratory rate greater than 60/min)
    - Nasal flaring
    - Expiratory grunting
    - Retractions
    - Labored breathing with prolonged expiration
    - Fine crackles on auscultation
    - Cyanosis
    - Unresponsiveness, flaccidity, and apnea with decreased breath sounds (manifestations of worsened RDS)
  - Laboratory tests
    - Culture and sensitivity of the blood, urine, and cerebrospinal fluid
    - Blood glucose and serum calcium
  - Diagnostic procedures
    - ABGs reveal hypercapnia (excess of carbon dioxide in the blood) and respiratory or mixed acidosis.
    - Chest x-ray

Patient-Centered Care

- Nursing Care
  - Suction the newborn's mouth, trachea, and nose as needed.
  - Maintain thermoregulation.
  - Provide mouth and skin care.
  - Correct respiratory acidosis with ventilatory support.
  - Correct metabolic acidosis by administering sodium bicarbonate.
  - Maintain adequate oxygenation, prevent lactic acidosis, and avoid the toxic effects of oxygen.
  - Decrease stimuli.
- Medications
  - Beractant (Survanta)
  - Classification
    - Lung surfactant
  - Intended effect
    - It is prescribed for newborns who are premature and have RDS. It restores surfactant and improves respiratory compliance.
  - Nursing considerations
    - Perform a respiratory assessment including ABGs, respiratory rhythm, and rate and color before and after administration of agent.
    - Provide suction to the newborn prior to administration of the medication.
    - Assess endotracheal tube placement.
    - Avoid suctioning of the endotracheal tube for 1 hr after administration of the medication.
- Miscellaneous
  - Factors that can accelerate lung maturation in the fetus while in utero include increased gestational age, intrauterine stress, exogenous steroid use, and ruptured membranes.

PRETERM NEWBORN

Overview

- A preterm newborn's birth occurs after 20 weeks of gestation and before 37 weeks of gestation. This may occur once the cervix has dilated to 4 cm.
- Preterm newborns are at risk for a variety of complications due to immature organ systems. The degree of complications depends on gestational age. There is a decreased risk for complications the closer the newborn is to 40 weeks of gestation.
  - Respiratory distress syndrome – decreased surfactant in the alveoli occurs, regardless of a newborn's birth weight
  - Bronchopulmonary dysplasia – causes the lungs to become stiff and noncompliant, requiring a newborn to receive mechanical ventilation and oxygen, and it is sometimes difficult to remove the newborn from ventilation and oxygen after initial placement

○ Aspiration – a result of a newborn who is premature not having an intact gag reflex or the ability to effectively suck or swallow

○ Apnea of prematurity – a result of immature neurological and chemical mechanisms

○ Intraventricular hemorrhage – bleeding in or around the ventricles of the brain

○ Retinopathy of prematurity – disease caused by abnormal growth of retinal blood vessels and is a complication associated with oxygen administration to the neonate, and it can cause mild to severe eye and vision problems

○ Patent ductus arteriosus – occurs when the ductus arteriosus reopens after birth due to neonatal hypoxia

○ Necrotizing enterocolitis (NEC) – an inflammatory disease of the gastrointestinal mucosa due to ischemia, and it results in necrosis and perforation of the bowel (short-gut syndrome may be the result secondary to removal of most or part of the small intestine due to necrosis)

○ Additional complications include infection, hyperbilirubinemia, anemia, hypoglycemia, and delayed growth and development.

  ▪ Goals include meeting the newborn's growth and development needs, and anticipating and managing associated complications such as RDS and sepsis.

  ▪ The main priority in treating newborns who are preterm is supporting the cardiac and respiratory systems as needed. Most newborns who are preterm are cared for in a neonatal intensive care unit (NICU). Meticulous care and observation in the NICU is necessary until the newborn can receive oral feedings, maintain body temperature, and weighs approximately 2 kg (4.4 lb).

Risk Factors

• Maternal gestational hypertension

• Multiple pregnancies that are closely spaced

• Adolescent pregnancy

• Lack of prenatal care

• Maternal substance use, smoking

• Previous history of preterm delivery

• Abnormalities of the uterus

• Cervical incompetence

• Premature rupture of the membranes

• Placenta previa

• Premature labor

• Premature rupture of membranes

Assessment

- Objective Data
  - Physical assessment findings
    - A Ballard assessment shows a physical and neurological assessment totaling less than 37 weeks of gestation.
    - Periodic breathing consists of 5- to 10-second respiratory pauses, followed by 10- to 15-second compensatory rapid respirations.
    - Manifestations of increased respiratory effort and/or respiratory distress include nasal flaring or retractions of the chest wall during inspirations, expiratory grunting, and tachypnea.
    - Apnea is a pause in respirations longer than 10 to 15 seconds.
    - The newborn has a low birth weight.
    - The newborn has minimal subcutaneous fat deposits.
    - The newborn's head is large in comparison with his body, and fontanels are small.
    - The newborn has wrinkled features with abundance of lanugo covering back, forearms, forehead, and sides of face, and few or no creases on soles of feet.
    - The newborn's skull and rib cage feel soft.
    - The newborn's eyes are closed if he is born at 22 to 24 weeks of gestation.
    - The newborn has a weak grasp reflex.
    - The newborn has an inability to coordinate suck and swallow; and a weak or absent gag, suck, and cough reflex; weak swallow.
    - The newborn has hypotonic muscles, decreased level of activity, and a weak cry for more than 24 hr.
    - The newborn is lethargic, is experiencing tachycardia, and has poor weight gain.
    - Evidence of infection
      - Observe the newborn for findings of dehydration or overhydration (resulting from IV nutrition and fluid administration).
      - Dehydration
        - Urine output less than 1 mL/kg/hr
        - Urine-specific gravity more than 1.015
        - Weight loss
        - Dry mucous membranes
        - Absent skin turgor
        - Depressed fontanel
      - Overhydration
        - Urine output greater than 3 mL/kg/hr
        - Urine-specific gravity less than 1.001
        - Edema
        - Increased weight gain
        - Crackles in lungs
        - Intake greater than output

- ○ Laboratory tests
  - ▪ CBC shows decreased Hgb and Hct as a result of slow production of RBCs
  - ▪ Urinalysis and specific gravity
  - ▪ Increased PT and aPTT time with an increased tendency to bleed
  - ▪ Serum glucose
  - ▪ Calcium
  - ▪ Bilirubin
  - ▪ ABGs
- ○ Diagnostic procedures
  - ▪ Chest x-ray
  - ▪ Head ultrasounds
  - ▪ Echocardiography
  - ▪ Eye exams

Patient-Centered Care

- Nursing Care
  - ○ Perform rapid initial assessment.
  - ○ Perform resuscitative measures if needed.
  - ○ Monitor the newborn's vital signs.
  - ○ Assess the newborn's ability to consume and digest nutrients. Before feeding by breast or nipple, the newborn must have an intact gag reflex and be able to suck and swallow to prevent aspiration.
  - ○ Monitor the newborn's I&O, and daily weight.
  - ○ Monitor the newborn for bleeding from puncture sites and the gastrointestinal tract.
  - ○ Ensure and maintain thermoregulation in a newborn who is premature by using a radiant heat warmer.
  - ○ Administer respiratory support measures, such as surfactant and/or oxygen administration.
  - ○ Administer parental or enteral nutrition and fluids as prescribed (most premature newborns who are less than 34 weeks of gestation will receive fluids either by IV and/or gavage feedings). Provide for nonnutritive sucking, such as using a pacifier while gavage feeding.
  - ○ Minimize the newborn's stimulation. Cluster nursing care. Touch the newborn very smoothly and lightly. Keep lighting dim and noise levels reduced.
  - ○ Position the newborn in neutral flexion with his extremities close to his body to conserve body heat. Prone and side-lying positions are preferred to supine with body containment using blanket rolls and swaddling, but only in the nursery under monitored supervision.
  - ○ Protect the newborn against infection by enforcing hand hygiene and gowning procedures. Equipment should not be shared with other newborns.
- Medications
  - ○ Betamethasone (Celestone)

- Classification
  - Glucocorticoids
- Intended Effect
  - It is administered for a 24-hr period prior to delivery to promote fetal lung development and increase surfactant in an attempt to prevent RDS.
- Health Promotion and Disease Prevention
  - Client education
    - Keep parents informed about and engaged in the care of their preterm newborn.

SMALL FOR GESTATIONAL AGE NEWBORN (SGA)

Overview

- Small for gestational age (SGA) describes a newborn whose birth weight is at or below the 10th percentile and who has intrauterine growth restriction.
- Common complications of newborns who are SGA are perinatal asphyxia, meconium aspiration, hypoglycemia, polycythemia, and instability of body temperature.

Risk Factors

- Congenital or chromosomal anomalies
- Maternal infections, disease, or malnutrition
- Gestational hypertension and/or diabetes mellitus
- Maternal smoking, drug, or alcohol use
- Multiple gestations
- Placental factors (small placenta, placenta previa, decreased placental perfusion)
- Fetal congenital infections such as rubella or toxoplasmosis

Assessment

- Objective Data
  - Physical assessment findings
    - Weight below 10th percentile
    - Normal skull, but reduced body dimensions
    - Hair is sparse on scalp
    - Wide skull sutures from inadequate bone growth
    - Dry, loose skin
    - Decreased subcutaneous fat

- Decreased muscle mass, particularly over the cheeks and buttocks
- Thin, dry, yellow, and dull umbilical cord rather than gray, glistening, and moist
- Drawn abdomen rather than well-rounded
- Respiratory distress and hypoxia
- Wide-eyed and alert, which is attributed to prolonged fetal hypoxia
- Hypotonia
- Evidence of meconium aspiration
- Hypoglycemia
- Acrocyanosis
  - Laboratory tests
    - Blood glucose level for hypoglycemia
    - CBC will show polycythemia resulting from fetal hypoxia and intrauterine stress.
    - ABGs may be prescribed due to chronic hypoxia in utero due to placental insufficiency.
  - Diagnostic procedures
    - Chest x-ray to rule out meconium aspiration syndrome

Patient-Centered Care

- Nursing Care
  - Support respiratory efforts, and suction the newborn as necessary to maintain an open airway.
  - Provide a neutral thermal environment for the newborn (isolette or radiant heat warmer) to prevent cold stress.
  - Initiate early feedings. (A newborn who is SGA will require feedings that are more frequent.)
  - Administer parenteral nutrition if necessary.
  - Maintain adequate hydration.
  - Conserve the newborn's energy level.
  - Prevent skin breakdown.
  - Protect the newborn from infection.
- Health Promotion and Disease Prevention
  - Client education
    - Provide support to the newborn's parents and extended family, and encourage them to participate in caring for the newborn. Anticipate home care needs.

LARGE FOR GESTATIONAL AGE NEWBORN (LGA)/MACROSOMIC

Overview

- Large for gestational age (LGA) occurs in neonates who weigh above the 90th percentile or more than 4,000 g (8 lb, 12 oz).

- Neonates who are LGA may be preterm, postterm, or full-term. LGA does not necessarily mean postmature.

- Newborns who are macrosomic are at risk for birth injuries (shoulder dystocia, clavicle fracture or a cesarean birth, asphyxia, hypoglycemia, polycythemia and Erb-Duchenne paralysis due to birth trauma).

- Uncontrolled hyperglycemia during pregnancy (leading risk factor for LGA) can lead to congenital defects with the most common being congenital heart defects, tracheoesophageal fistula, and CNS anomalies.

Risk Factors

- Newborns who are postterm

- Maternal diabetes mellitus during pregnancy (high glucose levels stimulate continued insulin production by the fetus)

- Fetal cardiovascular disorder of transposition of the great vessels

- Genetic factors

- Maternal obesity

- A mother who is multiparous

Assessment

- Objective Data
  - Physical assessment findings
    - Weight above 90th percentile (4,000 g)
    - Plump and full-faced (cushingoid appearance) from increased subcutaneous fat
    - Manifestations of hypoxia including tachypnea, retractions, cyanosis, nasal flaring, and grunting
    - Birth trauma (e.g., fractures, shoulder dystocia, intracranial hemorrhage, and CNS injury)
    - Sluggishness, hypotonic muscles, and hypoactivity
    - Tremors from hypocalcemia
    - Hypoglycemia
    - Respiratory distress from immature lungs or meconium aspiration
    - Findings of increased intracranial pressure (dilated pupils, vomiting, bulging fontanels, and high-pitched cry)

- Laboratory tests
  - Blood glucose levels to monitor closely for hypoglycemia (less than 40 mg/dL).
  - ABGs may be prescribed due to chronic hypoxia in utero secondary to placental insufficiency.
  - CBC shows polycythemia (Hct greater than 65%) from in utero hypoxia.
  - Hyperbilirubinemia resulting from polycythemia as excessive RBCs break down after birth.
  - Hypocalcemia may result in response to a long and difficult birth.
- Diagnostic procedures
  - Chest x-ray to rule out meconium aspiration syndrome

Patient-Centered Care

- Nursing Care Prior to Delivery
  - Prepare the client for a possible vacuum-assisted or cesarean birth.
  - Prepare to place the client in McRoberts' position (lithotomy position with legs flexed to chest to maximize pelvic outlet).
  - Prepare to apply suprapubic pressure to aid in the delivery of the anterior shoulder, which is located inferior to the maternal symphysis pubis.
  - Assess the newborn for birth trauma, such as a broken clavicle or Erb-Duchenne paralysis.
- Nursing Care for a Newborn Who is LGA Following Delivery
  - Obtain early and frequent heel sticks (blood glucose testing).
  - Initiate early feedings or intravenous therapy to maintain glucose levels within the expected reference range.
  - Provide thermoregulation with isolette care.
  - Administer surfactant by endotracheal tube if indicated.
  - Identify and treat any birth injuries.

POSTTERM INFANT

Overview

- A newborn who is postterm is one who is born after the completion of 42 weeks of gestation. Postmaturity of the infant can be associated with either of the following:
  - Dysmaturity from placental degeneration and uteroplacental insufficiency (placenta functions effectively for only 40 weeks) resulting in chronic fetal hypoxia and fetal distress in utero. The fetal response is polycythemia, meconium aspiration, and/or neonatal respiratory problems. Perinatal mortality is higher when a postmature placenta fails to meet increased oxygen demands of the fetus during labor.
  - Continued growth of the fetus in utero because the placenta continues to function effectively and the newborn becomes LGA at birth. This leads to a difficult delivery, cephalopelvic disproportion, as well as high insulin reserves and insufficient glucose reserves at birth. The neonatal response can be birth trauma, perinatal asphyxia, a clavicle fracture, seizures, hypoglycemia, and/or temperature instability (cold stress).

- A newborn who is postmature may be either SGA or LGA depending on how well the placenta functions during the last weeks of pregnancy.

- Newborns who are postmature have an increased risk for aspirating the meconium passed by the fetus in utero.

- Persistent pulmonary hypertension (persistent fetal circulation) is a complication that can result from meconium aspiration. There is an interference in the transition from fetal to neonatal circulation, and the ductus arteriosus (connecting the main pulmonary artery and the aorta) and foramen ovale (shunt between the right and left atria) remain open, and fetal pathways of blood flow continue.

Risk Factors

- In most cases, the cause of a pregnancy that extends beyond 40 weeks of gestation is unknown, but there is a higher incidence in first pregnancies and in women who have had a previous postterm pregnancy.

Assessment

- Objective Data
  - Physical assessment findings
    - Wasted appearance, thin with loose skin, having lost some of the subcutaneous fat
    - Peeling, cracked, and dry skin; leathery from decreased protection of vernix and amniotic fluid
    - Long, thin body
    - Meconium staining of fingernails and umbilical cord
    - Hair and nails may be long
    - May demonstrate alertness similar to a 2-week-old newborn
    - May have difficulty establishing respirations secondary to meconium aspiration
    - Hypoglycemia due to insufficient stores of glycogen
    - Clinical findings of cold stress
    - Neurological manifestations that become apparent with the development of fine motor skills
    - Macrosomia
- Laboratory Tests
  - Blood glucose levels to monitor for hypoglycemia
  - ABGs secondary to chronic hypoxia in utero due to placental insufficiency
  - CBC may show polycythemia from decreased oxygenation in utero
  - Hct elevated from polycythemia and dehydration
- Diagnostic Procedures
  - Cesarean birth
  - Chest x-ray to rule out meconium aspiration syndrome

Patient-Centered Care

- Nursing Care
  - Monitor the newborn's vital signs.
  - Administer and monitor the newborn's IV fluids.
  - Use mechanical ventilation if necessary.
  - Administer oxygen as prescribed.
  - Prepare and/or assist with exchange transfusion if hematocrit is high.
  - Provide thermoregulation in an isolette to avoid cold stress.
  - Provide early feedings to avoid hypoglycemia.
  - Identify and treat any birth injuries.

NEONATAL INFECTION/SEPSIS (SEPSIS NEONATORUM)

Overview

- Infection may be contracted by the newborn before, during, or after delivery. Newborns are more susceptible to micro-organisms because of their limited immunity and inability to localize infection. The infection can spread rapidly into the bloodstream.

- Neonatal sepsis is the presence of micro-organisms or their toxins in the blood or tissues of the newborn during the first month after birth. Manifestations of sepsis are subtle and may resemble other diseases; the nurse often notices them during routine care of the newborn.

- Organisms frequently responsible for neonatal infections include: *Staphylococcus aureus*, *S. epidermidis*, *Escherichia coli*, *Haemophilus influenzae*, and streptococcus ß-hemolytic, Group B.

- Prevention of infection and neonatal sepsis starts perinatally with maternal screening for infections, prophylactic interventions, and the use of sterile and aseptic techniques during delivery. Prophylactic antibiotic treatment of the eyes of all newborns and appropriate umbilical cord care also help to prevent neonatal infection and sepsis.

Risk Factors

- Premature rupture of the membranes
- TORCH (toxoplasmosis, rubella, cytomegalovirus, and herpes)
- Chorioamnionitis
- Premature birth
- Low birth weight
- Maternal substance use
- Maternal urinary-tract infection
- Meconium
- HIV transmitted from the mother to the newborn perinatally through the placenta and postnatally through the breast milk

Assessment

- Objective Data
  - Physical assessment findings
    - Temperature instability
    - Suspicious drainage (eyes, umbilical stump)
    - Poor feeding pattern, such as a weak suck or decreased intake
    - Vomiting and diarrhea
    - Poor weight gain
    - Abdominal distention, large residual if feeding by gavage
    - Apnea, sternal retractions, grunting, and nasal flaring
    - Decreased oxygen saturation
    - Color changes such as pallor, jaundice, and petechiae
    - Tachycardia or bradycardia
    - Tachypnea
    - Low blood pressure
    - Irritability and seizure activity
    - Poor muscle tone and lethargy
  - Laboratory tests
    - CBC
    - Blood, urine, and cerebrospinal fluid cultures and sensitivities
    - Positive blood cultures, usually polymicrobial (more than one pathogen) indicates the presence of infection/sepsis
    - Chemical profile shows a fluid and electrolyte imbalance.

Patient-Centered Care

- Nursing Care
  - Assess infection risks (review maternal health record).
  - Monitor the newborn for clinical findings of opportunistic infection.
  - Monitor the newborn's vital signs continuously.
  - Monitor the newborn's I&O and daily weight.
  - Monitor the newborn's fluid and electrolyte status.
  - Monitor the newborn's visitors for infection.
  - Obtain specimens (blood, urine, stool) to assist in identifying the causative organism.
  - Initiate and maintain IV therapy as prescribed to administer electrolyte replacements, fluids, and medications.
  - Administer medications as prescribed (broad-spectrum antibiotics prior to cultures being obtained).

- Medications: A combination of ampicillin with an aminoglycoside or a third-generation cephalosporin (Rocephin) is the mainstay of therapy for treatment of newborns who have suspected sepsis.
  - Ampicillin (Principen)
    - Classifications
      - Antibiotic
    - Intended Effect
      - It is a broad-spectrum antibiotic that is bactericidal.
    - Nursing Considerations
      - Obtain cultures prior to administration of antibiotics.
  - Gentamicin sulfate (Garamycin)
    - Classification
      - Aminoglycoside antibiotic
    - Intended Effect
      - It is a bactericidal that causes cell death.
    - Nursing Considerations
      - Obtain cultures prior to administration of antibiotics.
      - Monitor the newborn's peak and trough levels as prescribed.
- Nursing Considerations
  - Initiate and maintain respiratory support as needed.
  - Assess IV site for evidence of infection.
  - Provide newborn care to maintain temperature.
  - Maintain standard precautions.
  - Clean and sterilize all equipment to be used.
- Health Promotion and Disease Prevention
  - Discharge instructions
    - Provide the family with education about infection control
      - Instruct them how to use clean bottles and nipples for each feeding.
      - Discard any unused formula.
      - Supervise hand hygiene
    - Promote adequate rest for newborn, and decrease physical stimulation.
    - Provide emotional support to the family.

BIRTH TRAUMA OR INJURY

Overview

- Birth injury occurs during childbirth resulting in physical injury to a newborn. Most injuries are minor and resolve rapidly. Other injuries may require some intervention. A few are serious enough to be fatal.
- Types of birth injuries
  - Skull (linear fracture, depressed fracture)
  - Scalp (caput succedaneum)
  - Intracranial (epidural or subdural hematoma, cerebral contusion)
  - Spinal cord (spinal cord transaction or injury, vertebral artery injury)
  - Plexus (brachial plexus injury, Klumpke's palsy)
  - Cranial and peripheral nerve (radial nerve palsy, diaphragmatic paralysis)

Risk Factors

- Fetal macrosomia
- Abnormal or difficult presentations
- Prolonged labor
- Precipitous labor
- Cephalopelvic disproportion
- Multifetal gestation
- Congenital abnormalities
- Internal FHR monitoring
- Forceps or vacuum extraction
- External version
- Cesarean birth

Assessment

- Objective Data
  - Physical assessment findings
    - Irritability, seizures within the first 72 hr, and a decreased level of consciousness are all manifestations of a subarachnoid hemorrhage.
    - Facial flattening and unresponsiveness to grimace that accompanies crying or stimulation, as well as eyes remaining open, are all findings to assess for facial paralysis.
    - A weak or hoarse cry is characteristic of laryngeal nerve palsy from excessive traction on the neck.
    - Flaccid muscle tone may signal joint dislocations and separation during birth.
    - Flaccid muscle tone of the extremities suggests nerve-plexus injuries or long bone fractures.
    - Limited motion of an arm, crepitus over a clavicle, and absence of the Moro reflex on the affected side are manifestations of clavicular fractures.

- A flaccid arm with the elbow extended and the hand rotated inward, absence of the Moro reflex on the affected side, sensory loss over the lateral aspect of the arm, and intact grasp reflex are all manifestations of Erb-Duchenne paralysis (brachial paralysis).

- Localized discoloration, ecchymosis, petechiae, and edema over the presenting part are seen with soft-tissue injuries.

  ○ Diagnostic Procedures

- Birth injuries are normally diagnosed by a CT scan, x-ray of suspected area of fracture, or neurological exam to determine paralysis of nerves.

Patient-Centered Care

- Nursing Care
  ○ Review maternal history to look for factors that may predispose the newborn to injuries.
  ○ Review Apgar scoring that might indicate a possibility of birth injury.
  ○ Perform frequent head-to-toe physical assessments.
  ○ Obtain vital signs and temperature.
  ○ Promote parent-newborn interaction as much as possible.
  ○ Administer treatment to the newborn based on the injury and according to the provider's prescriptions.
- Health Promotion and Disease Prevention
  ○ Discharge instructions
    - Educate the newborn's parents and family regarding the injury and the management of the injury.
    - Promote parent-newborn bonding.

HYPERBILIRUBINEMIA

Overview

- Hyperbilirubinemia is an elevation of serum bilirubin levels resulting in jaundice. Jaundice normally appears in the head (especially the sclera and mucous membranes), and then progresses down the thorax, abdomen, and extremities.
- Jaundice can be either physiologic or pathologic
  ○ Physiologic jaundice is considered benign (resulting from normal newborn physiology of increased bilirubin production due to the shortened lifespan and breakdown of fetal RBCs and liver immaturity). The newborn with physiological jaundice has no other manifestations and shows evidence of jaundice after 24 hr of age.
  ○ Pathologic jaundice is a result of an underlying disease. Pathologic jaundice appears before 24 hr of age or is persistent after day 7. In the term newborn, bilirubin levels increase more than 0.5 mg/dL/hr, peaks at greater than 13 mg/dL, or is associated with anemia and hepatosplenomegaly. Pathologic jaundice is usually caused by a blood group incompatibility or an infection, but may be the result of RBC disorders.
- Kernicterus (bilirubin encephalopathy) can result from untreated hyperbilirubinemia with bilirubin levels at or higher than 25 mg/dL. It is a neurological syndrome caused by bilirubin depositing in brain cells. Survivors may develop cerebral palsy, epilepsy, or mental retardation. They may have minor effects such as learning disorders or perceptual-motor disabilities.

Risk Factors

- Increased RBC production or breakdown

- Rh or ABO incompatibility

- Decreased liver function

- Ineffective breastfeeding

- Sibling with diagnosed jaundice

- Certain medications (maternal ingestion of aspirin, tranquilizers, and sulfonamides)

- Hypoglycemia

- Hypothermia

- Anoxia

- Prematurity

Assessment

- Objective Data

  - Physical assessment findings

    - Yellowish tint to skin, sclera, and mucous membranes.

    - To verify jaundice, press the newborn's skin on the cheek or abdomen lightly with one finger. Then, release pressure, and observe the newborn's skin color for yellowish tint as the skin is blanched.

    - Note the time of jaundice onset to distinguish between physiologic and pathologic jaundice.

    - Assess the underlying cause by reviewing the maternal prenatal, family, and newborn history.

    - Hypoxia, hypothermia, hypoglycemia, and metabolic acidosis can occur as a result of hyperbilirubinemia and may increase the risk of brain damage.

    - Clinical findings of kernicterus.

      □ Very yellowish or orange skin

      □ Lethargy

      □ Hypotonic

      □ Poor suck reflex

      □ Increased sleepiness

      □ If untreated, the newborn will become hypertonic with backward arching of the neck and trunk.

      □ High-pitched cry

      □ Fever

Q
S

○ Laboratory tests

■ An elevated serum bilirubin level may occur (direct and indirect bilirubin). Monitor the newborn's bilirubin levels every 4 hr until the level returns to normal.

■ Assess maternal and newborn blood type to determine whether there is a presence of ABO incompatibility. This occurs if the newborn has blood type A or B, and the mother is type O.

■ Review Hgb and Hct.

■ A direct Coombs' test reveals the presence of antibody-coated (sensitized) Rh-positive RBCs in the newborn.

■ Check electrolyte levels for dehydration from phototherapy.

○ Diagnostic procedures

■ Transcutaneous bilirubin level is a noninvasive method to measure a newborn's bilirubin level.

○ Treatment

■ Phototherapy is the primary treatment for hyperbilirubinemia. It is prescribed if a newborn's serum bilirubin is greater than 15 mg/dL prior to 48 hr of age, greater than 18 mg/dL prior to 72 hr of age, and greater than 20 mg/dL at any time.

Patient-Centered Care

• Nursing Care

○ Observe the newborn's skin and mucous membranes for jaundice.

○ Monitor the newborn's vital signs.

○ Set up phototherapy if prescribed.

■ Maintain an eye mask over the newborn's eyes for protection of corneas and retinas.

■ Keep the newborn undressed with the exception of a male newborn. A surgical mask should be placed (like a bikini) over the genitalia to prevent possible testicular damage from heat and light waves. Be sure to remove the metal strip from the mask to prevent burning.

■ Avoid applying lotions or ointments to the skin because they absorb heat and can cause burns.

■ Remove the newborn from phototherapy every 4 hr, and unmask the newborn's eyes, checking for inflammation or injury.

■ Reposition the newborn every 2 hr to expose all of the body surfaces to the phototherapy lights and prevent pressure sores.

■ Check the lamp energy with a photometer per facility protocol.

■ Turn off the phototherapy lights before drawing blood for testing.

○ Observe the newborn for effects of phototherapy.

■ Bronze discoloration – not a serious complication

■ Maculopapular skin rash – not a serious complication

■ Development of pressure areas

■ Dehydration (poor skin turgor, dry mucous membranes, decreased urinary output)

■ Elevated temperature

- Encourage the parents to hold and interact with the newborn when phototherapy lights are off.

- Monitor elimination and daily weights, watching for evidence of dehydration.

- Check the newborn's axillary temperature every 4 hr during phototherapy because temperature may become elevated.

- Feed the newborn early and frequently – every 3 to 4 hr. This will promote bilirubin excretion in the stools.

- Encourage continued breastfeeding of the newborn. Supplementation with formula may be prescribed.

- Maintain adequate fluid intake to prevent dehydration.

- Reassure the parents that most newborns experience some degree of jaundice.

- Explain hyperbilirubinemia, its causes, diagnostic tests, and treatment to parents.

- Explain that the newborn's stool contains some bile that will be loose and green.

• Administer an exchange transfusion for newborns who are at risk for kernicterus.

• Discharge Instructions

- Educate the parents regarding the newborn's plan of care.

CONGENITAL ANOMALIES

Overview

• Newborns can be born with congenital anomalies involving all systems. Anomalies are often diagnosed prenatally. A nurse should provide emotional support to the parents whose newborn is facing procedures or surgeries to correct the defects.

• When congenital anomalies are present at birth, they can involve any of the body systems. Major anomalies causing serious problems include the following:

- Congenital heart disease (atrial septal defects, ventricular septal defects, coarctation of the aorta, tetralogy of Fallot, transposition of the great vessels, stenosis, atresia of valves)

- Neurological defects (neural-tube defects, hydrocephalus, anencephaly, encephalocele, meningocele, or myelomeningocele)

- Gastrointestinal problems (cleft lip/palate, diaphragmatic hernia, imperforate anus, tracheoesophageal fistula/esophageal atresia, duodenal atresia, omphalocele, gastroschisis, umbilical hernia, or intestinal obstruction)

- Musculoskeletal deformities (clubfoot, polydactyly, developmental dysplasia of the hip)

- Genitourinary deformities (hypospadias, epispadias, exstrophy of the bladder)

- Metabolic disorders (phenylketonuria, galactosemia, hypothyroidism)

- Chromosomal abnormalities (Down syndrome [trisomy 21], which is the most common trisomic abnormality with 47 chromosomes in each cell)

• Congenital anomalies are generally identified soon after birth by Apgar scoring and a brief assessment indicating the need for further investigation. Once identified, congenital anomalies are treated in a pediatric setting.

Risk Factors

- Risk factors for congenital anomalies include genetic and/or environmental factors.
  - Maternal age greater than 40 years
  - Chromosome abnormalities such as Down syndrome
  - Viral infections such as rubella
  - Excessive body heat exposure during the first trimester (neural tube defects)
  - Medications and substance use during pregnancy
  - Radiation exposure
  - Maternal metabolic disorders (phenylketonuria, diabetes mellitus)
  - Poor maternal nutrition such as folic acid deficiency (neural tube defects)
  - Newborns who are premature
  - Newborns who are SGA
  - Oligohydramnios or polyhydramnios

Assessments

- Monitor the newborn for evidence of congenital anomalies:
  - Cleft lip/palate – failure of the lip or hard or soft palate to fuse
  - Tracheoesophageal atresia – failure of the esophagus to connect to the stomach, excessive mucous secretions and drooling, periodic cyanotic episodes and choking, abdominal distention after birth, and immediate regurgitation after birth
  - Duodenal atresia – common in newborns who have Down syndrome and is when the first part of the small bowel has not developed properly and is not open, and stomach contents are unable to pass; surgical intervention is required
  - Phenylketonuria (PKU) – the inability to metabolize the amino acid phenylalanine; can result in mental retardation if untreated; this will not be evident at birth, but will be identified with neonatal screening
  - Galactosemia – inability to metabolize galactose into glucose; can result in failure to thrive, cataracts, jaundice, cirrhosis of the liver, sepsis, and mental retardation if untreated; this will not be evident at birth, but will be identified with neonatal screening
  - Hypothyroidism – slow metabolism caused by maternal iodine deficiency or maternal antithyroid medications during pregnancy; can result in hypothermia, poor feeding, lethargy, jaundice, and cretinism if untreated
  - Neurologic anomalies (spina bifida) – a neural tube defect in which the vertebral arch fails to close, and there may be a protrusion of the meninges and/or spinal cord
  - Hydrocephalus – excessive spinal fluid accumulation in the ventricles of the brain causing the head to enlarge and the fontanels to bulge; sun-setting sign is common in which the whites of the eyes are visible above the iris
  - Patent ductus arteriosus – a noncyanotic heart defect in which the ductus arteriosus connecting the pulmonary artery and the aorta fails to close after birth; manifestations include murmurs, abnormal heart rate or rhythm, breathlessness, and fatigue while feeding

○ Tetralogy of Fallot – cyanotic heart defect characterized by a ventricular septal defect, the aorta positioned over the ventricular septal defect, stenosis of the pulmonary valve, and hypertrophy of the right ventricle; distinguished by respiratory difficulties, cyanosis, tachycardia, tachypnea, and diaphoresis

○ Down syndrome – oblique palpebral fissures or upward slant of eyes, epicanthal folds, flat facial profile with a depressed nasal bridge and a small nose, protruding tongue, small low-set ears, short broad hands with a fifth finger that has one flexion crease instead of two, a deep crease across the center of the palm frequently referred to as a simian crease, hyperflexibility, and hypotonic muscles

- Nursing assessments of newborns who have congenital anomalies

  ○ Newborn's ability to take in adequate nourishment

  ○ Newborn's ability to eliminate waste products

  ○ Vital signs and axillary temperature

  ○ Newborn-parental bonding, observing the parent's response to the diagnosis of a congenital defect, and encouraging the parents to verbalize concerns

Diagnostic and Therapeutic Procedures

- Prenatal screening for congenital anomalies may be done by ultrasound and multiple-marker screening (triple and quad screen).

- Confirmation of a diagnosis depends on the anomaly.

- Prenatal diagnosis or confirmation of congenital anomalies are often made by amniocentesis, chorionic villi sampling, or ultrasound.

- Routine testing of newborns for metabolic disorders (inborn errors of metabolism)

  ○ A Guthrie test for PKU is done to show elevations of phenylalanine in the blood and urine. It is not reliable until the newborn has ingested sufficient amounts of protein.

  ○ Monitor blood and urine levels of galactose (galactosemia).

  ○ Measure thyroxine (hypothyroidism).

  ○ Cytologic studies (karyotyping of chromosomes), such as a buccal smear, uses cells scraped from the mucosa from inside the newborn's mouth.

Patient-Centered Care

- Nursing Care

  ○ Nursing interventions for congenital anomalies are dependent upon the type and extent of the anomaly.

    ▪ Neurologic anomalies (spina bifida)

      □ Protect the membrane with a sterile covering and plastic to prevent drying.

      □ Observe for leakage of the cerebrospinal fluid.

      □ Handle the newborn gently by positioning him prone or to the side to prevent trauma.

      □ Prevent infection by keeping the area free from contamination by urine and feces.

      □ Measure the circumference of the newborn's head to identify hydrocephalus.

      □ Assess the newborn for increased intracranial pressure.

- Hydrocephalus
  - Frequently reposition the newborn's head to prevent sores.
  - Measure the newborn's head circumference daily.
  - Assess the newborn for manifestations of increased intracranial pressure, such as vomiting and a shrill cry.
- Patent ductus arteriosus
  - Educate the parents about surgical treatment.
- Tetralogy of Fallot
  - Conserve the newborn's energy to reduce the workload on the heart.
  - Administer gavage feedings, or give oral feedings with a special nipple.
  - Elevate the newborn's head and shoulders to improve respirations and reduce the cardiac workload.
  - Prevent infection.
  - Place the newborn in a knee-chest position during respiratory distress.
- Nursing interventions for congenital anomalies
  - Establish and maintain an adequate respiratory status.
  - Establish and maintain extrauterine circulation.
  - Establish and maintain adequate thermoregulation.
  - Administer medications as prescribed, such as thyroid replacement for hypothyroidism.
  - Educate the parents regarding preoperative and postoperative treatment procedures.
  - Provide adequate nutrition.
    - Cleft lip/palate – Determine the most effective nipple for feeding. Feed the newborn in the upright position to decrease aspiration risk. Feed the newborn slowly, and burp him frequently so that he does not swallow air. Cleanse his mouth with water after feedings.
    - Tracheoesophageal atresia – Withhold the newborn's feedings until esophageal patency is determined. Elevate the head of the newborn's crib to prevent gastric juice reflux. Supervise the newborn's first feeding to observe for this anomaly.
    - Duodenal atresia – Withhold the newborn's feedings until surgical repair is done and the newborn has begun to pass stools. Administer IV fluids as prescribed. Monitor the newborn for jaundice.
    - PKU – Special synthetic formula in which phenylalanine is removed or reduced. The mother should restrict meat, dairy products, diet drinks, and protein during pregnancy. Aspartame must be avoided.
    - Galactosemia – Give the newborn a soy-based formula because galactose is present in milk. Eliminate lactose and galactose in the newborn's diet. Breastfeeding is also contraindicated.
  - Encourage the parents to hold, touch, and talk to their newborn.
  - Ensure that the parents provide consistent care to the newborn.
  - Provide parents with information about parent groups or support systems.

APPLICATION EXERCISES

1. A nurse is called to the birthing room to assist with the assessment of a newborn who was born at 32 weeks of gestation. The newborn's birth weight is 1,100 g. Which of the following are expected findings in this newborn? (Select all that apply.)

_____ A. Lanugo

_____ B. Long nails

_____ C. Weak grasp reflex

_____ D. Translucent skin

_____ E. Plump face

2. A nurse is examining an infant who was just delivered at 41 weeks of gestation. Which of the following characteristics indicates that this infant is postterm?

A. Excess body fat

B. Flat areola without breast buds

C. Heels movable fully to the ears

D. Leathery skin

3. A nurse is caring for an infant who has a high bilirubin level and is receiving phototherapy. Which of the following is the priority finding in this newborn?

A. Conjunctivitis

B. Bronze skin discoloration

C. Sunken fontanels

D. Maculopapular skin rash

4. A nurse is caring for a newborn who is preterm and has respiratory distress syndrome. Which of the following should the nurse monitor to evaluate the newborn's condition following administration of synthetic surfactant?

A. Oxygen saturation

B. Body temperature

C. Serum bilirubin

D. Heart rate

5. A nurse is caring for a newborn who has suspected neonatal abstinence syndrome. Which of the following findings supports this diagnosis?

    A. Decreased muscle tone

    B. Continuous high-pitched cry

    C. Sleeps for 2 hr after feeding

    D. Mild tremors when disturbed

6. A nurse educator is reviewing hyperbilirubinemia with a newly hired nurse. What should the nurse educator include in this review? Use the ATI Active Learning Template: Systems Disorder to complete this item to include the following sections:

    A. Description of Disorder: Describe the difference between physiologic and pathologic jaundice and kernicterus.

    B. Assessment: Describe the procedure that can be used to verify the presence of jaundice.

    C. Nursing Care: Describe care of the infant receiving phototherapy.

APPLICATION EXERCISES KEY

1. A. **CORRECT:** Characteristics of a preterm newborn include the presence of abundant lanugo.

    B. INCORRECT: Long nails are findings in a newborn who is postterm.

    C. **CORRECT:** A weak grasp reflex is characteristic of a preterm newborn.

    D. **CORRECT:** Skin that is thin, smooth, shiny, and translucent is a finding in a preterm newborn.

    E. INCORRECT: A plump face would be observed in a newborn who is macrosomic.

    (N) NCLEX® Connection: Health Promotion and Maintenance, Aging Process

2. A. INCORRECT: Excess body fat is seen in a newborn who is macrosomic.

    B. INCORRECT: Flat areolas without breast buds is seen in a newborn who is preterm.

    C. INCORRECT: Heels that are movable fully to the ears is seen in newborn who is preterm.

    D. **CORRECT:** Leathery, cracked, and wrinkled skin is seen in a newborn who is postterm due to placental insufficiency.

    (N) NCLEX® Connection: Health Promotion and Maintenance, Aging Process

3. A. INCORRECT: Conjunctivitis is an important finding, but it is not the priority.

    B. INCORRECT: Bronze skin discoloration is an important finding, but it is not the priority.

    C. **CORRECT:** Using the safety and risk reduction framework, sunken fontanels is the priority finding. Infants receiving phototherapy are at risk for dehydration from loose stools due to increased bilirubin excretion.

    D. INCORRECT: Maculopapular skin rash is an important finding, but it is not the priority.

    (N) NCLEX® Connection: Physiological Adaptations, Alterations in Body Systems

4. A. **CORRECT:** Surfactant stabilizes the alveoli and helps increase oxygen saturation.

    B. INCORRECT: Surfactant administration has no direct effect on body temperature.

    C. INCORRECT: Surfactant administration has no direct effect on bilirubin levels.

    D. INCORRECT: Surfactant administration has no direct effect on heart rate.

    (N) NCLEX® Connection: Reduction of Risk Potential, System Specific Assessments

5. A. INCORRECT: Increased muscle tone is seen in a newborn who has neonatal abstinence syndrome.

    B. **CORRECT:** A continuous high-pitched cry is often an indication of CNS disturbances in a newborn who has neonatal abstinence syndrome.

    C. INCORRECT: A newborn who has neonatal abstinence syndrome can have sleep pattern disturbances and would have difficulty sleeping for 2 hr after feeding.

    D. INCORRECT: A newborn who has neonatal abstinence syndrome often has moderate to severe tremors when undisturbed. Many normal newborns have mild tremors when disturbed.

    Ⓝ NCLEX® Connection: Health Promotion and Maintenance, Aging Process

6. *Using the ATI Active Learning Template: Systems Disorder*

    A. Description of Disorder
    - Physiologic jaundice results from the breakdown of fetal RBCs and lack of liver maturity and appears after 24 hr of age.
    - Pathologic jaundice is caused by a blood incompatibility, infection, or a disorder of RBCs, and appears before 24 hr of age.
    - Kernicterus is a neurological syndrome caused by bilirubin deposits in brain cells when bilirubin levels are very high. It can result in long-term neurological problems.

    B. Assessment
    - Procedure to verify presence of jaundice
      ○ Press the newborn's skin on the cheek or abdomen lightly with one finger.
      ○ Then release pressure, and observe for a yellowish tint to the skin as the skin is blanched.

    C. Nursing Care
    - Care of the infant receiving phototherapy
      ○ Maintain an eye mask over the newborn's eyes.
      ○ Keep the newborn undressed. Place a mask (like a bikini) over the genitalia of a male newborn.
      ○ Remove the newborn from phototherapy every 4 hr, and unmask the eyes.
      ○ Reposition the newborn every 2 hr to expose all body surfaces to the phototherapy lights and prevent pressure sores.
      ○ Check the lamp energy with a photometer following facility protocol.
      ○ Turn off the phototherapy lights before drawing blood for testing.

    Ⓝ NCLEX® Connection: Physiological Adaptations, Alterations in Body Systems

Dudek, S. G. (2010). *Nutrition essentials for nursing practice* (6th ed.). Philadelphia: Lippincott Williams & Wilkins.

Grodner, M., Roth, S. L., & Walkingshaw, B. C. (2012). *Nutritional foundations and clinical applications: A nursing approach* (5th ed.). St. Louis, MO: Mosby.

Hockenberry, M. J., & Winkelstein M. L. (2013). *Wong's essentials of pediatric nursing* (9th ed.). St. Louis, MO: Mosby.

Lehne, R. A. (2013). *Pharmacology for nursing care* (8th ed.). St. Louis: Saunders.

Lowdermilk, D. L., Perry, S. E., Cahsion, M. C., & Aldean, K. R. (2012). *Maternity & women's health care* (10th ed.). St. Louis, MO: Mosby.

Perry, S. E., Hockenberry, M. J., Lowdermilk, D. L., & Wilson, D. (2010). *Maternal Child Nursing Care* (4th ed.). St. Louis, MO: Mosby Elsevier.

Pillitteri, A. (2010). *Maternal and child health nursing: Care of the childbearing and childrearing family* (6th ed.). Philadelphia: Lippincott Williams & Wilkins.

Wilson, B. A., Shannon, M. T., & Shields, K. M. (2013). *Pearson nurse's drug guide 2013*. Upper Saddle River, NJ: Prentice Hall.

| APPENDIX | ACTIVE LEARNING TEMPLATES |
| TEMPLATE | Basic Concept |

CONTENT_____ REVIEW MODULE CHAPTER _____

TOPIC DESCRIPTOR_____

Related Content
(e.g. delegation, levels of
prevention, advance directives)

Underlying Principles

Nursing Interventions
› Who?
› When?
› Why?
› How?

Appendix

CONTENT _____ REVIEW MODULE CHAPTER _____

TOPIC DESCRIPTOR _____

DESCRIPTION OF PROCEDURE:

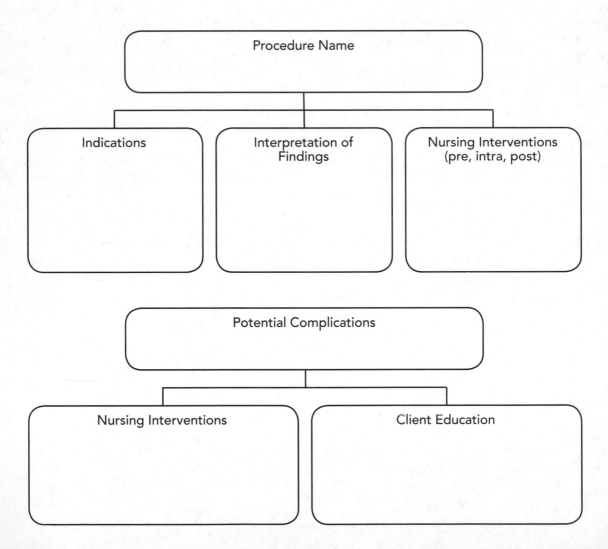

Procedure Name

Indications

Interpretation of Findings

Nursing Interventions (pre, intra, post)

Potential Complications

Nursing Interventions

Client Education

Appendix

CONTENT _____ REVIEW MODULE CHAPTER _____

TOPIC DESCRIPTOR _____

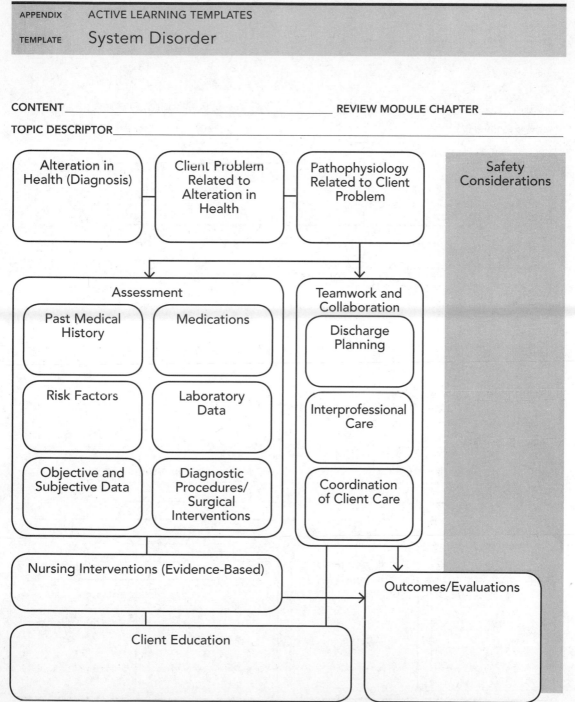

Alteration in Health (Diagnosis)

Client Problem Related to Alteration in Health

Pathophysiology Related to Client Problem

Safety Considerations

Assessment
- Past Medical History
- Medications
- Risk Factors
- Laboratory Data
- Objective and Subjective Data
- Diagnostic Procedures/ Surgical Interventions

Teamwork and Collaboration
- Discharge Planning
- Interprofessional Care
- Coordination of Client Care

Nursing Interventions (Evidence-Based)

Outcomes/Evaluations

Client Education

Appendix

CONTENT _____ REVIEW MODULE CHAPTER _____

TOPIC DESCRIPTOR_____

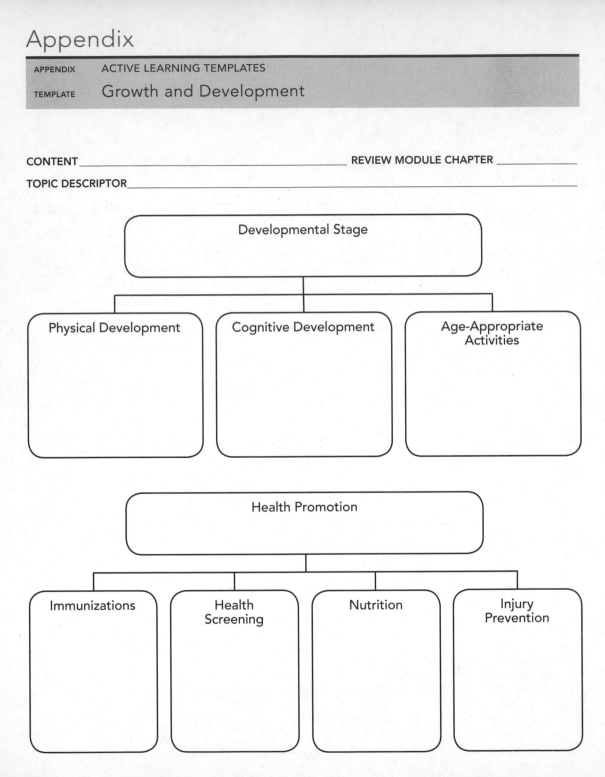

Developmental Stage

Physical Development

Cognitive Development

Age-Appropriate Activities

Health Promotion

Immunizations

Health Screening

Nutrition

Injury Prevention

CONTENT _____ REVIEW MODULE CHAPTER _____

TOPIC DESCRIPTOR _____

MEDICATION _____

EXPECTED PHARMALOGICAL ACTION:

```
                    ┌─────────────────────────┐
                    │     Therapeutic Uses     │
                    │                          │
                    └─────────────────────────┘
                                 │
              ┌──────────────────┴──────────────────┐
  ┌────────────────────────┐          ┌────────────────────────┐
  │     Adverse Effects     │          │  Nursing Interventions  │
  │                         │          │                         │
  └────────────────────────┘          │                         │
  ┌────────────────────────┐          └────────────────────────┘
  │    Client Education     │          ┌────────────────────────┐
  │                         │          │    Client Education     │
  │                         │          │                         │
  └────────────────────────┘          │                         │
  ┌────────────────────────┐          └────────────────────────┘
  │ Medication/Food         │
  │ Interactions            │
  │                         │
  └────────────────────────┘
  ┌────────────────────────┐          ┌────────────────────────┐
  │ Nursing Administration  │          │ Evaluation of Medication│
  │                         │          │ Effectiveness           │
  └────────────────────────┘          └────────────────────────┘
```

Appendix

CONTENT _____ REVIEW MODULE CHAPTER _____

TOPIC DESCRIPTOR _____

DESCRIPTION OF SKILL:

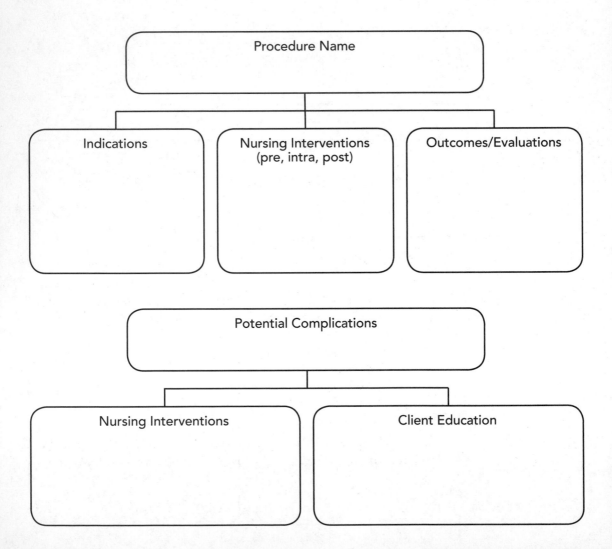

CONTENT_____ REVIEW MODULE CHAPTER _____

TOPIC DESCRIPTOR_____

DESCRIPTION OF PROCEDURE:

Procedure Name

Indications

Nursing Interventions
(pre, intra, post)

Outcomes/Evaluations

Potential Complications

Nursing Interventions

Client Education